POPULATION HEALTH POLICY

FIRST EDITION

Edited by Christine Cardinal

Sam Houston State University

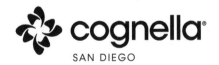

cognella®
SAN DIEGO

Bassim Hamadeh, CEO and Publisher
John Remington, Executive Editor
Gem Rabanera, Project Editor
Abbey Hastings, Associate Production Editor
Katie Zychowicz, Graphic Design Assistant
Trey Soto, Licensing Coordinator
Natalie Piccotti, Director of Marketing
Kassie Graves, Vice President of Editorial
Jamie Giganti, Director of Academic Publishing

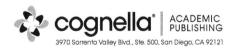

3970 Sorrento Valley Blvd., Ste. 500, San Diego, CA 92121

CONTENTS

INTRODUCTION

While the World Health Organization's (hereinafter WHO) definition of health policy is excellent and accurately explains that "health policy refers to decisions, plans, and actions that are undertaken to achieve specific health care goals within a society," it parses a subject so broad, that it is often hard for students to wrap their minds around the definition without extended consideration. One only has to review the history surrounding President Johnson's implementation of Medicaid and Medicare a half century ago, or President Obama's enactment of the Patient Protection and Affordable Care Act in recent years to appreciate the complexity and controversy surrounding the development of health policies. The substantial alterations made to both these pieces of legislation before Congress finally enacted them highlight the collaborative and interdisciplinary efforts required to craft health policy.

The creation of targeted, population-specific health policies that avoid negative, unintended consequences is an important goal that requires assessment, revision, and a commitment to quality at the micro and macro level. Federal and state health policy development is vital for sustainable, population health; however, it is also rife with obstacles such as budget restrictions and the timing of legislative sessions. Nonetheless, when enacted, these far-reaching health policies can serve as harbingers of change for good or ill of what's to come in the future of human health and as indicators of what we value as Americans. Breakthroughs in gene sequencing, consumer targeting, and online data are paving the way for increased specificity in how we can successfully modernize health policies, while longtime politically charged issues, such as health disparities and the environment, remain difficult to address. Nonetheless, while obtaining voter support for large-scale health policy change is very difficult, change is being seen on a smaller scale at local and organizational levels.

This book provides a series of editorials, selections, and case studies that are intended to engage the reader into examining the practical application of health policies and their resulting health care outcomes. The questions at the end of each chapter should be used to promote discussion and further investigation into the issues covered. While the chapters in this text are diverse, the common thread showcasing the impact of health policies on population health ties them together. I hope the readings foster an appreciation and respect for health policy as an academic discipline.

HEALTH POLICY BASICS

The Policy Process

William G. Weissert and Carol S. Weissert

One sister, Rosa, moved a few years ago to a beach town halfway down the long eastern coast of Florida. Unaccustomed to managed care and aware of its bad reputation among older people, Rosa initially opted to continue her fee-for-service Medicare coverage. After some persuasion from a friend in her bridge club, she and her husband agreed to call one of the local Medicare managed care firms and hear its pitch. They were amazed to find that the plan would charge no monthly premium, cover drug costs of up to $800 a month, and cover stays at either of the two nearby hospitals in their beach community. Clearly, coverage in the same federal program differed between fee-for-service and managed care, and it might be still different at a managed care firm other than the one Rosa and her husband chose.

When she had a small stroke a few days after joining the managed care plan, Rosa was very pleasantly surprised at the range of specialists who were quickly assigned to her case: a neurologist, a neurosurgeon, internists, and a physical therapist. After her first night in the hospital, she was visited by the managed care firm's medical director, who was taking a special interest in management of her potentially high-cost case. Had she remained in her fee-for-service plan, or had her stroke occurred a week earlier, before she'd made the switch, Rosa would have been worse off in several ways. She would have faced a one-day cost-of-hospital-care deductible, a daily copayment, a 25 percent copayment for drugs, a major gap in her drug coverage once she'd spent the limits of her coverage a few months after her stroke, and substantial copayments for ambulatory care visits to her physicians after leaving the hospital. She would have had a broader choice of physicians—not just those who were members of her plan—but the ones she had seemed fine and she liked the lower costs and referrals to specialists without searching for one herself.

Medicare notified Rosa and her husband a few months later that their managed care firm was losing its Medicare contract over some compliance issues. She and her husband went through another round of managed care plan visits and chose another one, and for the most part they were again satisfied, except with their primary care doctor. At the next open enrollment period a year later, they switched plans again in order to get a different primary care doctor. Luckily, she was assigned to a female internist whom she really liked. When she was again hospitalized, with lung cancer, she was attended by two hospitalists (specialists who practice only in the hospital, not in the community), a pulmonologist and a rehabilitation specialist. Managed care firms prefer hospitalists to manage their inpatient care to make sure things go well and don't become unnecessarily expensive. The two hospitalists managed all her hospital care, were very responsive to questions, went by their first names, and seemed to take a real interest in her personally. Ultimately, she did not opt for care by an oncologist because her cancer was too advanced for such care to do much good. She had been a lifelong smoker, and she failed to comply when her internists asked her to get an x-ray, but it was not for lack of excellent care. She did not have an excellent life style, of course, at least with respect to protecting her health.

Meanwhile, across the state, her sister Mae, not yet 65 and working for one of the thousands of service industry firms in Florida, needed back surgery—or at least was told she did, despite government warnings (based on government-sponsored research studies) that back surgery is often not very effective. With no health insurance and an income not close enough to poverty to qualify for Medicaid, Mae and her husband would not be able to pay for her hospital care or for the doctors who would do the surgery.

Were she to collapse at work, Mae might be able to claim workers' compensation coverage. If she were in a car accident and further injured her back, she might be able to get some of her medical expenses covered by the mandatory medical injury coverage that many states, including Florida, require auto insurance companies to include in their policies. Or if she were rushed to a hospital emergency department after such an accident, the federal EMTALA (Emergency Medical Treatment and Active Labor Act) law would require that her condition be diagnosed and stabilized by physicians and staff before they could send her home, but with no plans or obligations related to follow-up care that she might need. The EMTALA law doesn't cover that.

Of course, EMTALA would not stop the hospital from turning over the bill to a collection agency, which would dun Mae repeatedly and quite likely try to garnishee her wages to force her to pay the bill. In fact, Medicare and Medicaid agreements signed by the hospital would require it to go after her for payment—unless the hospital management wanted to adopt a policy of going after nobody who owed them money; Medicare and Medicaid want to be assured that their patients are not singled out for extra charges.

Mae's congressman heard about the problem of the bad debt collection policies of hospitals and was concerned that poor people were getting worse care than the nonpoor. She asked the administrator of the Centers for Medicare and Medicaid Services to testify before her House committee to explain how Medicare and Medicaid policies affected bad-debt collection by hospitals. The CMS administrator answered the committee's questions, many of which were written for the committee members by congressional staff who had read a report on the subject—most likely prepared by the Government Accountability Office, the Congressional Budget Office, or the Medicare Payment Advisory Commission.

For their research in preparing a report of this type, any or all of these agencies or individuals quite likely made use of the extensive Medicare and Medicaid data on use and cost provided by the hospitals, as well as cost reports covering all patients and all expenses and bad debts that hospitals must file regularly if they want to participate in Medicare or Medicaid. Or the researchers might have used one of the many surveys of hospital admissions, discharges, payment sources, and other features paid for with public funds.

If Rosa, the sister with Medicare coverage, had been discharged to a nursing home, Medicare might have paid for a few days' stay. A longer stay would have had to be paid for out of her own pocket, until she was poor enough to qualify for Medicaid to cover that portion of the bill that her Social Security and other funds could not pay each month. If either sister died during her hospital stay, state law would dictate whether the case had to be counted in some kind of published hospital mortality index, since the federal mandatory hospital death index was repealed some years ago and replaced in only a few cases, including Florida, by state law. (The new Obama health reform act contains another version of the death index.) And the federal Centers for Disease Control and Prevention would, of course, want to know about the death from a death certificate, so that mortality rates by cause of death and by state and county could be reported. The death might not result in an autopsy, since state laws vary on whether an autopsy is required in routine cases. Florida leaves the decision to the discretion of the state attorney, if that official thinks a crime may have been committed.

But the hospital might do an autopsy anyway, if it had the permission of the family, because the Joint Commission on Accreditation of Healthcare Organizations (JCAHO), a private group operated by hospitals, is a strong proponent of autopsies, and the hospital would not want to risk its state and local licenses to operate as a hospital, or lose its Medicare and Medicaid certification, by becoming careless and losing its JCAHO accreditation. Licensure and certification often require accreditation as one condition among many others. Furthermore, some states might require, as Florida does, that the deceased be transported from the hospital to a burial site under the direction of a funeral director, since the funeral industry has been successful in some states in lobbying the legislature to make it illegal to transport a corpse without involvement of a funeral director.

If neither sister died, after recovering at home they might go out and celebrate, vowing to give up smoking and go on a diet, especially after reading the antismoking, diet, exercise, and other health promotion materials prepared by the CDC and state public health agencies that their husbands had picked up for them in the hospital cafeteria. Driving home from the celebration, whoever was driving would want to be quite sober to avoid violating state driving laws aimed at preventing motor vehicle–related morbidity and mortality.

This is health care policy in the United States: who is and is not eligible to receive subsidized care; what share the individual pays; which types of health care and which services and procedures are covered; who can render care and get paid for rendering it; what government does and does not do when a person needs care but does not have the money to pay for it; who gets financial help with medical care training; what nurses can and cannot do for patients; how wide the doorways of hospital bathrooms should be; what data must be supplied to the federal and state governments; how federal tax policy and workers' protection laws interact with various health care laws; how federal agencies translate congressional intent into regulations affecting health care providers and patients; what records must be kept, how they must be kept, whom they can be shared with, and whom they must be shared with; what kinds of educational materials about healthy living are distributed and which behaviors are restricted or encouraged in the interests of improved health status—and much, much more.

Health care policies are not unique to government. Hospitals have their own private policies: some will not perform abortions; many operate as not-for-profits, while others operate for profit, many of them part of a chain of hospitals owned by investors; some have strong data system firewalls that protect medical records from unauthorized access, others weaker ones; bad debts are absorbed graciously or collected aggressively; infants under a certain weight at birth must be kept in the hospital until they gain weight at some hospitals but not others; one hospital does not operate a drug detoxification center, another does. Insurance companies, in the interest of reducing liability, may require of their nursing home clients that all residents be accompanied to the bathroom whether they need help or not. These private policies share many characteristics with public policies. They differ in that they do not usually have an explicit public purpose and are not compelled by public authority. People do not go to jail for violating a corporate policy (but they may be fired—for example, for violating corporate policy that forbids one worker to tell another worker his pay rate). The real difference, however, is that government policies are made by government and, as such, are the product of a political process in which public elections are a key determinant of who gets to make policy.

Chapter 1: Discussion Questions

1   Define policy legacies.

   a.   Give one example and describe its current impact on health in America.

2   Describe the pros and cons of incremental vs. comprehensive change in health policy.

   a.   What type of health policy change is more common and why?

3   Describe the framework progression of public policy.

   a.   Are four steps enough? Why or why not?

4   Define framing for health policy issues.

   a.   Give one example of a current health policy and how it is framed.

5   Define health disparities.

   a.   Describe two challenges disabled Americans face in getting and keeping insurance.

CHAPTER 2

GLOBAL HEALTH POLICY

Bridge to Care for Refugee Health

Lessons from an Interprofessional Collaboration in the Midwest

Ruth Margalit, Laura Vinson, Christine Ngaruiya, Kara Gehring, Pam Franks, Caci Schulte, Andrew Lemke, Joshua Blood, Tyler Irvine, Chelsea Souder, Deeko Hassan, Andrea Langeveld, Carolyn Corn, Thu Hong Bui, and Ann Marie Kudlacz

Abstract

The United States resettles tens of thousands of refugees annually, with hundreds placed in mid-sized Midwestern cities such as Omaha, Nebraska. Prior to resettlement, refugees have limited access to health services and arrive with inadequate knowledge on basic hygiene practices, general healthcare issues, and minimal understanding of the American healthcare system. Additionally, current training for healthcare practitioners in the United States on issues related to refugee populations and their unique health needs is insufficient. The enormous need coupled with inadequate preparation, poses great challenges for both newly resettled refugees and health professionals, and provides opportunities for improvement with creative initiatives. The Bridge to Care (BTC) project is a unique partnership between health professions students, leaders from city and state refugee service organizations, and refugee leaders. It is a student-led/community-engaged organization overseen by the Service Learning Academy (SLA) in the College of Public Health at the University of Nebraska Medical Center. The SLA facilitates campus wide interprofessional community-based experiences like Bridge to Care. Through BTC, students take the forefront in communicating directly with leaders from community organizations and engaging with refugee leaders to determine all relevant service activities. Bridge to Care provides opportunities for students to engage in experiences that are not otherwise available in their standard curriculum. While providing essential services, students are able to enhance cultural and communication skills and gain experience working with an interprofessional team, building an understanding of the vital role each profession plays within the full spectrum of care for patients and communities.

Keywords: Interprofessional education, refugees, health, community engagement

Introduction

According to the United Nations High Commissioner for Refugees (UNHCR), a refugee is defined as someone who "owing to a well-founded fear of being persecuted for reasons of race, religion, nationality, membership of a particular social group or political opinion, is outside the country of his nationality, and is unable to, or owing to such fear, is unwilling to avail himself to the protection of that country" (1). "Secondary Migrants" are those refugees who have originally resettled in one part of the country and have subsequently moved to another location. There are approximately 15 million refugees around the world (1).

Refugees begin the process of seeking resettlement after fleeing their home countries to seek safety in neighboring nations. When refugees arrive at the nation providing asylum or temporary residence, they face three possible endpoints, one of which is resettlement in a third country such as the United States (1). This process often times takes more than 5 years while refugees live in harsh conditions within the refugee camps (1). The President of the United States sets the ceiling for refugee admission to the United States (U.S.) each fiscal year (2), for which the U.S. averages more than 50,000 refugee resettlements per year (1). Many of these refugees choose to resettle in mid-sized Midwestern cities given low costs of living and low rates of unemployment (2). Refugees are also placed in locations where existing family ties are already established (2).

Refugee Resettlement in Nebraska

Currently, there are an estimated 25,000 refugees in Nebraska, with 15,000 in Omaha alone, according to Omaha resettlement agencies (personal communications) and federal resettlement reports (2, 3). In fiscal year 2013, there was a record high of 1,006 refugees resettled, and the number is expected to increase in 2014 (4). Over the years, refugees from Sudan, Somalia, Burma, Bhutan, Nepal, Iraq, Afghanistan, Ethiopia, Liberia, Congo, and Burundi have been resettled in Nebraska. As of 2006, it is estimated that over 50% of the Sudanese population in the U.S. settled in Nebraska (5, 6). In more recent years, the majority of resettled refugees are those who have fled to camps in Thailand from nearby Burma (Myanmar) (7).

The three primary refugee resettlement agencies that provide services to these refugees in Nebraska are Lutheran Family Services (LFS), Southern Sudan Community Association (SSCA), and Catholic Charities (4). The agencies provide various services such as: English classes, cultural orientation, employment assistance, fair housing education, financial literacy and household budgeting, as well as training programs for churches and civic organizations that wish to sponsor refugees and immigration legal assistance. Agencies also help coordinate access to healthcare services while in the U.S (8).

Refugee Health Issues

Prior to arrival in the U.S., the refugee receives inadequate preparation regarding health and health-related issues (3). Refugees also lack basic understanding about navigating the healthcare system, Western hygiene practices, preventive practices, and Western disease management (9). As a result of their circumstances, it is not unusual to find individuals with complicated health issues upon arrival and for years following resettlement. Past history of poor nutrition, poor sanitation, exposure to on-going violence and lack of adequate medical care also contribute to poor health (1).

One particular area of concern is the high rates of undiagnosed infectious conditions such as tuberculosis, malaria, hepatitis C, Human Immunodeficiency Virus (HIV), as well as skin and intestinal parasites (9–11). Mental health disorders also affect a large portion of the population including a high prevalence of depression, drug and alcohol abuse (7, 11). Individuals who experienced persecution, terrorization by violent groups, imprisonment, and torture, may suffer from somatization disorders, psychosocial distress, post-traumatic stress disorder, anxiety and depression (1,9–11). Another source of health concern is injury at the workplace (4). The majority of refugees in Omaha, Nebraska work in meat packing plants performing physically demanding jobs which puts them at high risk for injury (8).

Lastly, cultural differences distinguish America from many of the countries from which refugees originate, and these differences extend to healthcare (12). For example, in Somalia, only 2% of births take place in a health facility whereas in America, women are expected to deliver in the hospital. In addition, numerous Somali women have undergone female circumcision, which can make birthing more complicated (12).

Bridge to Care (BTC) was founded on principles of community-based participatory research (CBPR) and service learning after identifying a gap in refugee health and healthcare needs. In addition to the language barrier, numerous refugees lack the cultural constructs to understand life in this country. Timely, appropriate healthcare acculturation is frequently unmet and much needed (9, 10). Refugees receive inadequate preparation prior to resettlement regarding fundamentals such as running a 'Western home', family roles, job distribution, the legal system, and navigating the education system (2).

The program is designed to prioritize the vast needs of the refugee populations, link refugees to existing services, and increase provider competence for refugee care. When working with refugees, BTC refers to health as "a state of complete physical, mental and social well-being and not merely the absence of disease or infirmity" (13). Few other programs have been set up to address refugee health issues through collaboration with community organizations.

The purpose of the work described in this manuscript is to illustrate the unique setup between community, interprofessional health professions students and refugee leaders to enhance refugee health in Omaha and surrounding communities. With the number of interactions through BTC currently approaching 4,000 and continuing to grow, the organizational leaders seek to share this novel initiative to impact other communities that interact with refugee populations. The Institutional Review Board of the University of Nebraska Medical Center approved parts of this project that involve research, such as implementation of surveys for the health education sessions.

Methods

Bridge to Care (BTC) was established in April 2010 as an interprofessional organization supported by the interprofessional Service Learning Academy (SLA), College of Public Health at the University of Nebraska Medical Center (UNMC). It is a partnership involving students from the colleges of medicine, nursing, pharmacy, public health, and allied health, faculty, healthcare providers and community refugee service agencies. The goal is to facilitate positive healthcare outcomes for refugees by teaching them how to navigate the healthcare system, enhancing knowledge and cultural skills necessary for successful assimilation, and developing strong relationships with their communities.

This is achieved by: discerning group specific health needs from each refugee community; providing health education, linkage to healthcare and services; and improving cultural awareness and knowledge regarding resettled refugees among healthcare providers

BTC has three initiatives to accomplish this mission; monthly health education sessions, monthly mentoring sessions, and health fairs/linkage to care events. Each of these initiatives requires collaboration with the community. Table 2.1.1 lists the partners of this project.

Health education sessions

Health education sessions are developed with each refugee community (Sudanese, Somali, Burmese/Karen, and Bhutanese) for a period of three consecutive months. Health professions student leaders with respective refugee community leaders, work on building relationships, identifying health needs, planning the education opportunities in community settings and linking the refugee community to appropriate health services. Typically 15–40 participants attend each session.

Health education session topics have included pain management, hypertension, stroke, addiction, mental health, suicide prevention, immunizations, autism, healthy eating, using over the counter medications, and navigation of the U.S. healthcare system.

Table 2.1.1   Bridge to Care Partners

BTC Partners	Role
University of Nebraska Medical Center, College of Public Health, Service Learning Academy	Oversees the Bridge to Care program and assists in sustaining and expanding the program; Provides evidenced-based models of theory and community development, research methods for tracking and identifying evaluation process and outcomes
Southern Sudan Community Association (SSCA)	Resettlement Agency
Lutheran Family Services (LFS)	Resettlement Agency
Embrace the Nations	Faith-based organization providing cultural awareness training to Bridge to Care volunteers; Assists refugees in multiple areas of need and assists the public in better understanding and interacting with refugee populations
Omaha Public Schools, ESL Program	Partners for the mentoring program offered to refugee youth grades 5–12
Nebraska Department of Health and Human Services	Responsible for coordinating and administering the Refugee Resettlement Program on the state level
Alegent-Creighton Florence Clinic	Federally designated clinic assigned to provide initial health screenings/healthcare services to refugees; participates in annual health fair and various educational sessions, while linking refugees to long term healthcare
One World Community Health Center	Provides clinical supplies for health fairs and flu shots for multiple 'Flu Shot Clinics'
Douglas County Health Department	Providing health education resources and support
Walgreens Pharmacy	Provides clinical supplies and personnel for health fairs and flu shots for multiple 'Flu Shot Clinics'

When health needs are selected, refugee community leaders play an important role in identifying an appropriate session format (presentation by students or experts versus discussion groups), venue (faith gathering place—Church/mosque, community center, the familiar resettlement organization office), and time/day for the session, recruitment of interpreters, as well as recruitment of refugee community members to attend. The health education sessions occur once every 2–4 weeks in the community.

BTC leadership recruits health profession students to participate in the sessions.

The majority of students participating in health education sessions have no previous experience with refugees prior to their involvement with BTC. Hence, increasing the foundation of knowledge is important to foster appropriate interactions with and understanding of the populations being served. As an introduction, at every health education session prior to the arrival of the refugees, student and faculty volunteers are required to participate in cultural awareness training about refugees and their health needs. The training is designed to enhance cultural sensitivity, increase knowledge and ensure that participants are better equipped to effectively interact with the refugees. The training covers topics such as: the unique characteristics of the various refugee groups arriving in the U.S. and Omaha; the specific health needs of refugees; the importance of and tips on communicating effectively with various cultures regardless of race, ethnicity, culture or language proficiency.

Health-fairs/Linkage-to-care

In addition to health education and focused services (like flu-shot clinics for specific refugee communities), two major health fairs/linkage to care events are organized each year in response to the needs of the refugee community. These large events (up to 500 participants) offer a wide range of education opportunities, offering over 35 different resource booths in 2013, including information relating to proper hygiene, nutrition, immunizations, chronic disease management, and child health. Prescription and over the counter medication counseling is also available. Free preventative services like flu shots, screening for hypertension, diabetes, obesity, vision and dental services are also provided.

Mentoring program

In 2012, BTC expanded its engagement by adding the BTC Mentoring Program, partnering with Omaha Public School's English as a Second Language (ESL) program for refugee students. Younger, school-aged children often find it easier to acculturate into the American lifestyle and can act as a great resource for their families. Health professions students can become mentors following successful completion of a background check and training. Mentors are randomly assigned mentees and engage with them on selected Saturdays throughout the academic year, at least 12 times, covering topics concerning wellness and health. BTC has identified this venue as another way to improve communication with refugees. In Fall 2013, 352 refugee students participated with 20 health profession student mentors.

Results

Since the inception of BTC (April 2010), over 700 students and over 4,000 refugees engaged together to address health needs.

Unlike other venues for volunteering, Bridge to Care is a relatively new model of healthcare outreach in the community. The track record, albeit short, has been consistent and positive. Different refugee groups throughout the city have benefitted from relevant education sessions and services. While progressing through their rigorous programs of excellence, students acquire skills and knowledge that will help them excel in their field. Such skills as compassionate care, cross cultural communication and multi-cultural care, can impact their future patients who are likely to come from various cultural backgrounds. These skills are best learned through experiential real-life learning, and the unique setting provided by BTC undoubtedly forges the place for the learning while facilitating potential better care for refugee populations in the future. Table 2.1.2 presents qualitative data illustrating community partners, refugees and students' perspectives.

In addition to asking refugees about relevant health topics and appropriate logistics to facilitate BTC programming, refugees are all asked to provide feedback through systematic evaluations through all three BTC programs; health education sessions, mentoring sessions, and health fairs/linkage to care events. For example, following each health fair, refugees are asked to complete an oral evaluation. Of the 350 refugees who attended the past Fair, 131 completed the survey of which 99% indicated that the event was 'most useful' (rated 10 on a scale of 1–10 the usefulness of the health fair—1 being least useful and 10 being most useful), and that the information was presented in a way that they could understand. Additional responses from the refugees include the desire to have more clinical services offered and an indication of the variety of 'favorite booths' such as, basic health screenings, nutrition, over-the-counter medication, free vaccinations, dental care and vision screening with eye glasses.

Student perspectives

With each health education session, students take part in a pre/post assessment to determine knowledge, skills, comfort, and beliefs of the student's cultural competency.

The aggregate analysis of the pre and post assessments, administered to a total of 29 students over three consecutive sessions in 2013 with the Bhutanese population concluded the following in regard to knowledge, skills and cross cultural competence: following the cultural awareness training, 80% of students reported an ***increase in knowledge*** of cultural challenges that face refugees in U.S. and an ***increase in skills*** with student's ability to communicate effectively with different cultures regardless of race, ethnicity, culture or language (increase from 2 to 4 on a Likert scale [1-least, 5-most].

Students have also consistently reflected positively on their experiences through BTC. For example, following a Somali health education session, a student stated, "It has really opened my eyes to the refugee population in Omaha and the various challenges they face." Another student reflected "....It was a rewarding experience and I felt like I was doing something that really mattered for the community. The Bridge to Care organization is a great way to interact with the diverse community that lives within Omaha. It was very beneficial to learn about a different culture as well as use skills we have learned from our time at UNMC towards those in need. I will be able to use what I learned on Sunday for the rest of my career. I would encourage anyone to help out with a Bridge to Care event[s] because not only are you helping others, you are also bettering yourself as a person as well as a professional."

Table 2.1.2   Perspectives of partners in the Bridge to Care Program

	Community partner	Refugees	Student
Positive	"Thank you for providing information to a population that may have otherwise not received anything." "The partnership with the university helps us dream big and involve individuals that otherwise are not interested in refugees in our city." "The program provides services that we do not have resources for. At the same time students get to learn in a real-world setting. It's a win/win!" "Innovative; sustainable program!"	"My favorite part of the Fair is that my kids know more about health and healthy food." "I will tell my people to come and attend the next event." "The session helped me understand why I may need to have a flu-shot." "It's a really good experience for me to get to know more about health, improve my health." "I respect the students who care about me."	"It has really opened my eyes to refugees in Omaha to better understand the various challenges they face." "The most important part was to gain trust and build relationships with strangers: refugees and other health profession students." "I developed appreciation and awareness to the notion that nothing should be taken for granted." "I learned how important is cultural awareness and competent cultural practice."
Negative	"Shorten refugee evaluations they are hard to understand." "Make sure you use language that is simple and clear."	"They ran out of flu shots and I didn't get one!" "I want them to offer more dental care and glasses."	"I need more cultural training to be effective." "Needed interpreters, but lacked sufficient funding."

Discussion

The work with refugees has been often challenging, complex, and at the same time very rewarding. In various listening sessions during the past 2 years, refugees in Omaha identified the following needs: housing, health, employment, education, transportation and public safety/community awareness. Bridge to Care focused on healthcare issues, while taking into consideration the host of challenges the community face. The major lessons learned are listed below:

1   *Understanding of US healthcare system*—many members of the American society struggle to fully understand the ins and outs of the U.S. healthcare system, especially at a time of major changes in insurance coverage. Refugees have little foundational understanding of this complex system and often fall victims to misunderstandings and incur startling costs for minor services obtained outside of insurance coverage

or in an inappropriate manner (for example—use of ER for simple upper respiratory infection). Refugees hold a unique understanding of health and sickness, embracing a holistic approach to treatment of diseases (American medicine is deeply embedded upon scientific data and physical exam, when other cultures look at the environment, cultural customs and traditions, and rely heavily on healers for cures). The BTC program has to be both efficient in assisting with the understanding of the healthcare system while maintaining sensitivity to the traditional approach when presenting strategies for diagnosis and management of diseases.

2 *Understanding preventive care*—Students learned firsthand how individuals from diverse populations, cultural practices and beliefs have very different perceptions and understanding regarding health. A striking example was preventive health services, discussed at an education session as an important part of maintaining good health. Yet, 'preventive care', regarding cancer in the Bhutanese community, was found to be a new concept and a problematic one: "if you talk about or schedule screening for colon or cervical cancer you will bring it upon yourself". BTC has learned that more education and time is needed for preventive practices to be understood and embraced by refugees. This finding was an important one shared with the practice clinical community.

3 *Refugee participation in sessions:* Almost all refugees, regardless of geographic location, tend to avoid drawing attention to themselves. Asian refugees, especially, tend to be quite reserved. This means remaining silent rather than speaking up, not asking questions, not asking for clarification and essentially agreeing with whatever is said or done. Because time is limited in the education sessions, it is difficult to check for understanding, to assess how much of the presented material is comprehended, and how useful it was for the refugees. With consistent repetition of health topics presented at health education sessions, the hope is that the information will eventually be absorbed.

4 *Sensitive topics:* Another challenge has been the discussion of more sensitive topics such as women's health, torture and abuse, mental illness and subjects related to sex (i.e. sexually transmitted diseases). Generally speaking, these topics are discussed very little in the community or in the home and special measures must be taken in order to successfully address them. Due to matters of sensitivity and confidentiality, interpreters coming from the community are especially unsuitable when discussing these personal issues. The interpreters need to correctly communicate the health needs of their respective populations, and be of an appropriate age with adequate knowledge. Medically-certified interpreters are in very high demand, and as a result, are quite expensive and often unavailable. Finding competent medical interpreters was a challenge for BTC as it was for the practice community, and many of the sensitive topics could not be addressed. New initiatives designed to address mental health and other sensitive topics in group settings are currently being developed.

5   *Logistics of the program*—The general logistics for the BTC program have been a challenge and a great lesson to all involved. Scheduling planning meetings, session dates/times, session venues, refugee recruitment and selecting appropriate food have all required on-going open communication, flexibility, leadership and good problem solving skills. Refugees often work the first (7–4) and second (1–9) shifts 6–7 days a week, have limited access to transportation, and prefer gatherings in places of worship or at the housing complexes where most of the community members live. Since weekends tend to work best for the refugees, students, community organization leaders and faculty extended their commitment to meet these needs, scheduling most activities on the weekends. Several sessions have been held following the conclusion of an existing ESL class or after faith-based activities to reach a larger number of refugees. In addition, students from the various health professions, have to coordinate between the various professional curricula to ensure student participation (avoiding dates prior to major exams etc.). In addition, for each activity, interpreters need to be recruited. They are expected to disseminate information about the activity, recruit individuals to attend, and be present at the session. As stated earlier, interpreters are in high demand and need to be contacted long in advance.

    Timely communication has also been an enduring challenge; perhaps the different perception of 'time, the lack of access to electronic communication, or the difference in norms and expectations for follow-up and response. In any case, the expectation of prompt reply to phone messages and emails is unrealistic and adds another layer to coordination.

6   *Funding and sustainability*—Each of the BTC's activities, especially the bi-annual health fairs, require resources (i.e.: medical supplies, transportation, food, translated materials, and many other relevant items). Funding for BTC activities has been secured through an ongoing effort by the SLA, through applications to local and national grants and for in kind contributions. Since its inception in 2010, over $20,000 cash funding were secured with over $100,000 in-kind services. Although tedious and very time consuming, through this process, BTC has formed numerous partnerships with local businesses and service providers.

New opportunities: The Refugee Health Collaborative

As a direct result of the BTC program, the Nebraska Refugee Health Collaborative (RHC) was formed, with the goal to improve health of the refugees who are a part of the fabric of the community. Twelve organizations joined together: UNMC, College of Public Health, (including the Service Learning Academy and Bridge to Care), Southern Sudan Community Association, Lutheran Family Services, Embrace the Nations, Omaha Together One Community, the Institute of Public Life, Nebraska Department of Health and Human Services (Refugee Coordinator and Refugee Health Coordinator), Douglas County Health Department, Ready in Five, Alegent-Creighton

Florence Clinic, One World Community Health Centers, Omaha Public Schools, and to date, over 250 refugee leaders and key community members have participated in the monthly meetings.

Much like BTC, the larger RHC embraced the following goals: to develop mutual understanding and trust among the group, to determine major perceived barriers to service (i.e. economic, cultural, language, financial, organizational, navigation of the health system, insurance), to identify culturally appropriate methods of engagement and to determine priorities and opportunities for action.

The two sub-committees working under the RHC: The first is the Engagement Team, which looks at methods of engaging the refugee community in order to build capacity, improve existing and develop new services and empower the targeted populations to improve their own health. The second is the Data Team, which works a. to help clarify the number of refugees and their respective culture groups living in Omaha. Existing data sources were identified and will be linked to create a usable database that will support future activities including engagement and research; b. Since major funding is needed to ensure the sustainability of BTC and the RHC, the data team is working on developing scientific research grant applications. In addition, the RHC is diligently working to develop a community health worker program with the refugee communities. The RHC encourages refugee involvement at all levels including refugee leaders from all groups who are represented in the city. This is not merely a project; the RHC is committed to long-term goals and implementation. With diverse team players from academia, local refugee organizations and refugee community leaders, the potential for successful outcomes is promising.

As we identify and embrace the different refugee groups in Omaha NE, we can better understand health-related needs, develop effective interventions, enhance cultural sensitivity and track outcomes. All are bound to benefit from this endeavor.

Limitations

The limitations of this project center on the assessment of its effectiveness. Currently, due to language barriers, limited resources, slow coordination among agencies, and limited data-sharing agreements, we are unable to better track how the program is making a difference in the community. With a $50,000 grant recently obtained for linkage of data and the development of a comprehensive data system for the city, we hope to better capture the impact on health and other related outcomes in the near future.

Conclusion

The definition of Health as referred by the World Health Organization (WHO) is especially important when considering the refugee populations (13). Started in 2010 from an initiative of a caring student (author CN) the interprofessional student-led/community-engaged Bridge to

Care project expanded its activities into 2014. It created great ripples for further collaborative action and capacity building to improve the health of the refugee community. Students are rewarded with an exceptional real-life community based experience, while community needs are addressed, local capacity is built, and sustainability is built.

Acknowledgments

We are deeply grateful for the work of all of the Bridge to Care student leaders, the faculty volunteers who supervise and mentor the students, refugee community leaders; and to the refugee service organizations leaders who trust and nurture this partnership.

References

UNHCR: The UN Refugee Agency. A pocket guide to refugees 2008. URL: http://www.unhcr.org/pages/49c-3646c4b8.html

US Office of Refugee Resettlement. Refugee arrival data 2000–2012. URL: http://www.acf.hhs.gov/programs/orr/resource/refugee-arrival-data

US Department of State Refugee Resettlement in the United States 2013. URL: http://www.state.gov/j/prm/releases/factsheets/2013/203578.htm

Department of Health and Human Services-Nebraska, 2012–2013 Minority Health Initiative Annual Report. URL: http://dhhs.ne.gov/Pages/srd_srdindex.aspx

Lainof CA, Elsea SJ. From Sudan to Omaha: how one community is helping African refugees find a new home. Am J Nurs 2004;104:58–61.

Tompkins M, Smith L, Jones K, Swundell S. HIV-education needs among Sudanese immigrants and refugees in the midwestern United States. AIDS Behav 2006;10:319–23.

Benner MT, Townsend J, Kaloi W, Htwe K, Naranichakul N, Hunnangkul S, et al. Reproductive health and quality of life of young Burmese refugees in Thailand. Confl Health 2010;4:5.

Campbell DS. Health hazards in the meatpacking industry. Occup Med 1999;14(2):351–72.

World Health Organization. Overcoming migrants' barriers to health. URL: http://www.who.int/bulletin/volumes/86/8/08-020808/en/

Morris MD, Popper ST, Rodwell TC, Brodine SK, Brouwer KC. Healthcare barriers of refugees post-resettlement. J Commun Health 2009;34:529–38.

Carswell K, Blackburn P, Barker C. The relationship between trauma post-migration problems and the psychological well-being of refugees and asylum seekers. Int J Soc Psychiatry 2011;57:107–19.

Herrel N, Olevitch L, Dubois DK, Terry P, Thorp D, Kind E, el al. Somali refugee women speak out about their needs for care during pregnancy and delivery. J Midwifery Womens Health 2004;49:345–9.

World Health Organization. Preamble to the Constitution of the World Health Organization 1946. URL: http://www.who.int/about/definition/en/print.html

Israel BA, Schulz AJ, Parker EA, Becker AB. Review of community-based research: assessing partnership approaches to improve public health. Annu Rev Public Health 1998;19:173–202.

Museums and Art Galleries as Partners for Public Health Interventions

Paul M. Camic and Helen J. Chatterjee

Abstract

The majority of public health programmes are based in schools, places of employment and in community settings. Likewise, nearly all health-care interventions occur in clinics and hospitals. An underdeveloped area for public health-related planning that carries international implications is the cultural heritage sector, and specifically museums and art galleries. This paper presents a rationale for the use of museums and art galleries as sites for public health interventions and health promotion programmes through discussing the social role of these organisations in the health and well-being of the communities they serve. Recent research from several countries is reviewed and integrated into a proposed framework for future collaboration between cultural heritage, health-care and university sectors to further advance research, policy development and evidence-based practice.

Keywords: well-being; social inclusion; health promotion; health inequalities; museums; art galleries; community-based interventions

Cultural Heritage and Public Health

Most public health practitioners and researchers are probably not likely to consider the heritage sector, and specifically museums and art galleries, as venues for interventions focused on health and well-being, two areas directly related to public health policy and programming. This article begins with a rationale as to why museums and

Paul M. Camic and Helen J. Chatterjee, "Museums and Art Galleries as Partners for Public Health Interventions," *Perspectives in Public Health*, vol. 133, no. 1, pp. 66-71. Copyright © 2013 by SAGE Publications, Ltd. Reprinted with permission. Provided by ProQuest LLC. All rights reserved.

galleries offer the possibility to be good partners to carry out public health policy initiatives; this is followed by a discussion about the social role that museums/galleries can play in health care, along with some examples of recent research. We conclude by presenting a framework for museum and gallery involvement with recommendations about future engagement.

Throughout much of the world, health-care treatment is delivered in clinics and hospitals while health promotion and illness prevention activities mostly occur in schools, community organisations and the workplace. While these are suitable locations that reach a great many people, there are other organisations and sectors that could be approached as partners in public health research and practice development. One such potential partner is the cultural heritage sector, a segment of which comprises museums and art galleries. (The term 'museums' will be used here to encompass art galleries and museums.) There are over 19,300 museums throughout the European Economic Area (EU member states, Norway and Switzerland)[1] and about the same number in Canada and the USA,[2] which make these organisations well placed to reach a diverse population across rural and urban settings.

Museums have experienced a great deal of change in recent years and many have become more aware of the needs and interests of their local communities[3] while also expanding the types of activities offered, including the development of in-house programmes and outreach activities to those who are often socially excluded from participation due to a range of exclusionary practices and circumstances.[4,5,52] Possibly unknown to the health-care sector, numerous museums currently offer innovative programmes that seek to address challenging health-care problems, offer support to caregivers and provide education, often within an aesthetically pleasing environment. Some of these programmes, activities and research studies, for example, have addressed health and well-being issues such as mental health problems,[7,8] dementia,[9–12] cancer,[13,14] lifelong learning for older adults,[15,16] health education[17] and social capital.[18]

While museums can sometimes be intimidating places, they are nearly always non-stigmatising settings in that they are not institutions where diagnosis and treatment of medical and mental health problems occur, nor are they settings where one experiences embarrassment, shame or criticism for attending. Museums *can* be places that encourage people to learn about themselves, their culture and society, and the larger world around them. Many museums also have websites that provide continuous virtual access to objects and other cultural information from their collections, thus extending their boundaries worldwide and unrestrained by opening hours. In addition, when attending the majority of UK national and US federal museums no cost is incurred for regular admission, while in many other European countries entrance fees are reduced or free for children, students, older adults and those unemployed, making access less dependent on financial ability while also encouraging frequent attendance across all age groups; two ideal variables for public health programming.

Places of Cultural Activity, Engagement and Interaction

There is increasing evidence from quantitative and qualitative studies in different countries that arts-based and other cultural programmes can reduce adverse psychological[19] and physiological[20] symptoms and are positive determinants for survival,[21,22] well-being and quality of life[23] and self-reported health.[24,25] The process of cultural impact on health and well-being is complex, and beyond the scope of this article; however, recent research supports the importance of cultural stimuli that can engage people but 'who (also) need to be willing to open themselves up to the experiences involved'[26] and participate regularly to more fully realise the benefits. Public health-oriented programmes in museums need to consider that not all activities will be suitable for all people. They will also need to take into account how best to boost regular engagement, knowing that it is likely to have greater benefit than infrequent participation. Encouraging people to 'open themselves up' within the confines of a publically accessible cultural activity may be a tall order and will require thoughtful programme development by reflective and sensitive staff to the nuances of human differences.

Several authors have described the social role of museums,[6,27,28] particularly their importance as agents to increase social inclusion and reduce socially excluding practices across communities, by providing environments and processes to re-examine behaviour, attitudes and beliefs.[29]

Although not all museums concur that they should play a role to decrease social exclusion or improve health, some have chosen to do so. The Marmot Review[30] draws together a range of research that exemplifies a direct link between health and well-being and sociality:

> Individuals who are socially isolated are between two and five times more likely than those who have strong social ties to die prematurely. Social networks have a larger impact on the risk of mortality than on the risk of developing disease, that is, it is not so much that social networks stop you from getting ill, but that they help you to recover when you do get ill. (p. 138)

This notion ties in with many recent UK policy initiatives that recognise the growing importance of the involvement of third sector organisations in community-based health improvement programmes, and not least with the recent Health and Social Care Act 2012,[31] which will see radical reforms to health service delivery. Given the economic challenges facing the cultural, health and social care sectors, and an increased focus on community-based public health interventions as part of the current UK government's Big Society policy,[32] we argue that the time has never been more pertinent for a closer engagement between museums and health and social care providers.

Silverman[28] suggests that museums contribute to the pursuit of health and well-being in five major ways: (1) promoting relaxation; (2) an immediate intervention of beneficial change in physiology, emotions or both; (3) encouraging introspection, which can be beneficial for mental health; (4) fostering health education; and (5) acting as public health advocates and enhancing health-care environments. While these suggestions are possibly useful, one of the biggest challenges is to demonstrate the value of museum interventions in terms of recognised health and well-being outcomes. Some of the best evidence to date, of the health and well-being benefits afforded by museum interventions, has focused around museum object handling and viewing paintings.[7,8,10,29] The objects held by museums contain the stories of civilisation but they can also stimulate people to create their own stories or to weave the story of an object, real or imagined, into one's daily life. Object handling in museums, while once forbidden, is now increasingly a part of in-house and outreach programmes across different age groups as the biopsychosocial and neuroscientific aspects of touch and tactile interpretation become known.[33] Recently completed research with medical and psychiatric patients demonstrated the health-care potential of museum objects 'to assist with counselling on issues of illness, death, loss and mourning, and to help restore dignity, respect and a sense of identity.'[34]

Mack[35] has described objects as 'containers or memory' and several authors have noted that museum objects trigger memories in ways that other information-bearing materials do not.[13,36,37] For this reason many museums offer reminiscence and memory activities, and evidence suggests that these activities can affect mood, ideas of self-worth and general sense of well-being.[8,10,28,34,36] During such encounters participants report that object interactions help them recall memories and encourage interactivity. Furthermore, the intrinsic material properties and the significance of the objects are often highlighted as participants report a sense of privilege at being afforded the opportunity to touch precious objects. Some museums have taken the notion of memory and reminiscence interventions a step further and extended such activities to the training of health-care professionals who care for people with dementia and other cognitive disorders.[38] Numerous practice-based examples and research demonstrates how museum interventions contribute to emotional well-being; these outcomes are drawn together by Wood[39] but have also been cited by others.[7,40]

- Sense of connection, and belonging
- Human capital: using and improving skills
- Optimism and hope
- Moral values, beliefs
- Identity capital, self-esteem
- Emotional capital, resilience
- Opportunity for success
- Recognition of achievement
- Support
- Quiet, rest, sanctuary
- Social capital, relationships

- Meaningful pursuits
- Safe, rich museum environment
- Access to arts and culture

It is argued that when people interact with museums and their collections, the objects' material, physical and intrinsic properties trigger a variety of emotional and sensory responses, cognitive associations, memories and projections.[41] Pearce[42] suggests that such encounters lead to a process of symbolisation, while Gregory and Whitcomb[45] and Dudley[46] argue that the multi-sensory aspect of cultural encounters elicits ideas and meaning-making opportunities. Meaning making has emerged from other studies of museum interventions,[11,28,44,45] while other researchers (e.g. Lanceley et al.[13]) have drawn upon the psychoanalytic conception of Winnicott's[46] transitional object to explore how museum objects can offer an 'intermediate area of experience' (p. 2) between the self and not-me object, where the (museum) object becomes an externalised representation of unconscious wishes and desires.

The role and interplay of sensory modalities may help explain why kinaesthetic museum interventions afford well-being benefits. Thomson et al.[14] proposed that museum interventions draw upon Paivio's[47] 'dual coding' model, which suggests that verbal and visual material are connected in a short-term working memory store, and Baddeley's[48] modality effect, which proposes cognitive advantages to working memory when auditory and visual modalities are integrated. Thomson et al.'s[14] research also highlighted the interplay of touch in the multi-sensory museum experience and they infer that since three senses are at play during museum interventions (touch, auditory and visual), a triple-coding model could help explain the cognitive advantages that lead to health and well-being outcomes. Camic,[49] in a study looking at the use of 'found objects' in a non-clinical adult population across eight countries, identified 'a *found object process* that involves the interaction of aesthetic, cognitive, emotive, mnemonic, ecological, and creative factors in the seeking, discovery, and utilization' of finding and using material objects (pp. 87–8).

Despite an enhanced understanding of the possible cognitive and psychosocial evidence regarding the benefits of arts- and health-focused interventions in museums/galleries, research is still in an early stage and tends to lack control or comparison groups that would better allow assessment of impact and health economic analysis. Notwithstanding this, numerous examples of well-described cases and small-scale empirical studies exist, some of which are outlined above, and these can be used to confer the multifarious health and well-being benefits of museum interventions.

A 'Culture and Health' Framework for Museum and Gallery Involvement

In order to assist professionals from both the heritage and public health sectors to make the best use of museums as complementary partners in public health work, it would be useful to have an overarching framework from which to consider the values, assumptions, practices, problems and populations that could be best served from museum involvement. One such framework, we suggest, would involve cultural involvement (with museums) and the public health activities of health promotion and health education[50] while addressing the problems of well-being[51] and social exclusion[52] (Figure 2.2.1). Rather than attempting to address all known health and well-being concerns, a more productive and strategic approach would involve museums developing partnerships with local health-care authorities, health-care funders and other local museums and galleries to coordinate resources, knowledge and expertise. While some museums have developed partnerships with health and social care services in the UK and elsewhere, this is far from the norm. As a key element of the framework, these partnerships would provide the fundamental structure for supporting programme development, outreach to communities and research. Partnership working also suggests an avenue for further health behaviour research about those who currently attend and do not attend museums/galleries so that health promotion/education can be more focused and evidenced based within these settings.

While valuing their independence and unique focus as distinct cultural organisations, local *and* shared coordination of museum-based public health services—'culture and health planning'—can enhance the variety of programmes offered and also increase their sustainability;[23,53] two exemplars of this type of framework are seen through health-care and museum networks in Boston, Massachusetts[54] and the northwest of England.[41] The public health implications for such an expanded network of partners is highly significant. Throughout Europe, for example, in large market towns or medium-sized cities, one is likely to find local history and culture museums, perhaps a science/natural history museum and specialty museums, and one or two art galleries, along with a health authority and health-care delivery organisations. Coordinating arts and health initiatives through the suggested framework would likely be challenging, however, as different ways of working (e.g. the differences in the medical and social models of health and illness),[55] dissimilar organisational cultures and indeed, vastly disparate business rationales would need to be addressed and bridged in the early planning stages. The benefits of working with a 'culture and health framework', however, could see a radically different way to engage local public health offices, regional governments and museums/galleries to best address the needs of local communities, reduce overlap of programmes, share resources and deliver health intervention and promotion activities. Museums have the potential to develop a type of 'arts on prescription' scheme as advocated by O'Neill[26] and similar to the social prescribing research Stickley and Hui have reported.[56] O'Neill's referral-ready museum service recommends a system that links staff from the health service and/or voluntary organisations with staff in cultural organisations, so that the former can refer their patients/clients/members to the latter, in a similar way that we have suggested in the culture and health framework.

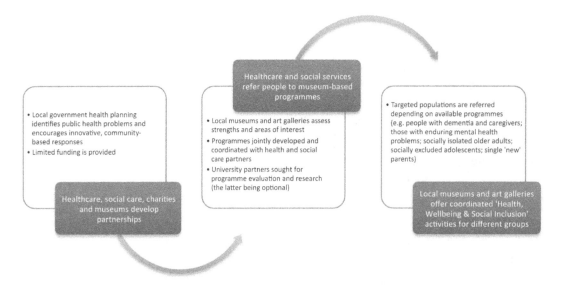

Figure 2.2.1   Culture and health framework for museum and gallery involvement in public health

Another benefit of the framework would be to provide research opportunities to coordinate the development of improved evaluation strategies using similar assessment tools[14,57,58] that could help shape future programme improvements. A further advantage of collaboration and co-ordination between the heritage and health-care sectors could lead to the development of new research partnerships with universities, further adding to the growing evidence of the impact of cultural activities on health,[59,60,61] a goal that Clift[62] has forcefully argued for in order to support and encourage more evidence-based practice.

Conclusion

Innovative health-care and public health intervention programmes have demonstrated that they can be delivered in alternative venues and through a variety of means, some of which have been discussed in this article within the cultural heritage sector of museums and art galleries. Museums and art galleries are obviously structured differently from health-care organisations and both have traditionally been focused on distinctly separate and divergent purposes. Yet, these differences in purpose, scope and structure can also be drawn upon to help address some of the problems related to health promotion, illness prevention, well-being and quality of life for people across a range of age groups, with different risk factors, and from different socioeconomic and ethnic groups, only some of which we have cited above. Large-scale epidemiological population surveys in Sweden, Norway, the UK and the USA have demonstrated strong positive correlations between cultural activities and health. Medium- and smaller-scale quantitative and qualitative studies involving museums, art galleries and material objects in Australia, Canada, the UK and the USA, among other countries, have begun to build an evidence base to address specific problems and issues that are ideally suited for public health interventions and programmes. Although much more needs to be done, a foundation has been laid that encourages the further development of evidenced-based practice in this area. Future research would greatly benefit from a systematic or structured literature review that focused on health and well-being research within a museum and art gallery context. Additional research should also use social comparison and control groups in order to more rigorously assess the impact of the overall museum/art gallery experience, but also in relation to measuring specific health and social outcomes.

References

1 European Group on Museum Statistics (EGMS). *Museum Statistics*. Available online at http://www.egmus.eu (accessed November 2012)

2 American Alliance of Museums (AAM). http://www.aam-us.org/Canadian Heritage. *Interesting Facts about Canadian Museums*. Available online at http://www.pch.gc.ca/special/jim-imd/canada_dyk-eng.cfm (Last accessed November 2012)

3 Jung Y. The art museum ecosystem: A new alternative model. *Museum Management and Curatorship* 2011; 26: 321–38

4 Coffee K. Cultural inclusion, exclusion and the formative roles of museums. *Museum Management and Curatorship*, 2008; 23: 261–79

5 Sendell R, Nighingale E (eds). *Museums, equality and social justice*. London: Routledge, 2012

6 Classen C. *The book of touch*. Oxford: Berg, 2005

7 Shaer D et al. The role of art therapy in a pilot for art-based information prescriptions at Tate Britain. *International Journal of Art Therapy* 2008; 13: 25–33

8 Roberts S, Camic PM, Springham N. New roles for art galleries: Art-viewing as a community intervention for family carers of people with mental health problems. *Arts & Health: An International Journal for Research, Policy and Practice* 2011; 3: 146–59

9 Rosenberg F. The MoMa Alzheimer's project: Programming and resources for making art accessible to people with Alzheimer's disease and their caregivers. *Arts & Health: An International Journal for Research, Policy and Practice* 2009; 1: 93–7

10 Eeckelaar C, Camic PM, Springham N. Art galleries, episodic memory and verbal fluency in dementia: An exploratory study. *Psychology of Aesthetics, Creativity and the Arts* 2012; 6: 262–72

11 Stephens A, Cheston R, Gleeson, K. An exploration into the relationships people with dementia have with physical objects: An ethnographic study. *Dementia: The International Journal for Social Research and Practice* 2012. DOI: 10.1177/1471301212442585

12 MacPherson S, Bird M, Anderson K, Davis T, Blair A. An art gallery access programme for people with dementia: 'You do it for the moment'. *Ageing & Mental Health* 2009; 13: 744–52

13 Lanceley A, Noble G, Johnson M, Balogun N, Chatterjee HJ, Menon U. Investigating the therapeutic potential of a heritage-object focused intervention: A qualitative study. *Journal of Health Psychology* 2012. DOI: 10.1177/1359105311426625

14 Thomson L, Ander E, Lanceley A, Menon U, Noble G, Chatterjee HJ. Enhancing cancer patient well-being with a non-pharmacological, heritage-focused intervention. *Journal of Pain and Symptom Management* 2012; 44: 731–40

15 Grut S. Seniors as museum visitors. Lifelong Learning and Museum Conference 2011, The Open and Learning Museum, Tempere, Finland

16 Goulding A. Lifelong learning for people 64+ within the contemporary art gallery context. *Educational Gerontology* 2012; 38: 215–27

17 Wikström B-M. Nursing education at an art gallery. *Journal of Nursing Scholarship* 2000; 32: 197–9

18 White M. *Arts development in community health: A social tonic.* Oxford: Radcliffe, 2009

19 Stuckey HL, Nobel J. The connection between art, healing, and public health: A review of the current literature. *American Journal of Public Health* 2010; 100: 254–63

20 Clow A, Fredhoi C. Normalisation of salivary cortisol levels and self-report stress by a brief lunchtime visit to an art gallery by London city workers. *Journal of Holistic Healthcare* 2006; 3: 29–32

21 Bygren LO, Konlaan BB, Johansson E. Attendance at cultural events, reading books or periodicals, and making music or singing in a choir as determinants for survival: Swedish interview survey of living conditions. *British Medical Journal* 1996; 313: 1577–80

22 Glass TA, de Leon CM, Marottoli, RA, Berkman, LF. Population based study of social and productive activities as predictors of survival among elderly Americans. *British Medical Journal* 1999; 319: 478–83

23 Galloway S, Hamilton C, Scullion A. *Quality of Life and Well-Being: Measuring the Benefits of Culture and Sport.* Glasgow: Scottish Government report, University of Glasgow

24 Wilkinson AV, Waters AJ, Bygren LO, Taro AR. Are variations in rates of attending cultural activities associated with population health in the United States? *Public Health* 2007; 7: 226

25 Cohen GD, Perlstein S, Chapline J, Kelly J, Firth KM, Simmens S. The impact of professionally conducted cultural programs on the physical health, mental health, and social functioning of older adults. *The Gerontologist* 2006; 46: 726–34

26 O'Neill M. Cultural attendance and public mental health –from research to practice. *Journal of Public Mental Health* 2010; 9: 22–9

27 Sandell R. *Museums, society, inequality.* London: Routledge, 2002

28 Silverman LH. *The social work of museums.* London: Routledge, 2010, p. 51

29 Mittelman M, Epstein C. *Meet Me at MoMA Program. Research.* Available online at http://www.moma. org/docs/meetme/Resources_NYU_Evaluation.pdf (Last accessed November 2012)

30 Marmot M et al. *Fair Society, Health Lives: The Marmot Review.* Available online at http://www. instituteofhealthequity.org/ (accessed November 2012)

31 The National Archives. *Health and Social Care Act 2012.* Available online at http://www. legislation. gov.uk/ukpga/2012/7/contents/enacted (Last accessed November 2012)

32 Cabinet Office. *Big Society Overview.* Available online at http://www.cabinetoffice.gov.uk/content/ big-society-overview (Last accessed November 2012)

33 Chatterjee HJ (ed). *Touch in Museums.* Oxford: Berg, 2008

34 Chatterjee HJ, Vreeland S, Noble G. Museopathy: Exploring the healing potential of handling museum objects. *Museum and Society* 2009; 7: 164–77

35 Mack J. *The Museum of the Mind: Art and Memory in World Cultures.* London: The British Museum Press, 2003

36 Kavanagh G. *Dream Spaces: Memory and the Museum.* London: Leicester University Press, 2002

37 Philips L. Reminiscence: Recent work at the British Museum. In HJ Chatterjee (ed) *Touch in Museums: Policy and Practice in Object Handling.* Oxford: Berg, 2008

38 National Museums Liverpool. *House of Memories: National Museums Liverpool Evaluation Report.* Available online at http://www.liverpoolmuseums.org.uk/learning/documents/House-of-Memories-evaluation-report.pdf (accessed November 2012)

39 Wood C. *Museums of the Mind: Mental Health, Emotional Well-Being, and Museums.* Bude, Culture Unlimited, 2007

40 Davenport B, Corner L. *Review of Policy and Research Evidence Relating to the Ageing, Health and Vitality Project.* Available online at http://objecthandling.files.wordpress. com/2012/05/policy-re-search-review-for-ahv1. pdf (Last accessed November 2012)

41 Froggett L, Farrier A, Poursanidou K. *Who Cares? Museums Health and Well-Being: A Study of the Renaissance North West Programme.* Available online at http://gmartshealth.cubedev.co.uk/CubeCore/. uploads/For%20Cube/case%20studies%20 docs/Who%20Cares%20Report%20FINAL%20 w%20 revisions.pdf (Last accessed November 2012)

42 Pearce SM. *On Collecting: An Investigation into Collecting in the European Tradition.* London: Routledge, 1995

43 Gregory K, Whitcomb A. Beyond nostalgia: The role of affect in generating historical understanding at heritage sites. In SJ Knell, S MacLeod, SER Watson (eds) *Museum Revolutions: How Museums Change and Are Changed.* New York: Routledge, 2007

44 Dudley SH. Museum materialities: Objects, sense and feeling. In SH Dudley (eds) *Museum Materialities: Objects, Engagements, Interpretations.* London: Routledge, 2010

45 Dodd J, O'Riain H, Hooper-Greenhill E, Sandell R. *A Catalyst for Change: The Social Impact of the Open Museum.* Leicester: Leicester University Research Centre for Museums and Galleries, 2002

46 Winnicott DW. Transitional objects and transitional phenomena. In Winnicott DW (ed) *Through Paediatrics to Psychoanalysis: Collected Papers*. London: Brunner-Routledge, 1992

47 Paivio A. *Mental Representations: A Dual-Coding Approach*. New York: Oxford University Press, 1986

48 Baddeley AD. Working memory. *Science* 1992; 255: 556–9

49 Camic PM. From trashed to treasured: A grounded theory analysis of found objects. *Psychology of Aesthetics, Creativity and the Arts* 2010; 4: 81–92

50 Camic PM. Playing in the mud: Health psychology, the arts, and creative approaches to health care. *Journal of Health Psychology* 2008; 13: 287–98

51 Ander EE, Thomson LJ, Lanceley A, Menon U, Noble G, Chatterjee HJ. Generic wellbeing outcomes: Towards a conceptual framework for wellbeing outcomes in museums. *Museum Management and Curatorship* 2011; 26: 237–59

52 Sandell R. Museums as agents of social inclusion. *Museum Management and Curatorship* 1998; 17: 401–18

53 Wolfe G. Short term box-ticking projects do not change lives. *Museums Journal* 2010; 110/06: 16

54 Caulfield S. Art, museums, and culture. In PE Hartman-Stein, A La Rue (eds) *Enhancing Cognitive Fitness in Adults: A Guide to the Use and Development of Community-Based Programs*. New York: Springer, 2011

55 Gray L. *What have Art Galleries got to do with our Mental Health?* Available online at http://www.fullcirclearts.co.uk/features/what-have-art-galleries-got-to-do-with-our-mental-health/ (Last accessed November 2012)

56 Stickley T, Hui A. Social prescribing through arts on prescription in a UK city: Referrers' perspectives (part 2). *Public Health* 2012; 126: 580–6

57 Staricoff RL. Arts in health: The value of evaluation. *Journal of the Royal Society for the Promotion of Health* 2006; 126: 116–20

58 Angus J. *A Review of Evaluation in Community-Based Art for Health Activity in the UK*. London: Health Development Agency, 2002

59 Bygren LO, Johansson S-E, Konlaan BB, Gribovske AM, Wilkinson AV, Sjöström M. Attending cultural events and cancer mortality: A Swedish cohort study. *Arts & Health: An International Journal for Research, Policy and Practice* 2009; 1: 64–73

60 Cuypers KF, Knudtsen MS, Sandgren M, Krokstad S (eds). Cultural activates and public health: Research in Norway and Sweden. *Arts and Health: An International Journal for Research, Practice and Policy* 2011; 3: 6–26

61 Cuypers K, Krokstad S, Holmen TL, Knudtsen MS, Bygren, LO, Holmen J. Patterns of receptive and creative cultural activities and their association with perceived health, anxiety, depression and satisfaction with life among adults: The HUNT study, Norway. *Journal of Epidemiology and Community Health* 2012; 66: 698–703

62 Clift S. Creative arts as a public health resource: Moving from practice-based research to evidence-based practice. *Perspectives in Public Health* 2012; 132: 120–7

Chapter 2: **Discussion Questions**

1   Why might America have a harder time aligning incentives and expectations in health policy change than other countries?

   a.   Since Houston has one of the highest refugee populations in the nation, what unique health care services are necessary to maintain and improve the city's public health?

2   Give three examples of common refugee health problems that result from their past histories.

   a.   Which do you suspect is the most prevalent and why?

3   Why is assessment important in health interventions?

   a.   Was Bridge to Care successful in the assessment of their program?

4   How does venue impact health care?

   a.   List four benefits of holding health interventions at galleries and museums and rank them in importance (1, highest importance; 4, least importance)

5   How were the population groups listed in Figure 2.2.1 particularly suited for a health intervention located in a museum/gallery setting?

   a.   Suggest another target population to include in this type of program and explain why.

CHAPTER 3

EMPLOYER-SPONSORED INSURANCE AND WELLNESS

Health-Care Reform and Private Health Insurance

George E. Rejda

B efore proceeding, it is important to understand the major changes to individual and group medical expense coverages under the Affordable Care Act. [...]

The new health-care reform law will be phased in from 2010 through 2018. Some changes became effective in 2010 when the new law was enacted, while other major changes will become effective in 2014. Important provisions in the new law that affect individual and group coverages discussed in this chapter are summarized as follows:

- *Individual mandate.* Beginning in 2014, most people in the United States must have health insurance that meets certain minimum standards or else pay a tax penalty. Compulsory insurance reduces adverse selection against insurers and cost shifting by health-care providers for treating uninsured patients.
- *Elimination of lifetime limits.* Individual and group plans are prohibited from placing lifetime dollar limits on the value of the coverage.
- *Restrictions on annual limits.* Prior to 2014, the new law restricts and phases out any annual dollar limits on covered benefits that may be present in group plans and in individual health insurance as determined by the Secretary of Health and Human Services. Beginning in 2014, annual limits on coverage are prohibited.
- *Exclusions for pre-existing conditions for children not allowed.* Excluding coverage or denying claims for pre-existing conditions for children under age 19 and for adults beginning in 2014 is not allowed.
- *Retention of coverage for young adults until age 26.* Young adults must be allowed to retain coverage under their parents' policies until age 26.

- *Rescission of individual contracts not allowed.* Insurers are prohibited from rescinding individual insurance policies except in the case of fraud. Insurers earlier could deny claims on the basis of technical irregularities or mistakes in the application when the policy was first underwritten.
- *Restrictions on rating variables.* Beginning in 2014, variations in rating are allowed only for age, geographical area, tobacco use, and number of family members, and charging females higher premiums for their coverage is prohibited.
- *Benefit categories.* Applicants will have a choice of bronze, silver, gold, or platinum plans that cover 60 percent to 90 percent of the benefit costs, plus a separate catastrophic plan that will be offered through a Health Insurance Exchange, and in the individual and small group markets.
- *No cost-sharing provisions for preventive services.* New plans that start on or after September 23, 2010, and existing plans that make changes after that date cannot impose deductibles, coinsurance, and copayments on preventive services such as mammograms, colonoscopies, and cancer screenings.
- *Medical loss ratios.* Insurers are required to have a minimum loss ratio of 85 percent for plans in the large group market and 80 percent for plans in the individual and small group markets.
- *Premium credits to individuals and families.* Premium credits will be provided to eligible individuals and families with incomes of 133 percent to 400 percent of the federal poverty level to enable them to buy health insurance through the Health Insurance Exchanges. The premium credits are designed to limit the amount spent on health insurance from 2 percent to a maximum of 9.5 percent of income. This provision becomes effective in 2014.
- *Tax credits to small employers.* The new law provides tax credits to small employers that have fewer than 25 full-time equivalent employees and pay average annual wages of less than $50,000.
- *Employer penalties.* The new law does not require employers to offer health insurance to their employees. However, employers with 50 or more employees that do not offer coverage to their employees, where at least one employee is receiving a premium tax credit through a Health Insurance Exchange, will be assessed an annual fee of $2,000 for each full-time employee (in excess of 30 employees).

Individual Health Insurance Coverages

Millions of people are covered under individual health insurance plans. Many workers are laid off, fired, or retire early and need individual coverage; many unemployed workers are between jobs and need individual insurance; children who attain age 26 are no longer covered under their parents' plans and may need individual insurance; the self-employed who are not in group plans may require individual coverage; and a high percentage of people who are not in the paid labor force require individual protection. In addition, most workers need disability income insurance if they become sick or injured, and most retired persons need long-term care insurance. In this section, we discuss the following kinds of individual coverages.[1]

- Major medical insurance
- Health savings accounts
- Disability income insurance
- Long-term care insurance

Major Medical Insurance

Most individual medical expense plans sold today are major medical policies. Major medical insurance is a plan that pays a high percentage of covered expenses incurred by insured individuals when they have a catastrophic illness or injury. The primary purpose is to relieve the insured of the crushing financial burden of a catastrophic loss. A typical individual major medical policy sold today has the following characteristics:

- Catastrophe benefits
- Broad range of benefits
- Deductible
- Coinsurance
- Out-of-pocket limits
- Exclusions

Catastrophe Benefits

Major medical insurance is not designed to pay first-dollar coverage, but to pay catastrophic medical bills that can cause great economic insecurity. Because of the high cost of medical care, it is not uncommon for patients to incur medical bills of $50,000, $100,000, $500,000, or even higher amounts. Major medical policies are designed to pay a large part of these expenses. As stated earlier, lifetime dollar limits on benefits are no longer permitted. This limitation applies to both existing and new major medical plans.

Broad Range of Benefits

Major medical policies provide a broad range of benefits. New major medical plans must meet minimum benefit standards to be sold on the various exchanges. Benefits typically include the following:

- *Inpatient hospital services.* Inpatient services include room and board charges for the hospital room, meals, routine nursing care, and other services. Other covered inpatient services include charges for the operating room, surgical dressings, drugs, lab tests, X-rays, and radiology services.

- *Outpatient services*. Coverage for outpatient services typically includes surgery as an outpatient in a hospital or separate outpatient facility; pre-admission tests given prior to admission into the hospital as an inpatient; outpatient chemotherapy and radiation therapy; outpatient services provided in an emergency room; and other services as well.
- *Physicians' services*. Major medical plans typically cover office visits to physicians, consultation with specialists, surgeons' fees, cost of anesthesia services, and services provided by chiropractors, physician assistants, nurse practitioners, physical therapists, and other therapists.

  Surgeons and other physicians are commonly reimbursed on the basis of reasonable and customary charges, which vary by insurer. For example, an insurer may consider a surgeon's fee to be reasonable and customary if it does not exceed the 80th or 90th percentile for a similar procedure performed by other surgeons in the same area. In most cases, the surgeon's actual fee will be substantially above the reasonable and customary charge. *The allowable charge, however, is the lower of the surgeon's actual fee or the reasonable and customary charge.* With the exception of managed care plans discussed later, the insured must pay that portion of the fee that exceeds the upper limit.

- *Outpatient prescription drugs*. Outpatient prescription drug coverage is another important benefit. There are two ways to provide coverage for prescription drugs.[2] First, under the *integrated approach*, charges for prescription drugs are subject to the same deductible and coinsurance charges that apply to other covered medical expenses. Second, under a separate *drug card program*, prescription drugs are subject to their own deductible and copayment charges. The drug card program is usually administered by a third-party administrator, such as a benefit pharmacy manager. A three-tier or four-tier system of pricing is commonly used. For the first tier, the copayment charge is the lowest for generic drugs. For the second tier, the copayment charge is higher for brand-name drugs on an approved list (called a formulary). For the third tier, the copayment charge is even higher for brand-name drugs that are not on the formulary. Finally, for the fourth tier, some plans may include coverage for very expensive drugs; copayments and coinsurance charges are substantially higher for drugs in this category.

Deductible

A major medical policy typically contains a deductible that must be satisfied before any benefits are paid. Deductibles in policies sold today are much higher than in policies sold in previous years. The insured usually has a choice of deductibles. Typical deductibles are $500, $1,000, $1,500, $2,000, or some higher amount. *The purpose of the deductible is to eliminate small claims and the high administrative cost of processing them.* By eliminating small claims, insurers can provide high limits and still keep the premiums reasonable.

Most major medical policies have a calendar-year deductible. *A calendar-year deductible is an aggregate deductible that has to be satisfied only once during the calendar year.* All covered medical expenses incurred by the insured during the calendar year can be applied toward the deductible. Once the deductible is met, no additional deductible has to be satisfied during the calendar year. To avoid paying two deductibles in a short time, most plans have a carryover provision, which means that unreimbursed medical expenses incurred during the last three months of the calendar year and applied to that year's deductible can be carried over and applied to following year's deductible.

Finally, under the new health-care reform law, deductibles and other cost-sharing provisions do not apply to preventive services. All new individual and group health plans must provide first dollar coverage for preventive services. This provision became effective in 2010.

Coinsurance

Major medical policies contain a coinsurance provision, which requires the insured to pay a certain percentage of eligible expenses in excess of the deductible. Coinsurance should not be confused with copayment. *Coinsurance* refers to the percentage of the bill in excess of the deductible, which the insured must pay. *Copayment* is a flat amount that the insured must pay for certain benefits, such as $25 for a visit to a primary care physician, or a $10 copayment fee for a generic drug.

Coinsurance provisions typically require the insureds to pay 20 percent, 25 percent, or 30 percent of covered medical expenses that exceed the deductible. For example, assume that an insured person has covered medical expenses of $10,000, the calendar year deductible is $1,000, and the coinsurance percentage is 20 percent. In addition to the $1,000 deductible, the insured pays 20 percent of the excess, or $1,800 (20 percent x $9,000). The insurer pays the remainder, or $7,200.

The coinsurance provision has two basic purposes: (1) to reduce premiums, and (2) to prevent overutilization of plan benefits. Coinsurance has a powerful impact on reducing premiums, and the insured are less likely to demand unnecessary services if they pay part of the cost.

Annual Out-of-Pocket Limits

Major medical policies also contain an *annual out-of-pocket limit* (also called a *stop-loss limit*) by which 100 percent of the covered medical expenses in excess of the deductible are paid after the insured pays a certain annual amount of out-of-pocket expenses. The purpose of the annual out-of-pocket limit is to reduce the crushing financial burden of a catastrophe loss. The insured is usually given a choice of annual out-of-pocket limits when the policy is purchased, such as $3,000, $4,000, or some higher amount. Out-of-pocket limits for family policies are substantially higher.

Exclusions

All individual major medical policies contain exclusions. Some common exclusions are as follows:

- Expenses caused by war
- Elective cosmetic surgery
- Eyeglasses and hearing aids
- Dental care, except as a result of an accident
- Expenses covered by workers' compensation and similar laws
- Unnecessary treatment or experimental medical treatment
- Services furnished by governmental agencies unless the patient has an obligation to pay
- Expenses covered by Medicare or other government medical expense programs
- Expenses resulting from suicide or self-inflicted injury

Major Medical Insurance and Managed Care

Many individual major medical policies sold today are part of a managed care plan. Managed care is a generic term for medical expense plans that provide benefits to insured individuals in a cost-effective manner. There is heavy emphasis on controlling costs and providing benefits to plan members in a cost-effective manner. For example, a *preferred provider organization (PPO)* is a popular type of managed care plan for both individual and group health insurance plans. A PPO contracts with physicians, hospitals, and other health-care providers to provide medical services to the members at discounted fees. People insured under a PPO have a strong financial incentive to receive care from preferred providers because of lower deductibles and coinsurance charges. Those who receive care outside the network must pay higher out-of-pocket costs because of substantially higher deductibles and coinsurance charges. [...].

Individual major medical policies today have incorporated many elements of managed care in the plan design. For example, the plan may require precertification and approval for nonemergency admission into a hospital; certain types of surgery must be done on an outpatient basis; and an insured may be required to use health-care providers who are part of the network or pay higher-out-of pocket costs for the benefits received. [...].

Health Savings Accounts

A *health savings account (HSA)* is a tax-exempt or custodial account established exclusively for the purpose of paying qualified medical expenses of the account beneficiary who is covered under a high-deductible health insurance plan. Health savings accounts have two components: (1) a high-deductible health insurance policy that covers catastrophic medical bills, and (2) an investment account from which the account holder can withdraw money tax free for qualified medical expenses.

- *Eligibility requirements*. Several eligibility requirements must be fulfilled to receive favorable tax treatment. First, the insured must be under age 65 and be covered by a high-deductible health plan and must not be covered by any other qualified high-deductible plan. This requirement does not apply to accident insurance, disability insurance, long-term care insurance, auto insurance, and certain other coverages. Second, the individual must not be eligible for Medicare. Finally, the insured must not be claimed as a dependent on another person's tax return.

- *High-deductible health plan.* For 2011, the annual deductible must be at least $1,200 for an individual and $2,400 for family coverage. The deductible cannot be applied to preventive services and is indexed annually for inflation.

  There is a maximum limit on annual out-of-pocket expenses. For 2011, annual out-of-pocket expenses, including the deductible and other cost-sharing provisions, cannot exceed $5,950 for an individual and $11,900 for a family. The annual out-of-pocket limits are adjusted each year for inflation. In addition, an HSA may also have a coinsurance requirement. Although some HSA plans pay 100 percent of the covered expenses exceeding the deductible, many individuals prefer to pay a lower premium for a policy with a coinsurance requirement. The coinsurance percentage is typically 20 percent, 25, percent or 30 percent of the covered costs in excess of the deductible up to some maximum annual limit. If the insured person receives care outside of a preferred provider network, coinsurance and copayment charges are substantially higher.

- *Annual contribution limits.* HSA contributions can be made by the insured, his or her employer, and family members. For 2011, annual contributions for individual coverage are limited to $3,050 for individual coverage and $6,150 for family coverage. These amounts are adjusted annually for inflation. Insured individuals age 55 or older can make an additional catch-up contribution of $1,000.

- *Favorable income-tax treatment.* The investment account in a qualified HSA plan receives favorable income-tax treatment. Annual premiums are income-tax deductible up to the limits described earlier. The deduction is "above the line," which means the insured person does not have to itemize deductions on the tax return to receive the deduction. In addition, investment earnings accumulate income-tax free, and distributions from the account are not taxable if used to pay qualified medical expenses. If the distributions are used for nonmedical purposes, they are taxable as ordinary income, and a 10 percent penalty must also be paid. Once the insured person attains age 65, additional contributions cannot be made, but the funds can still be used to pay for qualified medical expenses. The funds can be used for nonmedical purposes, however, but the money used is taxable income.

- *Rationale for HSAs.* Proponents present several arguments for HSAs: (1) if consumers must pay more for health care out of pocket, they will be more sensitive to health-care costs, avoid unnecessary medical services, and shop around for health care; (2) health insurance will be more affordable because of lower premiums; (3) if not needed for medical expenses, funds in an HSA can be used for retirement; and (4) HSAs are portable, which means workers can keep their insurance if they change jobs or become unemployed.

Critics of HSAs, however, present the following counterarguments: (1) HSA premiums are lower only because a significant part of the initial medical bill is shifted to the insured; (2) low-income persons and many middle-income workers and families cannot afford to pay the high annual deductible and coinsurance payments until coverage begins; (3) shopping around for less expensive health care is not practical or even possible for sick or injured persons, who may require immediate medical care, and easily accessible and reliable cost information may not be available; and (4) because of lower premiums, HSAs are more appealing to younger and healthier people who may opt out of coverage in traditional plans, which dilutes the number of healthy people in the insurance pool and raises premiums for unhealthy members.

Disability Income Insurance

Disability income insurance provides monthly cash benefits to an insured individual who is totally disabled due to sickness or injury. The objective is to replace part of the loss of earnings due to the disability. The probability of becoming disabled before retirement is higher than is commonly believed. According to the Social Security Administration, studies show that a 20-year-old worker has a 3 in 10 chance of becoming disabled before reaching retirement age.[3]

In cases of long-term disability, earned income is lost, medical expenses must be paid, savings are often depleted, employee benefits may be lost or reduced, and someone must care for a permanently disabled person. Unless there is adequate replacement income during the period of disability, considerable economic insecurity is present.

Individual disability income policies have several key characteristics. The most important are summarized as follows:

- *Meaning of disability.* There are several definitions of total disability. Disability can be defined as (1) the inability to perform all duties of the insured's own occupation; (2) the inability to perform the duties of any occupation for which the insured is reasonably fitted by training, education, and experience; (3) the inability to perform the duties of any gainful occupation, which may be found in policies that insure hazardous occupations; and (4) a loss-of-income test, which considers the actual loss of earned income as an objective measure of disability.

    Many policies combine the first two definitions. For some initial time period, such as two to five years, total disability is defined in terms of the insured's own occupation. After the initial period of disability expires, the second definition applies. For example, assume that a dentist can no longer practice because of severe arthritis in his or her hands. For the first two years, the dentist would be considered totally disabled. However, after two years, if the dentist could work as a research scientist, or as an instructor in a dental school, or in a similar occupation, he or she would no longer be considered disabled because these occupations are consistent with the dentist's training, education, and experience.

Finally, the policy may also contain a definition of *presumptive disability*. Total disability is presumed to exist if the insured suffers the total and irrevocable loss of sight in both eyes, or the total loss or use of both hands, both feet, or one hand and one foot.

- *Partial disability.* Some disability income policies may pay partial disability benefits. Partial disability is defined as the inability of the insured to perform one or more important duties of his or her occupation. Partial disability benefits are paid at a reduced rate for a shorter period. Partial disability benefits generally must follow a period of total disability. For example, a person may be totally disabled for several months after a serious auto accident. If the person recovers and goes back to work on a part-time basis to see if recovery is complete, partial disability benefits can be paid.

- *Residual disability.* Newer policies may contain a residual disability definition, rather than a partial disability provision, or coverage for residual disability can be added as an additional benefit with a higher premium. *Residual disability* means that a pro rata disability benefit is paid to an insured person whose earned income is reduced because of an accident or sickness. For example, if the insured's earned income is reduced 25 percent during some measurable time period because of sickness or injury, 25 percent of the monthly disability benefit will be paid.

- *Benefit period.* The insured has a choice of benefit periods, such as 2, 5, or 10 years, or up to age 65 or 70. The vast majority of disabilities are under two years. However, this does not mean that a two-year benefit period is adequate. The longer the disability, the less likely the disabled person will recover. For example, 10 percent of the people who are disabled for at least 90 days will be disabled for 5 or more years.[4] Thus, because of uncertainty concerning the duration of disability, a longer benefit period is desirable—ideally, one that pays benefits to age 65 or 70.

- *Elimination period.* Disability income policies are typically sold with an elimination period (waiting period) during which time benefits are not paid. Insurers offer a range of elimination periods, such as 30, 60, 90, 180, or 365 days. The longer the elimination period, the greater is the reduction in premiums. However, an elimination period beyond six months is not advisable, because the reduction in premiums is relatively small.

- *Waiver of premium.* Most policies contain a waiver-of-premium provision, by which premiums are waived if the insured is totally disabled for at least 90 days. If the insured recovers from the disability, premium payments must be resumed.

- *Rehabilitation provision.* The insurer and insured may agree on a vocational rehabilitation program. To encourage rehabilitation, part or all of the disability income benefits are paid during the training period. At the end of training, if the insured is still disabled, benefits continue as before. If the individual is fully rehabilitated and is capable of returning to work, the benefits will terminate.

- *Accidental death, dismemberment, and loss-of-sight benefits.* In the case of an accident, some policies pay accidental death, dismemberment, and loss-of-sight benefits. The maximum amount paid is called the principal sum, and the amounts paid are based on a schedule. For example, the principal sum may be payable for the loss of both hands and both feet or sight of both eyes.
- *Optional disability income benefits.* Several optional benefits can be added to a disability income policy by payment of higher premiums. They include the following: (1) a cost-of-living rider by which disability benefits are periodically adjusted for increases in the cost of living; (2) option to purchase additional insurance by which disability benefits can be increased at specific times in the future with no evidence of insurability; (3) Social Security rider by which an additional amount is paid if the insured is turned down for Social Security disability benefits; and (4) return of premiums rider by which part of the premium is refunded, such as 80 percent of the premiums paid, less any claims, after 10 years.

Notes

1 This section is based on George E. Rejda, *Principles of Risk Management and Insurance.* 11th ed. (Boston: Pearson Education, 2011), pp. 316–327.

2 AHIP Center for Policy and Research, "Individual Health Insurance 2009: A Comprehensive Survey of Premiums, Availability and Benefits." Washington, DC, October 2009, p. 26.

3 Social Security Administration, *Disability Benefits.* SSA Publication no. 5 05–10029, August 2010, ICN 456000.

4 Thomas P. O'Hare and Burton T. Beam, Jr., *Individual Health Insurance Planning: Medical, Disability Income, and Long-Term Care* (Bryn Mawr, PA: The American College, 2008), p. 12.3. Data are from the Society of Actuaries, Commissioner's Individual Disability Table A.

The Affordable Care Act and the Politics of Health Care Reform

Donald A. Barr

The headlines in March 2010 just about said it all. On March 22, a *New York Times* editorial declared, "Health Care Reform, at Last." Two days later, the *New England Journal of Medicine* announced, "Historic Passage—Reform at Last" (Iglehart 2010b). President Barack Obama had signed the Patient Protection and Affordable Care Act (ACA)—the most significant reform of our health care system since the 1965 enactment of Medicare and Medicaid under President Lyndon Johnson. After what Bruce Vladeck, administrator of the Health Care Financing Administration under President Bill Clinton, characterized as "the epochal, exhausting, and contentious task of enacting comprehensive health care reform" (Vladeck 2010, p. 1955), the tumultuous process that had begun more than a year before with the release of President Obama's first federal budget proposal had finally come to a conclusion.

The passage of reform legislation over the unanimous and strident opposition of congressional Republicans was assuredly a major step in the evolution of health care in America. ACA has extended publicly funded health insurance coverage to millions of formerly uninsured adults whose income falls near or below the federal poverty level (FPL). ACA has also made affordable health insurance available to millions more Americans who are not poor, yet who previously could not afford the cost of acquiring health insurance in the private marketplace.

As it moved through Congress, the proposed health care reform legislation exposed deep divisions among politicians and within the US population over core issues of health policy. Do Americans have a right to health care? What should the role of government be in financing or regulating health care and health insurance? To what extent should we rely on the private marketplace as the source of health insurance?

How much should the government pay for health care? Perhaps even more important, how much can the government *afford to pay* for health care?

The passage of ACA did not provide definitive answers to these questions. We may well be discussing and debating them again in the not-too-distant future. In light of the likelihood of this ongoing discussion and debate, it is appropriate to look more closely at the process by which Congress and the president enacted the reforms included in ACA and then to place that reform process in the considerably broader context of the history of health care reform efforts in the United States.

Health Care Reform and the 2008 Presidential Election

The presidential election scheduled for November 4, 2008, began in earnest with the primary elections in January and February of that year. Before the first vote was cast, health care reform was an important issue in the minds of most voters. A series of public opinion polls conducted between 1994 (the year the Clinton health reform proposals collapsed) and 2007 showed that "about 90% of Americans were fairly consistent in agreeing that the U.S. health care system should be completely rebuilt or required fundamental changes" (Jacobs 2008, p. 1881).

In January 2008, Robert Blendon and his colleagues published the results of a series of opinion surveys of likely primary voters from thirty-five states with early presidential primaries (Blendon et al. 2008b). They found widespread awareness of problems inherent to health care in the United States among both Republicans and Democrats. While Republicans and Democrats were in general agreement on the need to enact some type of health care reform, however, they were divided on what the reform should look like. Among Democrats, 65 percent favored providing health insurance to "all or nearly all of the uninsured" and were willing to accept substantially increased government spending to accomplish this goal. By contrast, 42 percent of Republicans supported extending coverage "to only some of the uninsured," with an additional 27 percent preferring "keeping things basically as they are now" (p. 420). Before the first vote was cast in the presidential primaries, our country was divided largely along political party lines as to how we should address health care reform.

In November 2008, Blendon and colleagues reported a second series of opinion polls, this time comparing those who had voted for John McCain in the primary with those who had voted for Barack Obama (Blendon et al. 2008a). Consistent with the earlier polls, most Obama voters wanted the government to take responsibility for extending health insurance to the uninsured, while McCain voters were of the view that responsibility for acquiring health insurance should rest with the individual consumer. Obama voters favored a larger, more comprehensive reform plan, while McCain voters favored a more limited, smaller-scale approach. Before President Obama was to take office, a substantial polarization of views between Democrats and Republicans was already in place.

Shortly after his inauguration, President Obama released his first budget proposal. In it, he called on Congress to work collaboratively with the White House to design major reform of the health care system. It was clear, though, that Obama had learned the lesson of the failed Clinton reform proposals of 1993–94 [...]. Rather than defining the specifics of the reform proposals himself, President Obama wanted Congress to take the lead in developing reform legislation.

Within a few months of Obama's budget message, Congress had begun to work on reform legislation. The process of developing the actual legislation fell to five separate congressional committees: two in the Senate and three in the House of Representatives. A consensus began to emerge that the most promising approach to expanding health insurance coverage would be through requiring all US residents to carry health insurance (individual mandate) while also requiring most US employers to offer health insurance to their employees (employer mandate). This approach mirrored reforms that had been adopted in Massachusetts a few years earlier.

It did not take long in this process for the political divide evident in preelection polls to resurface. Mandating health insurance coverage would require creating a place for individuals and employers to go to acquire coverage. As part of its mandate program, Massachusetts had created a central clearing house to connect insurance companies offering coverage options with individuals or employers seeking coverage. Fairly quickly, leaders of the Senate committees dealing with reform agreed to adopt a model similar to that in Massachusetts. They would establish health insurance "exchanges" through which those seeking insurance could select from among the insurance options various companies had available.

As chair of the Senate Finance Committee, Senator Max Baucus (D-Montana) initially proposed that among the insurance options available through these health insurance exchanges would be a "public option," an insurance plan analogous to Medicare, organized and administered by the federal government. Almost immediately, Senate Republicans condemned the public option approach. Senator John Cornyn (R-Texas) criticized the public option approach as "a Washington-directed unfair-competition plan" (quoted in Iglehart 2009a, p. 2386). Senator Charles Grassley (R-Iowa) argued that the Democrats' approach "would cause us to slide rapidly down the slope towards increasing government control of health care" (Grassley 2009, p. 2397).

President Obama countered these criticisms in a *New York Times* Op-Ed. He argued that the Democrats' plan "is not about putting the government in charge of your health insurance. I don't believe anyone should be in charge of your health care decisions but you and your doctor—not government, not bureaucrats, not insurance companies" (Obama 2009b). With substantial majorities in both houses of Congress, Democratic leaders pushed for a comprehensive expansion of the existing health insurance system to include most of those who were without insurance. The federal government would take principal responsibility for organizing and financing this expansion. Republicans, on the other hand, with substantial support from the health insurance industry, argued for a more limited approach. As described by Karen Ignagni, CEO of America's Health Insurance Plans (a leading industry group), Congress should instead focus on "building on the strengths of the present public-private health care system rather than replacing it" (Ignagni 2009, p. 1134).

By the fall of 2009, the debate over health care reform had hit an impasse. There was a line drawn in the congressional sand separating Democrats from Republicans. It appeared there was no room for compromise—Democrats would not accept the approach supported by Republicans, and Republicans were equally unwilling to consider seriously the Democrats' proposals. It seemed to many that, once again, health care reform might end in failure.

At this point, President Obama chose to take decisive action, addressing a joint session of Congress in front of a prime-time viewing audience. Chiding both sides of the aisle for their impasse, Obama stated, "now is the season for action." He indicated that, from that point on, he was going to assert his leadership in the effort to enact health care reform. He identified three overarching goals for the reform effort: (1) expanding health insurance coverage to those who lacked it, (2) constraining the rising cost of health care, and (3) improving the security of coverage for those with chronic illness (Obama 2009a).

With a great deal of political maneuvering, carried out in the face of substantial public confusion, each house of Congress enacted health care reform legislation: the House of Representatives on November 7 and the Senate on December 24. While each bill had many things in common, each had unique features. Some form of compromise between the two versions would need to be agreed upon. Usually this process would involve the creation of a House-Senate Conference Committee, made up of members of both houses. The compromise struck by the Conference Committee would then be taken back for final approval in each house before being forwarded to the president for his signature.

This process turned out not to be an option, though. Senator Ted Kennedy of Massachusetts, a leader of Senate Democrats and for more than four decades a leading voice in the US Senate for health care reform, died of cancer. A special election in Massachusetts to fill his seat resulted in a Republican being elected, thereby giving the Republicans the forty-one votes needed to mount and sustain a filibuster in the Senate. With unanimous Republican opposition to passage of any health reform bill approved by Democrats, there was no chance for compromise legislation coming out of a House-Senate Conference Committee to gain passage in the Senate. Nor was there any chance the Senate would simply approve the reform bill passed previously by the House. There was only one option open to the Democrats: for the House of Representatives to approve the bill passed by the Senate, even though the Senate bill had several provisions to which House Democrats were opposed. Following House passage of the Senate bill, however, the House and Senate could then agree on a series of modifications to the bill under a special provision referred to as "reconciliation."

Not being a scholar of the intricacies of the legislative process, I will leave it to others to describe in more detail the history, purpose, and intended use of the reconciliation process in Congress (Herszenhorn 2010; Iglehart 2010a). As I understand it, the reconciliation process was established by Congress in 1974 as a simplified means of changing federal programs or policies to align them more closely with previously established budget policy. If legislation is passed that is inconsistent with the budget guidelines set by Congress, or, similarly, if an existing program is inconsistent with those guidelines, Congress can change the programs or policies to align them with the budget. Making these changes under the reconciliation process requires a simple majority vote in both houses of Congress—and therefore is not subject to a filibuster in the Senate.

Congress had previously used the budget reconciliation process at various times and for various purposes. One of the best known instances of reconciliation is the Consolidated Omnibus Budget Reconciliation Act, passed by Congress in 1986 and best known by its acronym, COBRA. COBRA gives employees who have lost their jobs the right to continue their previous group health coverage for a period of time. People frequently talk of their "COBRA benefits."

Sensing a potential procedural impasse, on February 25 President Obama convened an urgent summit meeting of leading Democrats and Republicans to discuss, and in front of a national television audience to debate, competing perspectives on health care reform. The political impasse that preceded Obama's summit was still there after it was over. All Republicans in Congress remained opposed to the bills that had been passed by the House and the Senate. President Obama and Democratic leaders had no choice but to invoke the budget reconciliation process. In an all-day session on Sunday, March 21, the House approved the health reform bill previously passed in December by the Senate, and on March 23 President Obama signed it into law. Then, on March 25, both the House and the Senate passed, by simple majority vote, the reconciliation bill that made a series of changes to the original bill that bridged the divisions between the original House and Senate bills. In essence, the reconciliation process replicated what the House-Senate Conference Committee process is intended to do: to find a middle ground between similar bills passed in the House and the Senate, and then to gain final approval of both houses of the compromise bill.

As Congress completed passage of ACA, the rhetoric on both sides made clear the continued deep divisions between Democrats and Republicans over how health care in the United States should be organized and financed, and the role government should play in the health care system. On the day he signed ACA, President Obama hailed the historic step that had been taken: "Today, after almost a century of trying ... health insurance reform becomes law in the United States of America.... We have now just enshrined the core principle that everybody should have some basic security when it comes to their health care" (Obama 2010).

Republicans were not so sanguine. Representative Marsha Blackburn (R-Tennessee), following the House vote in favor of the ACA legislation, remarked, "Freedom dies a little bit today." Carl Hulse, reporting on the House's approval of ACA, stated that "Republicans were outraged, characterizing the legislation as a major step toward socialism and an aggressive government takeover of the health care system" (2010, p. A17). These comments echoed those made a few months earlier by Representative Michele Bachmann (R-Minnesota), that Democrats were pushing for "socialized medicine" and a "government takeover" of the American health care system (quoted in Herszenhorn 2009).

This continued polarization over what ACA represented for the United States—a new "core principle" assuring access to health care, or a "government takeover" and a step closer to "socialized medicine"—remained in the wake of the year-long health care reform process. It would be easy to point to President Obama and the political parties in Congress as the source of this polarization. It is fundamental to our understanding of US health care reform, however, to consider, again, what President Obama said when he signed the ACA: " Today, after almost a century of trying ... health insurance reform becomes law in the United States of America."

The health care reform process did not begin with the inauguration of President Obama. Nor did it begin with the presidential campaign leading up to his election. The United States had been arguing over health care reform for nearly a century before President Obama was elected. A review of the repeated efforts over that century for or against reform reveals a striking similarity between what was proposed in 2009–10 and what had been proposed previously, as well as a striking similarity between the rhetoric of health care reform in the past and the rhetoric of 2009–10.

A Century of Trying to Achieve Health Care Reform in the United States

Theodore Roosevelt first attempted to reform US health care during his presidential campaign in 1912. As part of the Progressive Party's platform, Roosevelt proposed a system of national health insurance, modeled after the German system, to be administered by a new National Health Department. Those supporting national health insurance viewed health care as a right of all members of our society, analogous to the recently recognized right to a publicly financed education for children. Teddy Roosevelt lost the 1912 presidential election to Woodrow Wilson, however, and health care reform had to wait for another day.

In 1927, a group of physicians, public health professionals, and others concerned with national health care issues came together to form the Committee on the Costs of Medical Care (CCMC) (Ross 2002). CCMC was an in de pen dent group and was supported by a number of foundations. Committee members set in motion a five-year project to study and report on the economics and organization of health care in America. On March 10, 1931, the *New York Times* carried an article titled "Family Health Bill Put at $250 a Year" in which the CCMC was cited, stating that "the average family of five in an American city" spent $250 per year on medical care, a figure that raised serious concerns about the rising costs of medical care in a time of economic hardship. The committee's majority report, issued in 1932, recommended shifting the delivery of most medical care to a model that emphasized organized medical groups and prepayment of health costs through either insurance premiums or taxation. The American Medical Association (AMA), however, was stridently opposed to this approach, labeling such prepaid medical groups "medical soviets" and suggesting that "such plans will mean the destruction of private practice … . They are, in a word, 'unethical' " (American Medical Association 1932, p. 1950). The AMA's House of Delegates unanimously approved a motion to oppose the majority report of the CCMC, and to mount "an intensive campaign … among the medical profession and the public" to prevent adoption of the CCMC's recommendations. A follow-up report to the House of Delegates reported that "all the facilities of the American Medical Association have been used to oppose this trend and the propaganda in support of it" (American Medical Association 1934b, p. 2200). The AMA prevailed in its efforts to block the recommendations of the CCMC's report, and the report was shelved.

Franklin Roosevelt took up the issue of health care reform in 1934 as part of his initial proposals for old age security and unemployment insurance for workers. In response to Roosevelt's early proposals to include national health insurance as part of Social Security, the AMA House of Delegates passed a resolution reiterating its position that "all features of medical service in any method of medical practice should be under the control of the medical profession. No other body or individual is legally or educationally equipped to exercise such control" (American Medical Association 1934b, p. 2200). When it appeared as though health insurance might be added to the pending legislation for creation of the Social Security system, the AMA House of Delegates met in special session to reiterate its "opposition to all forms of state medicine" and to "reaffirm its opposition to all forms of compulsory sickness insurance" (American Medical Association 1935, pp. 750–51). Once again, AMA opposition to government involvement in health care was effective, and when Roosevelt signed the Social Security Act in 1935, health insurance was not part of it.

Roosevelt continued to support the creation of a system of national health insurance and appointed an "Interdepartmental Committee to Coordinate Health and Welfare Activities," charging it with studying the issue of extending Social Security benefits to include health care. At a national conference held in July 1938, the committee proposed a series of changes to US health care, including "a ten year program providing for the expansion of the nation's hospital facilities" and "a comprehensive program designed to increase and improve medical services for the entire population" (Interdepartmental Committee to Coordinate Health and Welfare Activities 1938, p. 433).

One month later, the AMA convened an emergency meeting of its House of Delegates to respond to the government's "campaign for some radical changes in medical practice" (American Medical Association 1938, p. 1192). The speaker of the House of Delegates reminded the delegates that the AMA had consistently "opposed legislation which would have the effect of vesting in some governmental agency power to enforce its decrees on patients and doctors" (p. 1192). The AMA president then addressed the delegates, stating that "the Association has constantly opposed the adoption of any form of state medicine by any definition of that term" (p. 1194).

It is interesting to note that at this special session, the leaders of the National Medical Association (NMA) — the national association of black physicians, most of whom were prevented from joining the AMA because of their race—were (after majority vote of the AMA delegates) invited to address the meeting. The past president of the NMA voiced his support for the position of the AMA, arguing that "if we have socialized medicine in America, I am very sure, as you must be sure, that the standards of medical practice will degenerate … and the patients again will suffer as they have suffered in Europe" (American Medical Association 1938, p. 1211).

Once again, fears that "governmental agency power" over the financing of health care would lead to "state medicine" and "socialized Medicine" were sufficient to derail Roosevelt's efforts. Health care reform would have to wait another decade before it was back on the table.

In January 1948, President Harry Truman asked Oscar Ewing, one of his senior administrators, to prepare a report on the status of health care in the United States. Released in September of that year, the Ewing Report outlined a series of steps the federal government should take to make health care more available. As Roosevelt's Interdepartmental Committee did in 1938, this report recommended extensive new hospital construction and a compulsory "system of Government prepayment health insurance" (Furman 1948) that over a period of three years would provide universal insurance for both hospital care and physician care, as well as coverage of certain prescription medicines.

The response of the AMA to the Ewing proposals is interesting. The AMA first went through a formal procedure to adopt the following definition: "*Socialized medicine*—Socialized medicine is a system of medical administration by which the government promises or attempts to provide for the medical needs of the entire population or a large part thereof" (American Medical Association 1948, p. 685). A few weeks later, Morris Fishbein, the longtime editor of the *Journal of the American Medical Association*, published a special editorial in which he warned physicians that the profession of medicine was "at a point of decision which may well determine the nature and the freedom of medical practice for many years in the future" (Fishbein 1948, p. 1254). Responding to politicians who denied that President Truman's proposals for national health insurance constituted "socialized medicine," Dr. Fishbein argued that "nations that embark on such programs move inevitably into a socialized state in which … practically all public services become nationalized, private responsibility and owner ship dis appear, individual initiative is destroyed and the result is a socialized state" (p. 1256).

In 1948, the AMA hired a political consulting firm from California that had successfully defeated California governor Earl Warren's 1945 proposal for a statewide health insurance plan. With a budget of more than $1 million, funded largely by an assessment of $25 on every AMA member, the firm developed a national strategy with two principal goals, as cited by Lepore (2012): "1. The *immediate objective* is the defeat of the compulsory health insurance program pending in Congress. 2. The *long-term* objective is to put a permanent stop to the agitation for socialized medicine in this country" (p. 57). As reported by the *New York Times*, the AMA fought Truman's proposals "with all the vigor and manpower it [could] assemble" (Phillips 1949), with the result that, once again, the efforts at health care reform went down to defeat in Congress.

It would be seventeen years before Congress would take up health care reform again, this time under the leadership of President Johnson. With large majorities in both houses of Congress following the 1964 election, Johnson moved quickly to enact Medicare (health care for the elderly) and Medicaid (health care for the poor) as amendments to the Social Security system. Headlines in the *New York Times* announced, "A.M.A. Opens Bid to Kill Medicare" (Wehrwein 1965). Testifying before the Senate Finance Committee, Dr. Donovan Ward, president of the AMA, warned senators, "This may be your last chance to weigh the consequences of taking the first step toward establishment of socialized medicine in the United States" (American Medical Association 1965, p. 16).

In 1965, Congress was not swayed by claims that government financing of health care for the elderly and the poor constituted a government takeover of the health care system. It was swayed even less by claims that the proposed Medicare and Medicaid programs would be "the first step toward establishment of socialized medicine in the United States." By substantial margins, both houses of Congress passed the Social Security Act of 1965, establishing the Medicare and Medicaid programs. President Johnson flew to the Missouri home of Harry Truman to sign the legislation in the presence of the former president.

Of course, providing government payment for health care for the elderly and the poor was only a partial fulfillment of earlier proposals for universal health insurance. As monumental an accomplishment as it represented, the passage of Medicare and Medicaid left substantial segments of the American population without the means to pay for health insurance. [...] [T]he aggregate cost of health care began to rise sharply in the years following the enactment of Medicare and Medicaid. By 1970, both President Richard Nixon and Senator Ted Kennedy were calling for expanded health insurance coverage to help individuals and families offset the rising costs of care. Nixon's plan called for private financing through what we today would call an employer mandate. Kennedy's plan called for direct government financing of care. Neither plan gained approval, and any further steps toward health care reform were lost in the wake of the Watergate scandal and President Nixon's resulting resignation.

Health care reform was again on the table in the early years of President Clinton's administration [...]. An effective national ad campaign by the health insurance industry, warning of a new, massive federal bureaucracy taking over American health care, coupled with a shift of congressional control from Democrat to Republican majorities, led to the defeat of the Clinton reform proposals. As many had warned, in the years following the defeat of the Clinton proposals health care costs continued their steep rise, and growing numbers of Americans became or remained uninsured against the cost of illness or injury—the situation confronting the candidates in the 2008 presidential election.

Placing the Obama Reforms in the Historical Context of Previous Reform Efforts

During the intensity of the yearlong debate over President Obama's proposals for health care reform, it was often difficult to gain a clear sense of what the core issues were. The heated rhetoric from all sides led to widespread confusion as to what the proposed reforms would or would not accomplish. A national poll (Kaiser Family Foundation 2010) taken two weeks after President Obama signed ACA showed that 55 percent of respondents were confused about what was in the new law. Support for the law fell largely along party lines, with 79 percent of Republicans having an unfavorable view of the law and 77 percent of Democrats having a favorable view.

Which view was correct? Would the law assure most Americans access to needed health care, as many people seemed to believe? Or would it mean the potential destruction of our health care system through a government takeover, as many others appeared to believe?

Taking a step back from this debate, it is informative to compare ACA and the political response to it with various proposals for health care reform made over the last century. As illustrated in table 3.2.1, there is a remarkable similarity between what ACA was intended to accomplish and what earlier proposals hoped to accomplish, and an equally striking similarity between the rhetorical opposition to ACA and the rhetoric in opposition to those earlier proposals.

In 1931, when the Committee on the Cost of Medical Care recommended programs to bring health care "within reach of persons of average means," the opposition predicted that the programs would "mean the destruction of private practice." When Franklin Roosevelt proposed "to increase and improve medical services for the entire population," the AMA labeled his proposals "socialized medicine" and predicted that, if Roosevelt's plan were implemented, "standards of medical practice will degenerate … and patients will suffer." Truman's proposal for "universal access to hospital and physician care" was predicted to lead to "a socialized state in which … practically all public services become nationalized." Johnson's proposal for Medicare and Medicaid would, the AMA predicted, "be the first step toward establishment of socialized medicine in the United States." President Obama's proposals were characterized by many Republicans as "a major step toward socialism and an aggressive government takeover of the health care system."

The history of health care reform in the United States is the history of our deep-seated divisions over core principles of health care delivery and of the role of government in the provision of health care. Is a basic level of health care a right of all Americans? If so, should the government enact and enforce the mechanism to ensure that right? Alternatively, is it inappropriate for government to interfere in the private provision of health services? Our society has struggled with these issues for a century. The kerfuffle surrounding the passage of ACA has simply been the latest episode in our attempts as a society to address these divisions.

Despite the confusion surrounding it, it is clear that ACA is bringing major change to our health care system. Among other things, it has:

Table 3.2.1   A history of arguments for and against health care reform

Year/president	Argument in favour	Argument opposed
1931 / Herbert Hoover	Modern medicine can be brought within reach of persons of average means. —Committee on the Cost of Medical Care	Medical soviets … such plans will mean the destruction of private practice. —American Medical Association
1934–38 / Franklin Roosevelt	Roosevelt A comprehensive program designed to increase and improve medical services for the entire population. —Committee to Coordinate Health and Welfare Activities	Opposition to all forms of state medicine. —American Medical Association If we have socialized medicine in America … standards of medical practice will degenerate … and patients will suffer. —National Medical Association
1948 / Harry Truman	A system of Government prepayment health insurance to provide universal access to hospital and physician care. —Ewing Report	Nations that embark on such programs move inevitably into a socialized state in which … practically all public services become nationalized. —American Medical Association
1965 / Lyndon Johnson	To improve health care for the American people, [I propose] hospital insurance for the aged under social security. —President Johnson, 1965 budget message to Congress	The President's proposal would be the first step toward establishment of socialized medicine in the United States. —American Medical Association
1993 / Bill Clinton	We must make this our most urgent priority: giving every American health security, health care that can never be taken away. —President Clinton, special address to Congress, September 1993	New government bureaucracies will cap how much the country can spend on all health care. —"Harry and Louise" TV ads, sponsored by the Health Insurance Association of America
2010 / Barack Obama	We have now just enshrined the core principle that everybody should have some basic security when it comes to their health care. —President Obama, on signing the health reform law	A major step toward socialism and an aggressive government takeover of the health care system. —Congressional Republicans

- Extended Medicaid coverage to more than 10 million people living in or near poverty who previously were ineligible for coverage
- Provided health insurance to an additional 11 million formerly uninsured people with low to moderate incomes through a combination of regulated insurance exchanges and tax subsidies for the cost of insurance
- Made a series of changes to regulations affecting companies that provide health insurance with the intent of making that insurance more affordable

- Made a series of changes in the Medicare program to reduce costs and improve benefits
- Created a series of new sources of tax revenues to support these programs

When Congress passed Medicare and Medicaid in 1965, our health care system was changed fundamentally. Yet those changes stopped short of solving many of the policy issues at the heart of our health care system. Nor did the passage of Medicare and Medicaid resolve our national ambivalence over what the role of government should be in our health care system.

When Congress passed ACA in 2010, our health care system was again changed fundamentally. Yet Congress again left unaddressed many continuing core questions. In future years, in future presidential elections, and in future Congresses, we will undoubtedly again be talking about health care reform. Rather than debating how to extend coverage to the uninsured, we likely will be debating what parts of ACA need to be changed and how to rein in the continuously rising cost of health care. When we have these discussions, the appropriate role of government will again be a topic of sharp debate.

References

American Medical Association. 1932. The committee on the costs of medical care (editorial). *JAMA* 99:1950.

American Medical Association. 1934b. Proceedings of the House of Delegates from June 12, 1934. *JAMA* 102:2199–2201.

American Medical Association. 1935. Minutes of the special session of the House of Delegates of the American Medical Association. *JAMA* 104:747–53.

American Medical Association. 1938. Minutes of the special session of the House of Delegates of the American Medical Association. *JAMA* 111:1191–1217.

American Medical Association. 1948. Report of the council on medical services. *JAMA* 138: 683–86.

American Medical Association. 1965. AMA urges defeat of Medicare. *JAMA* 192:15–17.

Blendon RJ, Altman DE, Benson JM, et al. 2008a. Voters and health care reform in the 2008 presidential election. *New England Journal of Medicine* 359:2050–61.

Blendon RJ, Altman DE, Dean C, et al. 2008b. Health care reform in the 2008 presidential primaries. *New England Journal of Medicine* 358:414–22.

Fishbein M. 1948. Health and Social Security. *JAMA* 138:1254–56.

Furman B. 1948. Truman gets report urging big 10-year health program. *New York Times,* September 3.

Grassley C. 2009. Health care reform—A Republican view. *New England Journal of Medicine* 361:2397–99.

Herszenhorn DM. 2009. An invitation to protestors. *New York Times*, November 5.

Herszenhorn DM. 2010. Budget reconciliation. *New York Times*, March 3.

Hulse C. 2010. Another long march in the name of change. *New York Times,* March 21.

Iglehart JK. 2009a. Building momentum as Democrats forge health care reform. *New England Journal of Medicine* 360:2385–87.

Iglehart JK. 2010a. The Democrats' last ditch—reconciliation or bust. *New England Journal of Medicine* 362:e39.

Iglehart JK. 2010b. Historic passage—reform at last. *New England Journal of Medicine* 362:e48, posted March 24, 2010, http:// content.nejm.org/cgi/content/full/362/14/e48.

Ignagni K. 2009. Health insurers at the table—industry proposals for regulation and reform. *New England Journal of Medicine* 361:1133–34.

Interdepartmental Committee to Coordinate Health and Welfare Activities. 1938. *JAMA* 111: 432–54.

Jacobs LR. 2008. All over again? Public opinion and health care. *New England Journal of Medicine* 358: 1881–83.

Kaiser Family Foundation. 2010. Kaiser health tracking poll, April, www.kff.org/kaiserpolls/upload/8067-F.pdf.

Lepore J. 2012. The lie factory—How politics became a business. *The New Yorker*, September 24, p. 50.

Obama B. 2009a. Remarks to a joint session of Congress on health care, September 9, www.whitehouse.gov/the_press_office/remarks-by-the-president-to-a-joint-session-of-congress-on-health-care/.

Obama B. 2009b. Why we need health care reform. *New York Times*, August 16.

Obama B. 2010. Remarks at the health care bill signing. *New York Times*, March 23.

Phillips C. 1949. Bitter debate begins over health program. *New York Times*, February 27.

Ross JS. 2002. The committee on the cost of medical care and the history of health insurance in the United States. *Einstein Quarterly Journal of Biology and Medicine* 19:129–34.

Vladeck BC. 2010. Fixing Medicare's physician payment system. *New England Journal of Medicine* 362: 1955–57.

Wehrwein AC. 1965. A.M.A. opens bid to kill Medicare. *New York Times*, January 27.

Worksite Wellness

Culture and Controversy

David B. Nash

In my previous column (see the Population Health column in the July/August issue of *JHM*), I wrote about the emergence of population health as a major trend on the American healthcare landscape. Over the past decade, we have witnessed the practical applications of population health tenets give rise to substantial changes in how healthcare is perceived, delivered, and financed. One such change is the fundamental shift in employer attitudes toward employee health.

Who among us hasn't felt a pain in the wallet as employers reacted to spiraling health insurance costs by reducing benefits coverage and increasing copayments and deductibles? Who hasn't considered the potential demise of our uniquely American system of employer-sponsored health insurance? But this is only a part of the ongoing change in healthcare.

Even before passage of the Affordable Care Act (ACA), employers had begun to recognize the value of a healthy workforce. As they adopted strategies to reduce costs of employee healthcare, large private employers and public agencies were beginning to create cultures of health and wellness in their workplaces.

A workplace culture of health and wellness is characterized by an environment, policies, and cues that encourage healthy choices; these choices, in turn, lead to reduced absenteeism and improved productivity, collective improvement in quality of life, and reduction in morbidity for the employee population.

Changing culture takes time, but a growing number of employers are implementing workplace programs that promote wellness and prevention to reduce the risk of chronic illnesses (e.g., diabetes, hypertension), reward healthy behaviors (e.g., smoking cessation, weight loss), and encourage employees to identify a patient-centered medical home for their overall healthcare.

The ACA encouraged workplace wellness by permitting employers to align group health plan premiums with employee participation in wellness programs. According to the U.S. Equal Employment Opportunity Commission (EEOC) (2013), 94% of employers with more than 200 employees and 63% with fewer employees currently use wellness programs to incentivize their staff to adopt healthier lifestyles.

Although the EEOC monitors the use of wellness programs, it has issued no regulations regarding the design or administration of these programs. Herein lay the seeds of controversy. In 2014 (Goff), the EEOC filed three federal lawsuits arguing that an individual employer's wellness program violates the Americans with Disabilities Act (ADA) or the Genetic Information Nondiscrimination Act (GINA).

1   *EEOC v. Orion Energy Systems* (filed August 20, 2014) alleges that the Wisconsin-based company's wellness program violated the ADA by requiring employees to submit to medical examinations that were not job related or consistent with business necessity. The company provided 100% health insurance coverage for participants in the wellness program; an employee who refused to participate was charged 100% of the premium cost plus an additional $50 per month.

2   *EEOC v. Flambeau, Inc.* (filed September 30, 2014) argues that the Wisconsin-based company's wellness program violated the ADA by requiring employees to submit to biometric screening and a health risk assessment in exchange for the employer's paying 75% of participants' health insurance premiums. The company's disciplinary actions for nonparticipants included terminating insurance coverage.

3   *EEOC v. Honeywell International, Inc.* (filed October 27, 2014) requests the court to issue a temporary injunction against the New Jersey-based company for imposing penalties as part of its wellness program.

Clearly, wellness programs must be carefully structured to comply with state and federal regulations. The ADA, the GINA, the Health Insurance Portability and Accountability Act (HIPAA), and state lifestyle discrimination laws all affect the design of a wellness program.

Nothing in the ADA bars employers from implementing wellness programs oriented toward health promotion and disease prevention; however, it does require employers to afford an equal opportunity for participation by employees with known disabilities. For instance, if the employer wishes to offer a premium discount to employees who achieve a specific score on a health risk assessment, the ADA requires the employer to make accommodations enabling employees with disabilities to participate. However, if the employer wishes to impose a surcharge on smokers, the ADA does not come into play because addiction to nicotine is an equal-opportunity risk.

Wellness programs rely heavily on health risk assessments for baseline and ongoing evaluations; however, employers need to keep in mind that the ADA prohibits them from making medical inquiries or requiring medical examinations unless they are job related and consistent with business necessity. The easiest route to compliance with HIPAA nondiscrimination rules is implementing wellness programs that are voluntary (e.g., encouraging prenatal care by waiving deductibles or copayments for visits to an obstetrician or by reimbursing the cost of a gym membership).

GINA limits an employer's ability to offer incentives that are linked to providing genetic information. Even a seemingly innocuous item such as family history on a health risk assessment can be construed as a violation if completing the form is tied program is unlikely to yield the expected outcomes of a healthier workforce, reduced medical expenditures, and lower insurance premiums in the first year or two. Achieving positive results requires cultural change, which occurs gradually. Looking at wellness programs over a 5-year period, the RAND Corporation (Mattke et al., 2013) found that participation was associated with lower healthcare costs (about $157 per employee) and a decrease in use of healthcare services.

As the controversy unfolds and these lawsuits make their way through the courts, employers are awakening to a new reality. Because the wellness programs they offer may soon be subject to new regulations that affect their design and scope, prudent employers will submit their wellness programs to review by legal counsel before rolling them out to employees.

On a positive note, the EEOC recently announced that employers may continue to use substantial financial rewards and penalties as encouragement for participation in workplace wellness programs. The EEOC also set forth some protective measures for employees (e.g., limits on the size of financial incentives, confidentiality of employee medical information, and prohibitions against firing employees or denying them access to the company's health plan for failure to participate in the wellness program). This bodes well for employers, employees, and the nascent culture of wellness in the United States.

References

Goff, A. (2014, December 15). EEOC cracking down on workplace wellness programs. Warner Norcross & Judd LLP. Retrieved from hrtp://www.wnj.com/Publications/EEOC-Crncking-Down-on-Workplace-Wellness-Programs

Manke, S., Liu, H., Caloyeras, J., Huang, C. Y., Yan Busum, K. R., Khodyakov, D., & Shier, V. (2013). Workplace wellness programs study: Final report. Santa Monica, CA: RAND Corporation. Retrieved from http://www.rand.org/pubs/research_reports/RR254 .html

U.S. Equal Employment Opportunity Commission (EEOC). (2013, May 8). Written testimony of Karen Pollitz, senior fellow, Henry J. Kaiser Family Foundation. Retrieved from http://www1.eeoc.gov//eeoc/meetings/5-8-13/pollitz.cfm?renderforprint=1

Chapter 3: **Discussion Questions**

1. Is there a health disparity between high and low income workers that is highlighted by their ability/inability to obtain good insurance benefits?

   a. Define adverse selection in insurance.

2. Now that the tax penalty for failing to purchase insurance (the individual mandate) has been voided to zero beginning in 2019, what impact might this have on the exchanges?

   a. Beyond the economic consequences, what additional impact will this likely have on public health in America?

3. How have different presidents addressed the issue of uninsured Americans? List two examples.

   a. How does socialized medicine fit into the health care debate of the past and today?

4. When shopping for a medical policy, several things can impact a patient's finances beyond the cost of the premium payment. What do you think has the most impact on most patients' pocketbooks? (annual out-of-pocket limits, coinsurance rates, deductible etc.)?

   a. Describe the difference between the effects of major medical insurance vs. disability income insurance on disabled populations.

5. List three barriers to successful employee wellness programs.

   a. Go online to find a company, other than Google LLC, that provides a great wellness program, list the features that stood out to you, and explain why.

CHAPTER 4

PUBLIC INSURANCE AND LONG-TERM CARE

Long-Term Care

Donald A. Barr

U p to this point, this book has talked mostly about the system of acute care in the United States. Most of the money spent on health care and most of the attention given to recent changes in health policy have focused on the care we provide to people with specific conditions that need treatment from a physician or at a hospital.

What happens, though, when elderly or disabled people are not sick enough to require hospitalization but, due to chronic illness or general frailty, are not able to take care of themselves? These types of people are provided assistance through our system of long-term care. As the name implies, this type of care is ongoing and has less to do with the treatment of a specific disease until it is cured than with care for chronic conditions for which there is no cure.

There are many reasons why people need long-term care. Most often, an elderly person will simply have physical difficulty undertaking normal daily activities such as dressing, bathing, eating, and going to the toilet. (Activities such as these are referred to as activities of daily living, or ADLs.) Alternatively, a person may have a serious mental impairment such as Alzheimer disease that necessitates continuous supervision. Some people may have both physical difficulty with ADLs and mental impairment.

Traditionally, the need for long-term care was met principally by the family. As people became frail and in need of assistance, younger family members often teamed together to provide care. Because the dynamics of the American family has changed over the years, however, more and more frail elderly patients need organized institutions or services to help them. For example, between 1982 and 1994, the proportion of people in need of long-term care who were cared for in their home by family members or friends dropped from 74 percent to 64 percent (Liu, Manton, and Aragon 2000).

The Growing Need for Long-Term Care Among Frail Elderly People

Most people over 65 years old are able to care for themselves without any need for long-term care services. The problem of long-term care is mainly a problem of frail elderly individuals. It is very old people—those over 85—who typically need long-term care. Half of all people in nursing homes and one-fourth of all people with long-term care needs living in the community are over 85. Of the 39.6 million people age 65 or over in the United States in 2009, about 14 percent were age 85 or older (data from U.S. Census Bureau website). As Figure 4.1.1 shows, the number of people over 85 is growing much more rapidly than the number of elderly overall.

In 2009, 5.6 million people in this country were 85 years old or older. By 2020, this number is projected to increase to 7.3 million; by 2040, the number will be 15.4 million. As a result of the baby boom generation moving into their elder years, those over 85 will grow from 12.2 percent of

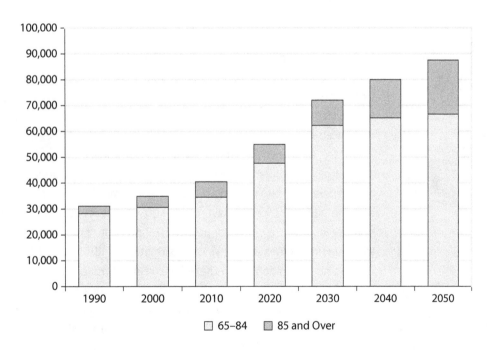

Figure 4.1.1   Projected Growth (in 1,000s) in the Elderly Population of the United States, 1990–2050.

Source: Data from U.S. Census Bureau

the elderly population in 2000 to 19.2 percent by 2040. Whatever problems our health care system has in providing and financing long-term care will be multiplied within a few decades. As stated in a 1998 report submitted to Congress by the U.S. General Accounting Office, "Increased demand for long-term care, which will be driven in part by the aging baby boom generation, will contribute further to federal and state budget burdens" (p. 2). The report went on to say that the increasing needs of the baby boom generation for long-term care "will lead to a sharp growth in federal entitlement spending that, absent meaningful reforms, will represent an unsustainable burden on future generations" (p. 3).

Nursing Home Care

If an elderly or disabled person is in need of long-term care that, for whatever reason, cannot be provided in the home, that person can receive care in a nursing home or other type of residential care facility. At any one time, about 5 percent of elderly Americans, or about 1.7 million people, are receiving long-term care in some sort of nursing facility.

The average age of people in nursing homes is about 84. Seventy-two percent are women. Three-fourths of these residents needed assistance with at least three ADLs. Seventy percent had severe memory loss (data from Kaiser Family Foundation 1999 and National Center for Health Statistics website).

Not all people in nursing homes, however, are there for chronic long-term care. Many people will spend time in a nursing home following an acute illness or injury, and then will return home after a short stay. As many as 1 in 5 elderly people will spend at least some time in a nursing home at some point. In 1999, the average length of stay for residents in nursing homes was about 29 months; however, 68 percent of residents discharged from nursing homes had stays of less than 3 months. About 20 percent of nursing home residents stay there for 2 years or more.

Many people have the impression that Medicare pays for most of the nursing home care needed by elderly people, but this is usually not the case. Medicare pays for about 12 percent of nursing home care. To qualify for Medicare payment, a patient must have an acute medical problem that requires skilled nursing care as part of the treatment program. Examples of skilled nursing care would be the administration of intravenous antibiotics or assistance with rehabilitation following

CONCEPT 4.1.1

The population group that is most in need of long-term care—those over 85 years old—is also the fastest-growing population group in the United States.

surgery or a stroke. In each case, a physician must certify that skilled care of this type is medically indicated. In most cases, the patient must have been in an acute care hospital just before entering the nursing home to qualify for Medicare payment. Even when a patient qualifies for skilled nursing care of this type, Medicare will pay the full cost only for the first 20 days. For skilled nursing care required beyond 20 days, the patient must pay $137.50 per day co-payment up to a maximum of 100 days of care. Any care required after 100 days is totally the responsibility of the patient, with no further coverage from Medicare.

Medicare distinguishes between *skilled nursing care* and *custodial nursing care*. Once a patient's medical condition has plateaued—that is, once he or she has attained the maximum level of healing or rehabilitation that can be expected in the short term—the patient no longer qualifies for Medicare's skilled nursing benefit. If the patient has to remain in the nursing home due to a need for assistance with ADLs, he or she is now considered to be receiving custodial care rather than skilled nursing care. Medicare does not pay for custodial care in nursing homes. Patients who need this type of care must find another way to pay for that care.

One of the advantages of Medicare's health maintenance organization (HMO) option has been a relaxation in Medicare policies pertaining to the use of skilled nursing facilities. A physician in a Medicare HMO is allowed to treat a patient in a skilled nursing facility at his or her discretion. It is not necessary that a patient be in a hospital first. The cost of skilled nursing care comes out of the overall yearly capitation received by the HMO, so there typically will be some type of control on the use of long-term care. The type of utilization control depends on the type of HMO, but it often involves a case manager—a nurse or social worker who supervises the overall process of care a frail elderly patient will receive. The patient still must require skilled nursing care to be eligible for nursing home payment under Medicare HMOs, however. If the patient needs ongoing custodial care, Medicare HMOs, like traditional Medicare, provide no coverage.

What does the person do, then, who no longer requires skilled nursing care but still needs constant assistance with ADLs? Consider the case, for example, of an elderly widow who has been living alone in her own home, but who has had a stroke and is partially paralyzed. Medicare will pay the costs of a short-term rehabilitation program, but after a few weeks the patient is no longer eligible for coverage. Returning home is not a realistic option, so the patient finds herself in a nursing home. The cost of that nursing home will typically be between $60,000 and $80,000 per

CONCEPT 4.1.2

Medicare pays very little of the cost of nursing home care. Patients who need long-term, custodial nursing home care are not eligible for Medicare payment.

year—often more. Who pays for the ongoing care this patient needs? There are three principal sources to pay for this care: out of pocket, Medicaid, and private insurance.

1. Payment out of pocket for nursing home care

Many patients find themselves with no way to pay for nursing home care other than to pay out of pocket. In 2002, patients and their families paid 25 percent of the overall cost of nursing home care from personal resources. About one in four patients pays for nursing home care out of pocket when she or he is admitted. At $60,000 a year or more, it does not take long to exhaust the patient's resources. Few seniors have sufficient assets to be able to generate an income of $60,000 a year on an ongoing basis. Nonetheless, in many cases there is no alternative for the patient but to exhaust her personal assets in paying for care.

2. Medicaid payment for nursing home care

Unlike Medicare, the Medicaid program will pay the costs of ongoing, custodial care in nursing homes for poor seniors. [...] [N]early 70 percent of Medicaid funds goes to pay for the care of elderly and disabled people who are also poor. Elderly, poor people who need long-term care in a nursing home or other type of custodial care facility are eligible to have Medicaid pay the full cost of their care. This is our country's final safety net to assure that no elderly or disabled person who needs custodial nursing care will be denied that care because he or she is unable to pay for it. About 60 percent of nursing home residents nationwide are covered by Medicaid.

An irony of our system of paying for nursing home care is the extent to which it causes people who were not originally poor to become poor. As described above, about one nursing home resident in four who needs ongoing custodial care will pay for that care out of pocket. For many of these people, it takes little time to completely exhaust one's life savings paying for nursing home care. Once a person, such as the elderly widow who is partially paralyzed, spends all (or nearly all) of her money paying for nursing home care, she then becomes eligible for Medicaid payment for any further care. She is allowed to keep up to $2,000 in a personal savings account, but otherwise she must sell all her assets and use all her funds before Medicaid will pay for her care. Of those patients who initially pay for their nursing home care out of pocket and end up staying in the nursing home for two to three years or more, half will become impoverished and become eligible for Medicaid payment for their care.

CONCEPT 4.1.3

Medicaid will pay the cost of long-term, custodial nursing care for those seniors who need it. However, before becoming eligible for Medicaid payment, seniors must exhaust nearly all their own resources by paying for care out of pocket.

What happens in the case of an elderly couple who have been living in their own home for years and one spouse sustains an illness or injury that requires long-term, custodial care in a nursing home? The spouse in the nursing home requires ongoing care, yet the healthy spouse is still able to stay at home and live independently. Historically, both spouses were required to spend all their money, including exhausting their combined savings *and* selling their house, and use the proceeds to pay for the nursing home care of the ill spouse. It was necessary for both spouses to become impoverished for the care of the ill spouse to be covered by Medicaid. The spouse remaining in the couple's home faced a heart-wrenching choice: either spend all the money, lose the home, and become poor, or divorce the spouse and sever legal responsibility for the cost of the nursing home care. For a number of years, the need to protect the financial independence of the healthy spouse was a major contributor to the divorce rate among elderly couples, many of whom had been married for decades.

Fortunately, Congress changed the rules on what has come to be called "Medicaid spend-down." Now, if a couple faces the need to have one spouse cared for in a nursing home, the other spouse is allowed to maintain assets sufficient to remain in the couple's home and live independently.

What if an elderly person—again, let's consider the partially paralyzed widow—has substantial personal assets and finds that she needs to be in a nursing home? Why not simply give all her money to her children, thus becoming poor and qualifying for Medicaid? When Congress changed the law to protect the remaining spouse from Medicaid spend-down, it also changed the law regarding giving away one's assets. There is now a "look-back" period, typically about three to five years, in which Medicaid can look to see if the patient gave away significant assets to children or other family members. If it is found that she did give away assets that she otherwise would have been required to spend before qualifying for Medicaid, the family members who received the gift s must first use those funds to pay for the needed nursing home care. Only after the gifted funds have been used will the patient qualify for Medicaid coverage for her long-term care needs.

3. Private long-term care insurance

A number of private insurance companies offer insurance specifically to cover the cost of long-term care. These types of policies are usually made available to large employee groups. Only those not currently in need of long-term care are eligible to obtain the policies. The cost of these policies can be prohibitive—more than $2,500 per year for someone who is 65 years old and more than $7,500 per year for someone 75 years old. As a result, few individuals can afford such coverage. About 7 percent of the elderly population is covered by private long-term care insurance, and about 7 percent of the cost of nursing home care is paid by these policies.

Home Health Care

A substantial number of elderly or disabled people in this country need help with ADLs on an ongoing basis but are not so ill that they need to be in a nursing home. If they are provided with a limited amount of assistance, these people are capable of remaining in their home. Many of them qualify for in-home, long-term care under either Medicare or Medicaid.

Typically, people who qualify for home care assistance will have a nurse visit them on a regular basis, checking on their situation and assuring that their basic needs are met. These nurses can provide services such as monitoring the patient's medications, assessing the patient's nutrition, and evaluating ongoing home safety. In addition, some of these patients may be eligible to have the assistance of a home health aide. An aide of this type is not a nurse but rather someone trained specifically in providing assistance with ADLs. The aide will visit the patient on a regular basis and help with such activities as bathing and meal preparation. (See Levine, Boal, and Boling 2003 for further discussion of the clinical aspects of home health care.)

In 2010, Medicare spent $20 billion on home health care (data from U.S. Centers for Medicare and Medicaid Services website). By comparison, in 2008 the Medicaid program, covering both elderly and nonelderly people in need of home health care, spent $47.8 billion (data from the Kaiser Family Foundation website).

The Medicare home health benefit was originally intended to be similar to the nursing home benefit: it would cover only a short period of care and only after hospitalization for an acute medical problem. In the 1980s, Congress modified the eligibility rules in two important ways:

1   They removed the requirement that the patient must be in the hospital before being eligible for home care services.

2   They removed the cap on the number of services an eligible patient may receive per year.

Now, any Medicare beneficiary who meets the following criteria is eligible for payment of home health services on an ongoing basis. If the patient meets these criteria, he or she is eligible to have Medicare pay for both the skilled care services and the custodial care services provided in the home. The criteria are that

- the patient is homebound
- the patient is under the care of a physician, who periodically reviews the plan for home care services
- the patient has an intermittent need for skilled care services from either a nurse or other care provider (for example, physical therapist)

READING 4.1 LONG-TERM CARE | 69

- the patient's care is provided by a home health agency that is a certified provider of services under the Medicare program

The costs associated with Medicare's home care program began to increase around 1980 when some of the initial program restrictions were relaxed. In 1989, there was a further loosening of eligibility requirements, and the costs of the program began to soar. In the nine years from 1980 to 1989, the cost of the program nearly tripled, from $662 million to $1.95 billion. A large part of the increase in the cost of the program was due to the increased frequency with which home care services were used over this time period. For most of the period from 1974 to 1989, those beneficiaries who qualified for Medicare home health services received about twenty-five visits per year. With the relaxation of eligibility requirements in the late 1980s, the average number of visits per home health care beneficiary jumped to nearly seventy-five per year.

The Medicare home health program was initially intended as a low-cost supplement to hospital care. In 1967, it accounted for less than 1 percent of all Medicare expenditures. Over the next thirty years, it became a major service program, accounting for nearly 5 percent of Medicare expenditures by 1997. In 2002, home health care accounted for 4.5 percent of overall Medicare expenditures.

[...] [T]he cost of home health care originally came out of the Part A Medicare trust fund. As Part A costs rose and the trust fund was facing potential insolvency, Congress modified Medicare's home health program in 1997 as part of the Balanced Budget Act. It re allocated most of the costs of the program to Medicare Part B and instituted new limitations on the use of home health services. These changes in eligibility and payment were successful in reducing costs, with a 12.9 percent decline in expenditures between 1997 and 1998.

Hospice Care

Consider the case of an elderly patient who discovers that he has cancer or some other terminal illness and is told by his doctor that he will most likely die within the next six months. Often this type of patient is not sick enough to be in the hospital, or alternatively, simply does not want to be in the hospital due to the futility of future attempts at treatment. It can be difficult for the family by itself to provide adequate care to a dying person,

CONCEPT 4.1.4

Medicare has become the principal source of payment for home health services for elderly and disabled people. Following a relaxation in eligibility guidelines in the 1980s, both the number of visits per homecare patient and overall program costs increased dramatically.

yet neither the patient nor the family wants placement in a nursing home. For this patient, a hospice may provide the best care available.

A hospice can be either a place for a person with a terminal disease to go for treatment or a team of professionals who assist the family to provide care to the terminally ill at home, or both. The hospice program focuses on relieving suffering rather than prolonging life. Hospice care involves a shift in the emphasis of care away from further attempts at cure to controlling the symptoms of the illness and providing emotional support during the dying process. Emotional support is offered both to the patient and to family members. Hospice care begins at the point that the inevitability of death is recognized and carries beyond the patient's death to help family members adjust to the loss.

The modern hospice movement, with an emphasis on symptom control and on dying as a process, began in England in the 1960s. The first modern hospice was named St. Christopher's and is described in the following quotation: "Several factors differentiate St. Christopher's from hospitals: allowing children to visit and play, personalized care, little patient-staff protocol, an informal social life, a continuum of care including home care, freedom to issue drugs and liquor as requested for symptom control, and follow-up with the family members after the patient's death" (Plumb and Ogle 1992, p. 812).

As it has developed in the United States over the past thirty years, a hospice program usually involves a health care team, often including a physician, a nurse, a social worker, a member of the clergy, trained home health aides, and community volunteers. The team will come to the patient's home and provide as much care as is feasible. Team members often will provide respite care for the family, relieving them for periods of time so they can take a break from the intense responsibilities of caring for a dying person. Some hospice programs will also have a care center, similar to that described for St. Christopher's. The patient who needs intensive assistance can stay in the facility, with family members visiting freely. Alternatively, the patient can split his or her time, spending part of the week in the hospice facility and part of the week at home with family members. As one might expect, hospice patients are three times as likely to die at home than in a hospital or nursing home when compared to patients who do not use hospice services.

Congress amended the Medicare program in 1982 to allow payment of hospice services for beneficiaries. To be eligible for hospice care, the beneficiary

- must be certified by a physician to have an incurable disease and be expected to live six months or less
- must agree to waive Medicare coverage for treatment of the illness provided outside the hospice program

Thus, a hospice patient under Medicare agrees to forgo further surgery or other types of therapy that are not intended for palliation and symptom relief. In return, the beneficiary is eligible for a substantially wider range of services than is available under traditional Medicare, such as drugs required for symptom relief, respite care at an in-patient facility, and bereavement counseling for the family.

An important study from 2010 evaluated the effect of receiving palliative care, such as that provided by hospice services, for patients with metastatic lung cancer—a condition that carries with it a grave prognosis. The patients in the study were not actually enrolled in hospice programs. They thus maintained the option of aggressive care, even as they neared the end of their life. Nonetheless, those patients receiving palliative care were less likely to choose aggressive care (33% as compared to 54% for those not receiving palliative care). Despite reduced use of aggressive care, the palliative care patients actually survived longer than patients not receiving palliative care (11.6 months as compared to 8.9 months) and reported a significantly better quality of life (Temel et al. 2010). An editorial accompanying the report of the study concluded "that life-threatening illness, whether it can be cured or controlled, carries with it significant burdens of suffering for patients and their families and that this suffering can be effectively addressed by modern palliative care teams. Perhaps unsurprisingly, reducing patients' misery may help them live longer" (Kelley and Meier 2010, p. 782).

The number of Medicare beneficiaries choosing to use hospice programs increased substantially during the 1990s, from 143,000 in 1992 to nearly 488,000 in 2000. During this same time period, the number of hospice programs providing care grew from 1,208 in 1992 to 2,244 in 2001 (data from U.S. Centers for Medicare and Medicaid Services website).

As the use of hospice programs and facilities expanded, the type of patient using hospice care changed somewhat. In 1992, 76 percent of all hospice patients were eligible for services because of a diagnosis of cancer. In 2008, this number had decreased to 31 percent. An increasing number of patients with diseases such as heart disease, lung disease, stroke, and Alzheimer disease had entered hospice programs. Despite this relative decline, nearly half of all Medicare patients who died of cancer were enrolled in a hospice program at the time of their death.

Although Medicare beneficiaries are eligible for a full six months of hospice care, the actual length of time in a hospice program before death is usually considerably shorter. In 1992, the median length of hospice service was twenty-six days. In 2000, the median had decreased to seventeen days. This means that half of all hospice patients in 2000 received fewer than three weeks of service.

Looking instead at the average length of stay, we find that it has risen somewhat, from forty-eight days in 2000 to seventy-one days in 2008. These data suggest that it is often difficult for physicians, patients, and family members to face the inevitability of death that confronts many patients, and to begin to plan for death in advance of the final stages of illness.

Life-Care Communities as an Alternative to Long-Term Care

The options for long-term care have expanded recently by the addition of a relatively new type of senior care facility—the life-care community. A life-care community offers a permanent place for seniors to live, in which their needs for assistance with living will be taken care of no matter how long they need them. Whatever level of services a resident needs will be provided for one fixed cost.

In a life-care community, different levels of care typically are available:

1. Independent Living

The life-care community provides individual apartments or condominiums for those residents capable of living alone. Residents in this level of care are fully independent, providing their own meals, and do not rely on assistance for any activities of daily living. They may, however, obtain meals from a central dining facility when desired, have assistance with transportation, and have someone always available for assistance in case of an emergency.

2. Assisted Living

Some residents are not fully capable of living independently but are not frail enough to require constant assistance. Typically, the life-care facility provides these residents with an apartment in a central facility that has staff immediately available. These residents can make the apartment their own home. They usually require little if any help with ADLs, although they may eat in a central dining room and may have assistance managing their medications and bathing. The apartments usually have call buttons and other surveillance devices, so if a resident ever needs assistance, it is immediately available. These facilities are staffed around the clock, usually with aides rather than nurses.

3. Custodial Care

Some residents in life-care communities have an illness or injury that necessitates round-the-clock assistance with ADLs or medical needs. This is the level of care that is usually provided in a nursing home. The life-care facility has a fully staffed nursing center available for these residents. They may need this level of care for only a short period of time, after which they can move back to their own home or apartment, or they may need this care for the rest of their life, in which case they will remain in the nursing center.

The unique aspect of life-care communities is that all these services are available for one fixed fee. The fee usually includes both a cash buy-in when the resident first enters the community and a monthly maintenance fee. In return for the buy-in and the monthly fee, residents are guaranteed whatever level of care they need, for the rest of their life. The only requirements are that the residents demonstrate sufficient income to assure lifetime payment of the maintenance fees, and that they enter the community at level 1 (that is, they are healthy enough initially to live independently).

Life-care communities offer an attractive alternative to many seniors who face the prospect of growing old alone at home and possibly ending their life in a nursing home. For a life-care community to work, however, seniors must plan for their remaining years when they are still relatively healthy. If they wait until they need extensive assistance, they are no longer eligible to enter these communities.

As one might imagine, it can often be very expensive to enter a life-care community, making them realistic alternatives for only the wealthiest seniors. A number of religious and other non-profit institutions have established life-care communities, however, making them available to people without a large number of assets.

Future Policy Issues in Long-Term Care

A number of policy questions remain to be answered regarding the future of long-term care in the United States. As difficult as the problems of the health care system are in general, the problems confronting our long-term care system are often even more vexing and are complicated by the relative lack of attention long-term care receives in the public health policy arena.

How Will We Provide Long-Term Care for the Growing Number of Frail Elderly People?

As discussed above, the number of people in this country over 85, the population most in need of long-term care services, is expected to more than triple in the next forty years, growing to 19 percent of the population. Many of these people will need nursing home care. Many states placed limits on the construction of new nursing home beds, leading to an 18 percent nation-wide decline between 1974 and 1994 in the number of beds per 1,000 people over 85. How will we build the nursing home facilities to meet the growing future need?

An alternative to building more nursing home beds is to develop more community-based services. In many cases a well-designed program of home health services can allow patients in need of substantial assistance to remain in the home with their families. For those without families to help them, smaller, community-based residential facilities that provide more of a homelike atmosphere can be an attractive alternative to traditional nursing homes.

How Will We Pay for Long-Term Care in the Future?

More challenging than simply building the facilities needed for care is the question of how we will pay for that care. Few will argue that the current system of financing long-term care is optimal. Many question whether the impoverishment of elderly, middle-class nursing home residents is a wise choice. Is the best option to ask people to pay for nursing home care out of pocket? Similarly, is the way we split responsibility between Medicaid and Medicare wise, with Medicaid paying for nursing home care and Medicare paying for home health care?

Long-term care can be seen as a broad social need that must be addressed through broad social policy. A system of social insurance, similar to the Medicare system of paying for acute care, could potentially meet the financing needs for long-term care. To do so, however, the system will need to be broadly financed by all taxpayers, not just those who need care. The American taxpayer has been especially reluctant in recent years to take on new social programs. Yet, a substantial portion of the financing burden of long-term care falls on middle-class families and individuals. Will the American taxpayer be willing to invest in long-term care now so that needed care is available in the coming decades?

How Will we Maintain the Quality of the Long-Term Care System?

For years there has been concern over the quality of long-term care services, especially care in nursing homes. As many as one nursing home in four has been found to have ongoing problems with quality (Feder, Comisar, and Niefeld 2000). Issues such as the appropriate level of staffing, the use of physical and chemical restraints, and the quality of the nursing services provided have led to continued federal and state oversight.

One of the issues contributing to these problems has been the relatively low level of Medicaid payment for nursing home care. As with acute medical care, Medicaid pays providers substantially less than private sources pay. With the large number of Medicaid beneficiaries in nursing homes, it has often been difficult for providers both to meet quality requirements and to maintain financial viability. The tradeoff between cost and quality will remain an important issue in long-term care.

Who Will Provide Medical Care for Frail Elderly People?

Good-quality long-term care requires the continuous participation and oversight of medical personnel. A number of physicians, however, are either unwilling or unable to provide active supervision of long-term care. Recent years have seen a reduction in interest in primary care among physicians. If the growing needs of the elderly are to be met, interest in primary care will have to expand and will need to include additional emphasis on geriatric care. This can be done either by including more involvement in geriatric care in the training of general internists and family physicians, or by increasing the number of physicians who focus their practice on geriatric care. As an alternative, nurse practitioners and other types of mid-level health care practitioners can assume a greater role in monitoring and supervising long-term care.

What Are the Ethical Issues Surrounding Care of Frail Elderly People?

In recent years, increased attention has focused on important ethical aspects of long- term care. The increasing role of advanced directives, such as living wills and durable power of attorney, has provided the opportunity for many elderly people to consider the appropriate level of care they wish to receive in the event that they become seriously ill. Issues of the autonomy and privacy of nursing home residents, especially those with cognitive impairment, are only beginning to be examined. The question of physician-assisted suicide has begun to receive increased attention as an option for patients facing inevitable death combined with intractable suffering. Future policy discussions will need to include consideration of these and other ethical issues that surround long-term care.

Summary

Policy issues pertaining to long-term care tend to receive less attention than those pertaining to health care more generally. Nonetheless, as the baby boom generation ages—especially as they move into their eighties—long-term care will become more of a central policy concern.

Care in nursing homes is one of the largest components of the long-term care system. Medicare provides only limited coverage and only for the cost of skilled nursing care. When frail elderly people or younger people with disabilities need assistance with basic ADLs such as dressing and bathing, they must either pay for it themselves or (after having exhausted most of their savings) go on Medicaid. A small but growing sector of the private market for health insurance provides some protection for the costs incurred when one must enter a nursing home.

Providing nursing and other support services in a person's home is another core component of the long-term care system. Medicare's coverage of home health care is substantially more extensive than its coverage of care in a nursing home. Other options for long-term care include life-care communities and, for those with a terminal illness, hospice care.

Finding ways to pay for the expected increase in the need for long-term care services will be one of the key policy challenges facing our country in coming years. Additional policy issues involve maintaining the quality of long-term care services and ensuring adequate personnel to provide these services.

The Affordable Care Act and Long-Term Care

There are relatively few changes to long-term care as a result of the Affordable Care Act (ACA). ACA establishes a "community living and assistance services and supports" (CLASS) program that will offer a new type of long-term care insurance to those who wish to purchase it. The benefits of the program may be used to purchase support services that allow individuals in need of assistance to maintain a residence in the community. It is expected that some employers will enroll in the plan and make it available to their employees on a voluntary basis.

ACA also establishes a series of new reporting requirements for skilled nursing facilities, covering issues such as ownership, accountability, expenditures, and quality data. This information will be posted to a website so Medicare enrollees can review it in order to compare facilities.

References

Feder J, Komisar HL, and Niefeld M. 2000. Long-term care in the United States: An overview. *Health Affairs* 19(3):40–56.

Kaiser Family Foundation. 1999. Long-term care: Medicaid's role and challenges. Publication No. 2172. www.kff.org/medicaid/2172-index.cfm.

Kelley AS, and Meier DE. 2010. Palliative care—a shifting paradigm. *New England Journal of Medicine* 363:781–82.

Levine SA, Boal J, and Boling PA. 2003. Home care. *JAMA* 290:1203–7.

Liu K, Manton KG, and Aragon C. 2000. Changes in home care use by older people with disabilities, 1982–1994: Executive summary. Washington, D.C.: AARP Public Policy Institute.

Plumb JD, and Ogle KS. 1992. Hospice care. *Primary Care; Clinics in Office Practice* 19(4):807–20.

Temel JS, Greer JA, Muzikansky A, et al. 2010. Early palliative care for patients with metastatic non-small-cell lung cancer. *New England Journal of Medicine* 363:733–42.

U.S. General Accounting Office. 1998. Long-term care: Baby boom generation presents financing challenges. Report No. GAO / T-HEHS-98-107. www.gao.gov/.

Chapter 4: **Discussion Questions**

1   Discuss the funding of long-term care through Medicare and Medicaid.

   a.   List the percentage of long-term care covered by each type of insurance.

2   Discuss out-of-pocket payments for long term care.

   a.   Are the baby boomers prepared for this financial burden?

3   Discuss how funding for home health benefits has changed from the 1980s.

   a.   Does Medicare or Medicaid cover these costs?

4   Define life care communities.

   a.   List two benefits and risks of this type of care for terminally ill adults.

5   Explain the dichotomy between patient autonomy and organizational liability in life care communities.

   a.   Describe the ideal environment for an average American during his or her last years of life either due to disease or age.

CHAPTER 5

ELDER CARE AND HEALTH POLICY

America's Eldercare Service Availability Faces Mounting Economic Issues

Marilyn Moon

Abstract The economic incentives present in our current healthcare system generate many obstacles to the development of a strong workforce for eldercare services. Low pay, inconsistent training opportunities, limited public resources, and limited financial resources by patients and their families restrict the opportunities for meeting workforce needs at a time when demand will be rising. Some modest improvements—such as better coordination of care, recognition of the role of family caregivers, and targeted support for near poor families—are possible, even in a political environment where larger, needed changes likely will not take place. | **key words:** *Medicaid, caregivers, unmet need, workforce, eldercare*

Lacking political will to fund a new LTC system, or effective changes to Medicare and Medicaid, only minimal change will occur in the eldercare workforce situation.

It is imperative that we align economic incentives to enhance our eldercare workforce. Demand for eldercare services will rise dramatically in the future, and the supply of such workers is not guaranteed in the current environment. The demand will be both for skilled workers and for caregivers who offer a broad array of supportive services. This article focuses on the latter category of caregivers—the direct care workforce (a less formal workforce), although the intersection between the two types of workforces also is important.

As the population of the United States ages, the demands for eldercare services will increase, although likely not until baby boomers are well into their seventies (Spetz et al., 2015). In addition to the growing share of older people in the population, other changes in family dynamics will increase demand. Baby boomers have fewer children and are less likely to live near other family members than did the generations before them. Also, groups such as Hispanics—a growing population segment that traditionally uses fewer services—may behave more like other Americans and begin using paid services to a greater extent.

Public and private policy addressing elder-care needs has resulted in a fragmented, hap- haz- ard system that complicates the creation of a stable workforce. Many considerations motivate decision making, including fear of public funding costs for long-term services and supports (LTSS). The problems are complex, involving the willingness to pay for services, and the question of how to ensure a reasonable supply of committed workers.

The Overarching Financial Issues

For those who need it, LTSS can be very expensive, largely because of the amount of care need- ed. And except for those with very low incomes, supportive services are not comprehensively covered by the two public programs older Americans rely upon for most of their healthcare needs—Medicare and Medicaid.

When informal care is included in estimates, contributions from private sources are much greater than from public programs. A 2013 study by the Congressional Budget Office (CBO) estimated this informal care at $234 billion—an amount much greater than from all other sources. (Other estimates of informal care are even higher; one estimate for 2009 pegged it at $450 billion.) When out-of-pocket spending and payments from private insurance on more formal services are added, private contribu- tions are more than twice as high as from public programs (see Figures 5.1.1A and 5.1.1B, below). (Private insurance in this article is treated as a part of contributions from individuals, because most long-term-care insurance is paid for by families or subsi- dized by employers.)

'Medicare provides only skilled services to those with long-term-care needs.'

Medicare provides only skilled services to those with long-term-care needs. So-called post- acute care services provided under Medicare totaled $68 billion, according to the CBO study, about 55 percent of which was for institutional care (skilled nursing, long-term hospital stays, and inpatient rehabilitation hospital stays) (CBO, 2013). The remainder was for home health services.

The other major public program is Medicaid, which covers medical and supportive services, but is limited to those with very low incomes or to people who have spent a large portion of their incomes and assets on care. In 2011, long-term-care spending for older adults was $60 billion—with two-thirds going to institutional care and the remainder to home- and communi- ty-based services (HCBS) (CBO, 2013). Most of these services would be supportive, particularly for those eligible for both Medicare and Medicaid.

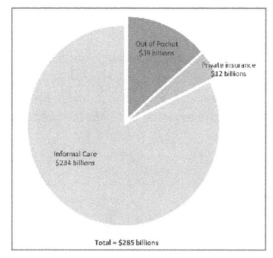

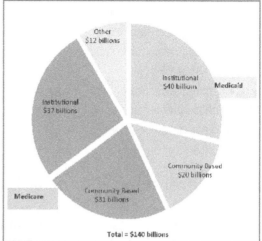

Figure 5.1.1A   Private Payment for LTSS, 2011

Figure 5.1.1B   Public Sources of Payment for LTSS, 2011

Source: CBO. 2013. Note: In Figure 5.1.1B, other is mainly public, with some private charitable contributions.

What does this mean? First, a substantial amount of money is spent by families and friends on caregiving, both out-of-pocket and through informal supports. The CBO study (2013) estimated that people ages 65 and older living in the community, with difficulty performing three or more activities of daily living (ADL), received on average, per day, seven hours of informal care and two hours of formal care. For those with cognitive challenges or who are older than age 65, the levels can be even higher. At $11 per hour for supportive services (see Dawson's article on page 38), the paid portion would total $8,030 per year, and if informal supports were replaced by paid care (or valued at the same level), the amount would be $36,135 annually. (Amounts spent by those on Medicaid who receive HCBS averaged $8,760, and for people in institutions, the amounts were much higher) (Medicaid and CHIP Payment and Access Commission [MACPAC], 2014.)

If the level of effort put forth at the informal care level is not sustained, all projections of future costs would have to be much higher than most people assume. If even a portion of that effort gets shifted to families buying services, the demand for formal eldercare services would skyrocket.

It also should be noted that those with long-term-care needs often spend a considerable amount on acute-care services as well. On average, about 87 percent of out-of-pocket spending by older adults is for acute-care services—or $4,129 per person in 2010. And, out-of-pocket spending steadily increases for all types of services for those with chronic conditions or restrictions on ADLs (Cubanski et al., 2014). Spending on services in 2010 (including long-term care) and premiums averaged $9,199 for those with three or more ADLs. Thus, anyone with long-term-care needs also will have substantial burdens from acute-care needs.

A substantial share of older Americans would have difficulty affording care if they needed LTSS. In particular, those with incomes too high to qualify for Medicaid but too low for the substantial resources needed to meet out-of-pocket expenses in the $10,000 range. (Eventually some of these individuals could spend enough on care to qualify for Medicaid in some states.) About 15 percent of older adults qualify for Medicaid, but about three-fourths of all elders have incomes below $50,000 (Moon, Wang, and Guo, 2016). Also, those with long-term-care needs have lower than average incomes (Kaye, Harrington, and LaPlante, 2010), so as many as two-thirds of all older adults likely would have difficulty obtaining paid care.

A major financing issue is whether or not better coordination of acute- and long-term-care services could lead to greater efficiencies—both through direct care workers taking on some skilled labor tasks, and by potentially reducing the overall number of services used. But most studies of care find considerable unmet need for supportive services, suggesting that a substantial reduction in overall services may not be feasible. Currently underway are demonstrations in which states are allowed to combine Medicaid resources with those available from Medicare to provide better coordination. The jury is still out on whether or not these efforts will be more efficient or merely result in skimping on care for patients (see MACPAC, 2014).

If direct care workers are expected to take over some skilled activities in the future, there is a strong need to provide better pay and training, and some efforts already are underway in this area. The going rate for direct care workers of about $11 per hour is for work that is demanding and critically important to the individuals receiving the care. This low rate of pay is the chief impediment to creating a larger and better-trained workforce. Also, the market for such help is fragmented: each state Medicaid program has its own approach (MACPAC, 2014), and the private market for care is largely informal, with little oversight or quality standardization.

'Those with long-term-care needs often spend a considerable amount on acute-care services as well.'

Economic Incentives Influencing Eldercare Workers and Services

Getting the economic incentives right means going beyond the issue of payment for services. In addition to paying higher wages, it will be essential to lessen the existing financial, cultural, and political barriers to a rational system of care. The challenges are many, and include the following:

- The medicalization of parts of eldercare services creates discontinuities in care and generates a two-class system that is inefficient and confusing.
- The division of services into silos by funding source and delivery site unnecessarily complicates care provision.

- Lack of agreement on training and education needs can create problems of quality and access.
- Poor coordination and communication about potential services preclude a well-functioning system. Lack of payment for coordination and the fragmented nature of services means that coordination is expensive, putting such services beyond many patients' means.
- Assuming there are unpaid caregivers to supplement services puts those without such support at greater risk, and generates burdens on those who provide such care.
- Housing, living arrangements, and transportation needs also complicate care provision. A lack of good public transportation contributes to the isolation of those individuals who need supportive services.

Which of these factors might benefit from public policy change? One of the most problematic barriers is the fear of overspending by public entities. This fear results in regulations and care limits that make sense within a budget context, but not for meeting patient needs. Consequently, there is a big gap in service availability for those not poor enough to qualify for Medicaid, but too poor to buy all needed care privately.

Medicare is nearly universally available to older adults and therefore represents a natural area for improving coverage, but policy makers are reluctant to expand its scope. Medicare consciously limits coverage to services deemed "medically necessary" as a way of restricting costs, resulting in the medicalization of certain services, and creating inefficiencies and complexity in obtaining care. Consequently, patients and their caregivers must interact with an array of workers and agencies. Finally, Medicare pays each type of service in a different way, creating silos within the Medicare program.

Some public services are available outside of Medicare and Medicaid. Social services such as meal delivery, and housing and healthcare programs are run by different segments of the government that often communicate poorly, if at all. And, housing and transportation programs seldom are discussed in the context of facilitating eldercare service provision, although they could help ease barriers to care. Eldercare workers may have a number of public sources to cover their services, but with many constraints and a great deal of variability.

Training is another area ripe for improvement. What types of training are needed and who will decide and formalize such activities? If public programs have a role in providing such services, they may determine what types of certification or training are needed. It will be important not to make these areas overly prescribed, but some minimal level of training and certification of workers (with appropriate background checks) could provide additional stability and help to those seeking to hire individuals privately. It might be appropriate to divert resources from other more professional training programs.

How Do Patients Meet and Interact with Direct Care Workers?

In our fragmented system, patients and their caregivers often must decide whether to work through intermediary agencies or to try to hire direct care workers on their own through a variety of means, including websites that serve as clearinghouses, care managers who recommend individuals, advertising, or word of mouth. Workers who operate through agencies often have little job security or guarantee of work. They tend to be hourly employees working only when the demand is there. It is not uncommon for the agency to charge customers about twice what they pay workers, but the patient benefits from some assurance that a worker will show up and that there has been some level of pre-screening.

Contracting privately allows patients and their families to screen workers themselves and assure consistency in staffing of needed services. Eliminating the agency as middleman can make care more affordable. But when families act as employers, it can be time-consuming and subject to quality and reliability issues. The highly personal nature of the work and its variability make it difficult to find good matches. Workers who are employed directly by families also can be exploited because their pay, benefits, and working conditions may not be what were promised initially.

Geriatric care managers are springing up to help families cope with service needs; skilled managers are adept at matching services and needs. But again, this is an area in which the quality can vary enormously. For people with substantial resources, a geriatric care manager is likely to be able to establish a reasonable care arrangement. But many older adults will not be able to afford such help, and these workers generally are not eligible for compensation from public sources. Some governmental support services are similar to care management, but it can be difficult to find or access such services, and they vary substantially.

There are some promising events that could help to protect workers and foster a more professional structure, going forward. As the U.S. labor force shifts from the traditional model of workers and employers to the gig economy in which people are independent contractors, changes will be needed in order to protect workers. It is evident in recent rulings concerning homecare workers and their rights that the courts are beginning to recognize this.

We could give credit to those who have informal caregivers, reducing copayments for other services.

What Improved Incentives Are Needed?

People who are near poor and those in the lower middle class who cannot afford to pay privately for services are the most likely to face unmet needs. Public resources to fill in the gaps in long-term supportive services for such families are needed—either by expanding Medicare benefits, or Medicaid eligibility. Improving quality and access to eldercare services and facilitating a more professional workforce would be easier to accomplish with expanded public support. However, no major expansions are likely. It is more realistic to assume only marginal expansions. The proposals below are put forth in that spirit.

First, better coordination across agencies in the public sector to package services could help stretch resources and simplify access. Medicare's effort to bundle post–acute care services is promising if it allows flexibility and does not leave decision-making responsibility to hospitals, where there is a high level of medical intensity, such that only skilled services are offered or the care becomes overly prescribed. We likely will see other demonstrations designed to improve care or coordination. But any program that begins with the goal of saving money will be a problem. While there could be savings from eliminating unnecessary services or providing care at a less intensive level, there also are substantial unmet needs that may swamp other savings.

One way to offer additional services through Medicare would be to make supportive services available, but use substantial copayments tied to income level. This would provide a clearinghouse for care that could offer more oversight and quality assurance. While this could become a new benefit track for Medicare (see Moon et al., 2015), it also could be implemented on a smaller scale with the main goal to jumpstart better coordination of services and an improved market for care. The following are some likely strategies for establishing such an approach:

- Offer explicit compensation to some entity to coordinate care and assure that services are of high quality and are appropriate. A care manager should be in a setting separate from service providers to avoid a conflict of interest and assure services take place in the right setting.
- A care plan should be developed in consultation with the patient and reflect the care manager's recommendations and the care recipient's needs and wishes.
- Consider the role of informal caregivers. It is always tempting to presume family caregivers will play a critical role. This helps cut the need, but not everyone has such help and for those who do, caregiver burden is substantial. One approach would be to give credit to those who have informal caregivers, reducing copayments for other services. This could reduce caregiver burden and encourage families to provide at least some care.
- Workers need training and some type of certification system to become more professional. This should include opportunities for obtaining benefits and protections of their rights. Compensation to entities, perhaps at the state level, to represent workers and organize supply could help jumpstart this effort.

Conclusion

Over the years, there have been many suggestions for improvements in Medicare and Medicaid—and even proposals for a new stand-alone long-term-care system. Though there is no lack of imagination about what could be done, there is no political will to fund such an effort. Until (or unless) this central issue is addressed, making improvements in the supply of eldercare workers will be a makeshift and haphazard effort—reflecting the current dysfunctional system.

References

Congressional Budget Office (CBO). 2013. *Rising Demand for Long-Term Services and Supports for Elderly People*. Washington, DC: CBO.

Cubanski, J., et al. 2014. *How Much Is Enough? Out-of-Pocket Spending Among Medicare Beneficiaries: A Chartbook*. Kaiser Family Foundation. http://kff.org/health-costs/report/how-much-is-enough-out-of-pocket-spending-among-medicare-beneficiaries-a-chartbook/. Retrieved February 19, 2016.

Kaye, H., Harrington, C., and LaPlante, M. 2010. "Long-Term Care: Who Gets It, Who Provides It, Who Pays, and How Much?" *Health Affairs* 29(1): 11–21.

Medicaid and CHIP Payment and Access Commission (MACPAC). 2014. *June 2014 Report to the Congress on Medicaid and CHIP*. Washington, DC: MACPAC.

Moon, M., et al. 2015. "Serving Older Adults with Complex Care Needs: A New Benefit Option for Medicare." *Issue Brief* 23: 1–11. New York: Commonwealth Fund.

Moon, M., Wang, Y., and Guo, J. 2016. *How Social Security and Medicare Reduce Inequality*. Washington, DC: American Institutes for Research Center on Aging.

Spetz, J., et al. 2015. "Future Demand for Long-term-care Workers Will Be Influenced by Demographic and Utilization Changes." *Health Affairs* 34(6): 936–45.

Rehabilitation Counselor Ethical Considerations for End-of-Life Care

Jan C. Case, Terry L. Blackwell, and Matthew E. Sprong

Among the changes in the 2010 revised *Code of Professional Ethics for Rehabilitation Counselors* of the Commission on Rehabilitation Certification (CRCC) are standards and guidelines addressing end-of-life care for clients who are terminally ill. The CRCC standards provide guidance in three key areas: (1) Counselor competency for working with end-of-life clients; (2) counselor scope of practice regarding end-of-life clients; and (3) counselor choices pertaining to confidentiality in cases where terminally ill clients are considering hastening their own deaths. In this article we discussed the *Code of Professional Ethics for Rehabilitation Counselors* (Commission on Rehabilitation Certification [CRCC], 2010) that addresses end-of-life care for clients who are terminally ill. Practical ramifications of the standards are discussed and potential dilemmas presented. Practice implications for rehabilitation counselors are outlined.

Among the changes in the 2010 revised *Code of Professional Ethics for Rehabilitation Counselors* (Commission on Rehabilitation Certification [CRCC], 2010) are standards and guidelines addressing end-of-life care for clients who are terminally ill. The CRCC standards provide guidance in three key areas: 1) counselor competency for working with end-of-life clients (A.9.a); 2) counselor scope of practice regarding end-of-life clients (A.9.b); and 3) counselor choices pertaining to confidentiality in cases where terminally ill clients are considering hastening their own deaths (A.9.c). A. 1 .a, A.2.a, A.4.a., B. 1 ,b., B. 1 .c., B. 1 .d., B.2.a., 1.1 .b). With these new guidelines, rehabilitation counselors must now anticipate and consider potential dilemmas that may arise when applying CRCC (2010) Standard A.9 in conjunction with other ethical standards and seek resources to resolve such dilemmas. This article seeks to (1) explore some considerations and implications that Standard A.9 may present for the rehabilitation counseling practitioner, (2) to familiarize rehabilitation counselors with other portions of the Code that will assist their ethical implementation of A.9, and (3) to provide initial best practice considerations.

End-of-Life Issues

Consider the following case scenario:

> You prepared yourself for the inevitable phone call from a client, but it still jolted you when it did finally come: "I knew it was really only a matter of time, and now my doctors think it's probably going to be only a few months until I pass on. I have enjoyed my job so much, and the last few months they have even let me do most of my work out of my parents 'home. But now I feel like I am becoming a drag on everyone, and maybe it's time I just gave up trying. My options are limited. Maybe it's time I did something to move my death along. Have you had any experience with this type of thing? I need your advice. I have always admired your wisdom, so I wanted to get together with you about this."

The term "end-of-life" is understood to mean the developmental period in a person's life when approaching death colors the content of many of their decisions and actions (Papalia & Martorell, 2014). This period of time may differ widely from person to person, and could consist of days, weeks, or months. A person who enjoys good health will be unable to live forever, and by their 70's or 80's, end-of-life becomes a part of almost everyone's thought process. People in good health often complete living wills or personal care directives, and for those with severe medical issues or with a terminal diagnosis, being able to assure themselves that existential, spiritual, familial, and emotional aspects of their care are also going to be addressed are often cited among the most important concerns of patients (Greisinger, Lorimor, Aday, Winn, & Baile, 1997). Those whose health is less steady or who have progressive disabilities and received terminal diagnoses are even more apt to be preoccupied with end-of-life concerns (Smart, 2012). End-of-life is not limited to the medical aspect of death; it may include areas such as financial and legacy decisions, creating memorials, attaining a comfortable spiritual acquiescence, and saying goodbye to family and friends. End-of-life concerns impact each theater of a person's life including work roles, educational roles, family roles, and community roles.

Not everyone who is seen by a rehabilitation counselor will need nor seek counseling at end-of-life. Many may find their needs met by pastoral, rabbinical, or monastic counseling; others will confide in, and receive guidance from, their healthcare professionals, including physicians, nurses, or hospice staff. People with disabilities however, especially those with severe disabilities, may also benefit from specialized expertise from a rehabilitation and/or mental health counselor who has knowledge and skills to serve people who are approaching death. Wadsorth, Harley, Smith, & Kampfe (2008) asserted that rehabilitation counselors may be the initial point of contact for employees from diverse cultural backgrounds or employees with a disability who face barriers to accessing hospice and other end-of-life resources. Additionally, clients who have difficulty with end-of-life issues may experience changes in productivity and interpersonal conflicts with co-worker and supervisor relationships. In addition, rehabilitation counselors may find themselves involved with end-of-life issues through participation in case management, ethics, research, and administrative committees in which decisions regarding end-of-life practices can occur.

Rehabilitation Counseling Scope of Practice

The Scope of Practice for Rehabilitation Counseling identifies assumptions, underlying values, and specific rehabilitation counseling modalities that are extremely pertinent to clients in end-of-life times. As the Scope of Practice states: "Rehabilitation counseling is a systematic process which assists persons with physical, mental, developmental, cognitive, and emotional disabilities to achieve their personal, career, and independent living goals in the most integrated setting possible through the application of the counseling process." (CRCC, 2010, p. 1). This same systematic process of service can bring important services to the person who is facing end-of-life decisions. Furthermore, the Scope of Practice reminds counselors that their underlying values as rehabilitation practitioners include:

Facilitation of independence, integration, and inclusion; the belief in the dignity and worth of all persons; commitment to equal justice; and emphasis on the holistic nature of human function; recognition of the importance of focusing on the assets of a person; and commitment to models of service delivery that emphasize integrated, comprehensive services, (p. 1)

These underlying values are also pertinent to the content and the delivery of services to persons in end-of-life times. Finally, the Scope of Practice reiterates the differentiation between a professional scope of rehabilitation counseling practice and an individual scope of practice. While these may overlap, an individual's scope of practice is more specialized and is based on one's own knowledge of the abilities and skills that have been gained through a program of education and professional experience. This insight underscores the importance of continuing education, and suggests that many fellow rehabilitation practitioners may have developed specific expertise in working with clients regarding end-of-life issues. These rehabilitation practitioners have abilities and skills that can assist other rehabilitation practitioners in the effective delivery of their own respective services to clients who face end-of-life transitions and decisions.

Standard A.9

Although there are a variety of informative articles published on specific counseling techniques and considerations in working with end-of-life clients (e.g., Werth & Crow, 2009), much of the literature concerning end-of-life counseling, although valuable and perceptive, does not specifically address the unique roles of rehabilitation counselors and the unique challenges rehabilitation counselors face in formulating and implementing best practice. The challenges in dealing with end-of-life issues are varied and can be quite complex. This fact is made all the more evident in the enumeration of a specific standard in the *Code of Professional Ethics for Rehabilitation Counselors* (CRCC, 2010) that calls attention to this precise issue.

Section A.9: Quality of Care

Counselors take measures that enable clients to:

1   obtain high quality end-of-life care for their physical, emotional, social, and spiritual needs;

2   exercise the highest degree of self- determination possible; be given every opportunity possible to engage in informed decision-making regarding their end-of-life care; and, receive complete and adequate assessment regarding their ability to make competent rational decisions on their own behalf from mental health professionals who are experienced in end-of-life care practice (CRCCA.9.a).

The "Quality of Care" standard of the *Code* (A.9.a. 1) is poignant and impactful, because while traditionally the goal of rehabilitation counseling has been the optimization and promotion of the lives of those served, Standard A.9.a.2 extends to those wishing to enhance the experience of death. This standard spells out briefly what quality care for an end-of-life client would look like. First, it states that such care addresses physical and emotional health as well as social and spiritual needs. Addressing a client's biological, psychosocial, and spiritual needs is a tall order of business for a single counselor and suggests a team approach (Kaut, 2006; Smart, 2012). This team might include health care and mental health professionals, family, friends, or other support system members, and spiritual advisors. The rehabilitation counselor being guided by the *Code* might do well to take a case-management approach and become the one pulling together all the various components of the client's needs. For example, Olkin (1999) suggested that persons who are older and have disabilities "may have less education, more unemployment, lower income, higher levels of poverty,…, increased need for support from family or service agencies, higher medical costs, and more costs associated with assistive devices and modifying the environment to increase accessibility" (p. 154). Moreover, Olkin stated that a decrease in functioning may occur sooner for persons with disabilities and result in being more susceptible to injury, and a quicker onset of fatigue, while cognitive abilities will also begin to diminish (Smart, 2012). For example, the ability to process and retrieve information decreases, working memory deteriorates in speed and function, and speech is slowed and disorganized due to a decline in word retrieval.

Next, standard A.9.a.3 states that clients should be helped to "exercise the highest level of self-determination possible". Self-determination is not easily defined either across cultures or within a single culture; every individual effectively has a sense of what self-determination means to him or her. For persons whose major identification is with the European American dominant culture, self-determination is usually equated with a high level of individual autonomy (Werth & Crow, 2009). Examined across cultures, Standard A.9.a.3. brings up several possible ethical dilemmas which will be discussed later in this paper, but it appears the main thrust of this standard is to attempt to insure that a client will not be influenced in life-and-death decisions by ill-considered or intrusive expressions of values on the part of caregivers or family members (Botsford & King, 2005; Longmore, 2005; Werth, 2005). This is a particularly cogent issue in caring for clients with cognitive disability who might often be easily swayed by the values of those around them (Botsford & King, 2005). Rehabilitation counselors need to be mindful of this and must be careful not to impose their values on the client. However, the ability to recognize that true autonomy or self-determination probably does not exist is beneficial as often times people who need to make these end-of-life decisions probably consult others (e.g., family members, friends) to seek guidance on their values and feelings.

When speaking of self-determination, the *Code* seems to be addressing such things as potential abuse of physicians' or others' authority in influencing persons with disabilities toward a value judgment that life with a severe disability is not worth living (Wachsler, 2007). For example, as discussed by Wachsler, "physicians often urge family members to sign Do Not Resuscitate orders (DNRs) when a child is born with a disability or a parent becomes disabled" (p. 9). Additionally, since self-determination for persons with disabilities cannot be taken for granted but must necessarily be advocated by rehabilitation counselors, facilitating decision making in the end-of-life stage for persons with disabilities is also important This issue also touches on counselor competency because, while it might be possible to ensure self-determination for clients who clearly can make decisions for themselves, it is not easy to do so at those times when the self-determination of an individual may be challenged by other individuals, as well-intentioned as those individuals may be. Given the complexities of beliefs, traditions and customs associated with death and dying, rehabilitation counselors must be willing to align themselves with other professionals or seek additional educational resources or professional supervision in an effort to function more competently as an advocate for dying clients (Blevins & Papadatou, 2005). In CRCC 2010 Ethical Standard A.9.a.2., deciding what is meant by "self-determination" and what it might look like in different social and cultural contexts is difficult because not every culture believes that the individual is the last resort in decision-making or that the individual's needs and desires should always trump those of family or society. For example, the Chinese culture believes that a dying person should not be given an exact prognosis because it may add additional stress (National Hospice and Palliative Care Organization, 2009). Muller (1992) reported the case of a dominant-culture White American physician who, in the interest of autonomy, seriously harmed the emotional well-being of a terminal patient's family by insisting against their wishes by having a discussion related to having a do-not-resuscitate order. Similarly, the Navajo culture believes that speaking of a person's death is bad luck and doing so will result in a self-fulfilling prophecy (Daitz, 2011).

Third, informed decision making, always a part of ethical counseling, is especially important with end-of-life clients whose decisions often leave no chance for reconsideration. Each person's decision-making is influenced by several issues, such as the presence of physical pain, co-existing psychological conditions, cognitive abilities, fear of loss and abandonment, values, and perceived quality of life. (American Psychological Association [APA], 2001). In addition, a client's capacity to make decisions may vacillate over time as a function of medical treatments or emotional distress that may impair cognitive abilities (Wadsworth et al., 2008). Informed decision making on the part of the client requires that rehabilitation practitioners attend to essential components such as knowledge, competence, and voluntariness on the part of the client (Blackwell & Patterson, 2003). Furthermore, empowering a client for such decision making necessitates the need for the client to consider utilizing a variety of resources in reaching informed decisions, and that these resources include those from both "outside" of the client (e.g., legal counsel, medical counsel, psychological counsel, family counsel, spiritual counsel) and those from "inside" the client (e.g., the client's own preferred method of making decisions, the perceived adequacy of such processes in helping to reach decisions in end-of-life matters).

Ensuring a truly informed decision process for a client exposed to moral values and information sources from widely varying points of view among family, friends, cultural leaders, and health care professionals, can be a difficult task for a rehabilitation counselor. At end-of-life, family members can become affected by grief to the extent that they may no longer be able to offer cogent advice, and it is the counselor's job to aid those so affected as well as the client; this is all a part of creating a climate in which the client can engage in true informed decision making. Here, as in the entire process, the rehabilitation counselor must carefully refrain from allowing the information presented to be affected by her or his own values and attitudes about death and the meaning of life. End-of- life informed decision making is vastly more complex than, for example, a clinical intake for vocational rehabilitation. Throughout history, much of human culture—literature, art, music, philosophy, and theology—has been concerned with the meaning of life and of death. The end-of-life counselor can use a vast array of information sources culturally and personally appropriate to the client with a disability to help access information for the client's personal decision process.

Finally, assessment for competency is a thorny tangle of competing medical, legal, and ethical areas. Traditionally, any individual who has considered ending their life has been viewed as incompetent (Olkin, 1999). Additionally, an array of services are in place to prevent suicide of persons without disabilities, but when a person with a disability requests assistance to commit suicide, services are available to assist in this request (Smart, 2009; as cited in Smart 2014). However, people with disabilities still encounter healthcare and other professionals who may assume that any person with a visible disability is, in fact, "incompetent." Within the medical model of disability, the disability itself is often regarded as "pathological." Under this model of disability, even a person with a mild cognitive impairment would be viewed as being unable to handle discussions of "serious" matters such as death (Smart, 2012). Much harm has occurred due to supposedly "experienced" mental health professionals hiding deaths from people with intellectual disability because the thought that extreme disorientation caused by a parent or family member "going on a long trip" is somehow less harmful than an open discussion of death (Botsford & King, 2005). Clearly this is a case where the professional's inability to come to terms with their values and existential dilemmas, yet in many such cases the assessment of client competence by such professionals would pass muster by the *Code* because the professional is considered "experienced in end-of-life care practice." Whether they are aware of it or not, even experienced professionals may allow the assessment process to be swayed by their own ethico-spiritual values. Although Standard A.9.a. implies that clients have a right to be assessed by "mental health professionals who are experienced in end-of-life care practice", experience *perse* might not be enough to ensure high-quality care, self-determination, or informed decision making. The standard states that it is the duty of the rehabilitation counselor to seek out and offer access to such professionals, but we take the position that this is not enough, that it is also the rehabilitation counselor's duty to advocate for the client's competency whenever possible and to attempt to create a well-balanced "climate of information" around a client who, because he or she is close to death, must take on the task of making decisions relating to their own end of life.

Rehabilitation Counselor Competence, Choice, and Referral

Rehabilitation counselors may choose to work or not work with terminally ill clients who wish to explore their end-of-life options. Rehabilitation counselors provide appropriate referral information if they are not competent to address such concerns (CRCC [2010] Code of Ethics A.9.b).

Vital to providing adequate and appropriate services to clients who are terminally ill, rehabilitation counselors must self-assess their desire and ability to provide counseling services. This choice however, is indicated in conjunction with guidelines regarding competency and referral. Basic competency about death and dying should be a primary consideration for rehabilitation counselors choosing to provide services (Allen & Jaet, 1982; Allen & Miller, 1988; Hunt & Rosenthal, 2006). Standard A.9.b deals with scope-of-practice for rehabilitation counselors and alludes to the idea of physician assisted suicide or hastening death. This standard may assist a rehabilitation counselor who feels inexperienced or has moral compunctions about working with clients who are making end-of-life decisions the option of choosing "...to work or not work with terminally ill clients who wish to explore their end-of-life options" (p. 6). This sentence gives rehabilitation counselors considerable freedom to opt out if their own value system cannot support a client choosing to end life. When a rehabilitation counselor feels unable to work effectively with such a client, it is stated: "... counselors provide appropriate referral information if they are not competent to address such concerns" (p. 6). Appropriate referral is a part of ethical practice in any area which a rehabilitation counselor feels is outside her or his scope of experience and practice. Yet, as many have noted (e.g., Cates, Gunderson, & Keim, 2012; Werth, Hastings, & Riding-Malon, 2010), referral, although the ethically correct thing to do, is not always possible in the modem world of managed care, especially in rural areas with few counseling resources, or for purposes of assuring continuity of care. Even though rehabilitation counselors are trained to regularly conduct self-assessment to determine if their values are being imposed on the clients they serve, death is one in which even competent counseling professionals may allow their strongly held spiritual, philosophical, or religious values to interfere with a self-judgment of lack of end-of-life competence. Referral thus becomes problematic for two reasons: (1) because the automatic response of a rehabilitation counselor who fears to tread in the end-of-life arena; and (2) because a rehabilitation counselor may feel altogether too much confidence and competence in this area due to preconceived moral values.

Confidentiality

Rehabilitation counselors who provide services to terminally ill individuals who are considering hastening their own deaths have the option of breaking or not breaking confidentiality on this matter, depending on applicable laws and the specific circumstances of the situation and after seeking consultation or supervision from appropriate professional and legal parties (CRCC [2010]).

Standard A.9.c. takes up confidentiality in relation to end-of-life options. Here an attempt is made to chart a neutral course between conflicting state laws, values, and other ethical codes, but the standard is asserting that a client who considers hastening their own death does not necessarily constitute "serious and foreseeable harm" and therefore is not subject to mandatory reporting (Kocet, 2006). Because Standard A.9.c gives the rehabilitation counselor the option of keeping or breaking confidentiality, in effect the decision rests with the rehabilitation counselor who will have to apply his or her own ethical decision making process here which would include legal and professional consultation. This section of the *Code* may not appear to offer much guidance to a rehabilitation counselor faced with an ethical dilemma about a terminal client contemplating suicide, but it does at least state that the rehabilitation counselor has a choice; the end result is to encourage and validate further investigation of the client's unique circumstances.

Rehabilitation counselors examining and applying the end-of-life care standards will recognize the ongoing significance of *principle* ethics (autonomy, beneficence, non-maleficence, justice, fidelity, veracity), and may struggle making decisions when conflict arises between these fundamental ethical principles. In addition, rehabilitation counselors will recognize the ongoing significance of *virtue* ethics (e.g., recognizing one's own values, recognizing one's own emotions, considering one's own culture, weighing the client's familial and community context), and may struggle in their application of these fundamentals as they serve in end-of-life situations. Dilemmas involving client autonomy, welfare, personal values, and professional competency in the area of death and dying are conceivable. Given the recent emergence of these new standards, it is likely many rehabilitation counselors have not been formally educated about death and dying or sound ethical end-of-life decision making (Wadsworth et al., 2008). Similarly, professional public and private rehabilitation services entities may have not yet adopted and accommodated for the standards to provide additional ethical guidance for counselors who encounter clients with disability seeking end- of-life counsel. Furthermore, as literature specific to rehabilitation counseling and ethical and effective end-of-life issues is seriously lacking (Zanskas & Coduti, 2006), it becomes even more imperative that the profession examine the applications and implications of section A.9.

The standards relating to end-of-life are a big step in the direction of ethical clarity. However, there are several places where problems could result if not approached with sensitivity, creativity, objectivity, and an awareness of possible discrimination against persons with disabilities. Rehabilitation counselors who have chosen to work with clients who are terminally ill need to be knowledgeable of the legal guidelines surrounding patients' rights to die within their state as well as the policies of employing organizations and agencies. Similarly, rehabilitation counselors choosing to work with terminally ill clients should accommodate for such guidelines within an informed consent addressing the end-of-life services provided and subsequent exceptions or stipulations.

End-of-Life and Client's Choice: Practice Implications for Rehabilitation Counselors

As previously discussed, the end-of-life care standards underscore the freedom of rehabilitation counselors to work or not work with clients who face end-of-life issues, particularly if the client chooses to explore their end-of-life options. At the same time, these standards reiterate the important role that the respective values of both clients and rehabilitation counselors play in making such decisions, and urge that such choices be made with knowledge, competence (capacity), and voluntariness—on the part of both the client and rehabilitation counselor.

The need for both client and rehabilitation counselor to possess adequate *knowledge* in making this choice raises such questions as: Do the client and rehabilitation counselor possess adequate knowledge regarding the specific illness (or illnesses), the course of the illness, possible treatments for the illness? Do the client and the rehabilitation counselor possess adequate self-knowledge (e.g., awareness of one's values, one's mental health)? Do the client and the rehabilitation counselor possess adequate knowledge regarding other resources that could be utilized to help make such decisions (e.g., community agencies, healthcare providers, spiritual consultants)? Do the client and the rehabilitation counselor possess adequate knowledge of pertinent laws? Does the rehabilitation counselor possess adequate knowledge of the Code of Ethics and opinions from their professional organization regarding these matters? Does the rehabilitation counselor possess a best practice framework to utilize in these matters, including adequate decision making models?

The need for both client and rehabilitation counselor to possess *competence (capacity)* in making this choice raises such questions as: Is the client or the rehabilitation counselor incapacitated by previous life experiences (e.g., personal and familial experiences with this issue, unresolved struggles with their grief) that may prevent them from making good decisions? An assessment of such factors as the robustness of family, community, and professional support networks is an essential component in the assessment process (Robinson, Phipps, Purtilo, Tsoumas, & Hamet-Nardozzi, 2006). Are rehabilitation counselors aware of their own values, but at the same time able to prevent their values from diminishing their competency to serve clients facing end-of-life decisions? Do rehabilitation counselors possess adequate time and flexibility in their schedules that may be required to competently serve? Have rehabilitation counselors adequately developed self-care networks, an awareness of the medical and cultural meanings of death, the ability to communicate about death, and appropriate outcome expectations (Wadsworth, et al., 2008)?

The need for both client and rehabilitation counselor to possess *voluntariness* in making this choice raises such questions as: Are the client and the rehabilitation counselor "free" to make such a decision, or are they burdened with a sense of guilt in making such a decision? Are they pressured in any way to make expedient decisions rather than good decisions? Are they overly concerned about what others may think of their decision, and, therefore, feel a need to compromise their choice in this matter? "Choice" necessitates that *both* the client and rehabilitation counselor fully examine these issues for themselves, and come to decisions that are, indeed, informed, made with adequate competence, and voluntary.

Competency

Because of the somewhat general nature of the *Code* and the large grey areas that remain even after the promulgation of the end-of-life standards, we believe it is imperative to outline some of the key rehabilitation counselor competencies in end- of-life work. A list of competencies might include: Experience in end-of-life care and/or personal experience of death and loss. The emotions and stages of grief resulting from a sudden loss or death can be set down, analyzed, and discussed, but there is no substitute for a rehabilitation counselor's having personally ex-perienced death. In order for the counselor to avoid imposing his or her values on a client, the practitioner must assess how these values are related to end-of-life decision making. Without personal experience of loss, a rehabilitation counselor may hold "book values" that he or she thinks would apply in an end-of-life situation (Wadsworth, et al., 2008). Dying will cause griev-ing, both in the client and family. Family members distracted by grief can make the end-of-life stage more difficult for clients (Werth & Crow, 2009).

A major rehabilitation counseling responsibility is to work for beneficence of the client by maximizing the adjustment of the surrounding family members (Millington & Marini, 2015). This should encompass competence in working with families as noted above, but also demands a thoroughgoing knowledge of the grieving process and appropriate interventions when grieving becomes dysfunctional. Olkin (1999) stated there are certain questions that arise for rehabilitation counselors related to physician-assisted suicide (P-AS), including "What are the counselor's beliefs regarding this issue? Can the rehabilitation counselor opt out of partici-pation if she or he works in a setting in which P-AS becomes available? If the counselor opts out, can the counselor still take referrals of elderly or seriously ill clients who may choose P-AS? What are the appropriate interventions with families facing loss of a member through P-AS? How should the issue of remaining minor children be handled? How are "voluntariness" and "capacity" best assessed, and by whom? How does the rehabilitation counselor assess for underlying treatable depression when many symptoms of serious or terminal illness overlap with those of depression?" (p. 267).

Knowledge of Family Systems Theory. Families must be taken into account in end-of-life situations (Lang & Quill, 2004). The client might not be in a conscious state, and to ignore the interplay of family systems and family decision making processes surrounding the client would amount to professional incompetence. No particular theoretical stance is being suggested here, merely that the rehabilitation counselor should acknowledge in his or her approach to counsel-ing that family and support group cannot be ignored when considering a therapy approach or counseling interventions (Millington & Marini, 2015).

Familiarity with Medical Issues. A rehabilitation counselor is required to be familiar with the medical side of disability, but end-of-life medical situations can be even more complex, often involving pain management and use of drugs that in other situations would be lethally addictive. Pharmaceutical knowledge, a good comprehension of the course of treatment for terminal diseases, and an ability to understand the physician's medical and ethical decision making process are all required. Additionally, a competent counselor must often become an advocate for her or his client with the client's health care providers (Smart, 2012). By being seen by the medical providers as competent to discuss the medical situation of a client, the rehabilitation counselor will increase his or her effectiveness in advocating for the client's right to self-determination and informed decision-making.

Client-Centered Skills. In keeping with the ethic of maximizing self-determination, it is especially necessary for the counselor to demonstrate objectivity. An essential component of helping clients is to create a non-judgmental and safe environment for the client to interact and speak freely (Ivey, Ivey, & Zalaquett, 2013). This is essential when the client's medical condition may preclude an easy expression of wishes and needs. The emotional turmoil that usually accompanies proximity of death will often make an easy expression of feelings, needs, and thoughts difficult for a client. The ability to always be listening, always be trying to understand the client's experience, is a valuable strength in an end-of-life rehabilitation counselor.

Knowledge of Applicable Laws. This is a highly desirable competency to help a rehabilitation counselor navigate the legal and moral morass of P-AS and mandatory disclosure laws. Every state has enacted their own laws governing disclosure of self-harm and several states have now legalized P-AS. Yet, as most physicians will acknowledge, de facto P-AS occurs everywhere (Barroso, 2012), has probably always occurred, whether it involves a patient demanding withdrawal of medical interventions or terminal sedation. Also, as Olkin (1999) has noted, there are complex laws governing end-of-life and do-not-resuscitate directives. For example, in 1997 there were two cases in which the U.S. Supreme Court rule that "P-AS is not a protected liberty interest under the constitution" ... "A person is guilty of promoting a suicide attempt when he knowingly causes or aids another person to attempt suicide" (U.S. Legal, 2010, para. 2). These court rulings resulted in the "failure to affirm a right to assisted suicide" (Olkin, p. 267). However, specific states have passed legislation (i.e., Oregon [1997], Washington [2009], and Vermont [2013]), that allows P-AS (Barone, 2014). Furthermore, Barone (2014) stated that in 2009, the state of Montana passed legislation establishing that doctors are protected if they prescribe lethal-medication at the request of a patient who is terminally ill, and the State of New Mexico passed legislation in 2014 that allowed people who are terminally ill to obtain aid in dying. California became the 5th state to pass legislation (October 5, 2015) that legalized P-AS (Pedroncelli, 2015).

Comfort with Spiritual Topics. Spiritual topics are an essential component of end-of-life care; discussion of death and existential concerns for most people cannot occur without reference to spiritual matters at some level (Manis & Bodenhom, 2006). A rehabilitation counselor need not share a client's spiritual or religious values, but a competent rehabilitation counselor must remain respectful of the client's beliefs (CRCC, Standard(s) A.2.a, A.3.c, D.2.a, D.2.b; ACA [2014], Standard A.4.b.). This should include at least a passing acquaintance with many different spiritual belief systems, but more important is the ability to listen respectfully and support the client's application of his or her own beliefs to the process of dying. Naturally, if the client is actively seeking such a contact, a referral to a spiritual adviser might be appropriate and a competent rehabilitation counselor will be open to this kind of action despite his or her personal belief system.

Referral Contacts for Assessment of Client Decision-Making Competency. Mental health professionals who are experienced, sensitive, caring, and competent to assess persons with disabilities are not easily found (Caldwell & Freeman, 2009). For example, Caldwell and Freeman pointedly note: Before educating others, rehabilitation counselors must first become more interdisciplinary and collaborative. A rehabilitation counselor should strive to develop such referral sources. Because, as noted above, the assessment process can be subject to imposition of values even by the most well-meaning professionals, the competent counselor must continually be assessing the assessors; matching the assessment professional to the particulars of the client's biopsycho- social situation may be necessary (Anastasi, 1982).

Well-Developed and Sensitive Counseling Skills with People of Diverse Backgrounds

End-of-life is an area where it is especially easy to encounter client-counselor spiritual value clashes and these may often be related to culture because every culture has widely varying ways of dealing with death. Therefore, multicultural counseling skills are required in end-of-life settings (Braun, Pietsch, & Blanchette, 2000) as spirituality may differ from the rehabilitation counselor's own beliefs. However, even if culturally based spiritual differences do not necessarily exist, there are often differences at the sub-cultural or even family level about the appropriateness of speaking about death and dying, disclosing prognosis to the dying person, or even speaking of the dying person and a competent rehabilitation counselor must become sensitive and open to all of this information.

Exploration of a Rehabilitation Counselor's Own Values Relating to the Meaning of Death and Toward Purposeful Ending of One's Own Life

Without such self-reflection, a rehabilitation counselor is in danger of unknowingly imposing his or her own value system on a client and may not be able to recognize when values clash or when a referral might be the ethical thing to do. Many rehabilitation counselors have experience working with suicidal clients (Rogers, Gueulette, Abbey-Hines, Carney, & Werth, 2001). Rehabilitation counselors are trained to value life, to protect the clients against self-harm, and yet this experience may paradoxically prevent them from coming to an unbiased moral stance toward an end-of-life client contemplating hastening their own death. Only by exploring their own conception of death, when it should be avoided and when it should be welcomed, can a rehabilitation counselor maintain a balanced stance when a client needs support at end-of-life. Even apart from the hastening of death, a rehabilitation counselor with his or her own unresolved issues toward death may not be able to offer effective counseling to a person in the end-of-life stage.

A Comprehensive Grasp of the Code of Ethics

Although the implementation of Standard A.9 of the Code may pose many challenges to rehabilitation counselors, other sections of the Code provide important guidance to rehabilitation practitioners that enhance their understanding of Standard A.9 and its efficient implementation. The Preamble of the *Code* reiterates this essential point when it states, "Each Enforceable Standard is not meant to be interpreted in isolation. Instead, it is important for rehabilitation counselors to interpret standards in conjunction with other related standards in various sections of the Code" (p. 2). It is, therefore, incumbent upon rehabilitation counselors to possess a comprehensive understanding of the *Code*. In studying the requirements and the application of A.9 consider significant *Code* sections such as these:

CRCC Code of Professional Ethics for Rehabilitation

- A.4   Avoiding Harm and Avoiding Value Imposition
- E.2   Consultation
- A.8   Termination and Referral
- E.3.b.   Interdisciplinary Teamwork
- A.7   Group-work (screening, protecting clients)
- A.6   Multiple clients
- Section J   Technology and Distance Counseling
- A.5.d.   Nonprofessional Interactions or Relationships other than Sexual or Romantic Interactions or Relationships
- H.6.   Responsibilities of Rehabilitation Counselor Educators
- L.2.c.   Conflicts between Ethics and Laws
- L.2.d.   Knowledge of Related Code of Ethics
- L.2.f.   Organization Conflicts

Counselors

It is also essential that rehabilitation counselors attend to CRCC Standard L.2.a. (Decision-Making Models and Skills) as they practice A.9. The Preamble of the *Code* also notes the importance of developing decision-making models for the enhanced application of A.9 and all other standards of the *Code:* "While there is no specific ethical decision-making model that is most effective, rehabilitation counselors are expected to be familiar with and apply a credible model of decision-making that can bear public scrutiny.

Tarvydas' (1998) Integrative Model for ethical decision making provides a nice, systematic framework for addressing dilemmas a rehabilitation counselor may encounter when providing end-of-life care. Application of this model first requires the counselor attend to four themes. These themes consist of: (1) Maintaining an attitude of reflection, (2) Addressing the balance between issues and parties to the ethical dilemma, (3) Paying close attention to the context(s) of the situation, and (4) Utilizing a process of collaboration with all rightful parties to the situation. The next step in the Integration Model requires the counselor to systematically review the situation in four stages. The stages are outlined as follows:

Stage I. Interpreting the Situation through Awareness

a. Enhance sensitivity and awareness.
b. Reflect, to determine whether dilemma or issue is involved.
c. Determine the major stakeholders and their ethical claims in the situation.
d. Engage in the fact-finding process.

Stage II. Formulating an Ethical Decision

a. Review the problem or dilemma.
b. Determine what ethical codes, laws, ethical principles, and institutional policies and procedures exist that apply to the dilemma.
c. Generate possible and probable courses of action.
d. Consider potential positive and negative consequences of each course of action.
e. Select the best ethical course of action.

Stage III. Selecting an Action by Evaluating Competing, Non-moral Values

a. Engage in reflective recognition and analysis of personal competing values.
b. Consider contextual influences on values selection at the collegial, team, institutional, and societal levels.
c. Select preferred course of action.

Stage IV. Planning and Executing the Selected Course of Action

a. Figure out a reasonable sequence of concrete actions to be taken.
b. Anticipate and work out personal and contextual barriers to effective execution of the plan of action, and effective countermeasures for them.
c. Carry out and evaluate the course of action as planned.

The utilization of this particular decision-making framework in the application of A.9 (perhaps in conjunction with other appropriate decision-making frameworks) could facilitate rehabilitation counselors in the identification of potential ethical dilemmas, the identification of pertinent resources in reaching ethical decisions, and the effective implementation of these decisions.

Other pertinent decision-making models are presented in the CRCC Desk Reference (2010). In addition to a comprehensive grasp of the *Code* and the implementation of effective ethical decision-making models, the aspiration to best practice (the best a counselor could be expected to do) in the implementation of A.9 suggests that the rehabilitation practitioner also consult with the CRCC and pertinent opinions that have been rendered by the CRCC with regard to A.9 or other pertinent Standards of the *Code*.

Best practice could also include a variety of continuing education endeavors regarding end-of-life issues, including volunteer experiences (perhaps with a hospital or a hospice program) in order to gain further awareness, knowledge, and skills regarding end-of life issues, resources, and practices. Continuing education experiences could also assist rehabilitation counselors become acquainted with other professionals and agencies in their communities who serve in end-of-life transitions. An enhanced knowledge of such individuals and agencies could also help rehabilitation counselors identify service opportunities for themselves through which they could enhance their knowledge and skills as they simultaneously contribute their own expertise as rehabilitation counselors.

End-of-Life Scenario

Consider the case scenario that was introduced at the beginning of this article. After reading the scenario, identify several pertinent issues that the scenario suggests. Formulate your preliminary responses to the scenario, and then consider the "Discussion Points" and "Sample of Related Standards" that are provided for your further consideration. What further "Discussion Points" would you raise? What other "Related Standards" of the *Code* come to mind?

Case Scenario

> *You prepared yourself for the inevitable phone call from a client, but it still jolted you when it did finally come: "I knew it was really only a matter of time, and now my doctors think it's probably going to be only a few months until I pass on. I have enjoyed my job so much, and the last few months they have even let me do most of my work out of my parents' home. But now I feel like I am becoming a drag on everyone, and maybe it's time I just gave up trying. My options are limited. Maybe it's time I did something to move my death along. Have you had any experience with this type of thing? I need your advice. I have always admired your wisdom, so I wanted to get together with you about this."*

Discussion Points
- What do you think the client meant when saying, "something to move my death along"? How would you explore this further with the client?
- How would you begin to explore the legal options that are available to the client?
- What are cultural considerations need to be evaluated?
- How would you engage the client in such an exploration?
- Would you attempt to include the client's family in this matter? Why? Why not? If you did so, how would you proceed to do so?
- What role does the ethical principle of "beneficence" play in this scenario?
- What role does the ethical principle of "veracity" play in this scenario?
- To what extent would your values play a role in your consultation with this client?

Sample of Related Standards
CRCC

- Preamble
- A.6 Multiple Clients
- B.7 Consultation

- A.4 Avoiding Harm and Avoiding Value Imposition
- B.1.b. Respect for Privacy
- L.2.c. Conflicts between Ethics and Laws

Decision Making Thoughts

Although each theme and each stage of the Integrative Model of Decision Making will likely be important in processing this scenario, consider the significance of these considerations of the Model:

1 Pay close attention to the context(s) of the situation. For example, the client appears to have been aware of this situation for a period of time and has likely been working in collaboration with a variety of specialists. Available treatment options have likely been explored, and have not been effective.

2 Enhance sensitivity and awareness. For example, you are described as being "jolted" by this news? As you strive to remain aware of the client's emotional reactions to this news, it may be equally important for you to remain aware of your own emotional reactions at this time.

3 Determine what ethical codes, laws, ethical principles, and institutional policies and procedures exist that apply to the dilemma. For example, are you aware of those state laws that govern "hastening one's death"?

4 Generate possible and probable courses of action. For example, what options are available to you now and in the days ahead? With whom could you consult further in order to more effectively weigh the implications and consequences of each option?

5 Engage in reflective recognition and analysis of personal competing values. For example, is the "hastening of one's death" compatible with your values? If not, would referral of your client be more in keeping with beneficence? With fidelity?

6 Anticipate and work out personal and contextual barriers to effective execution of the plan of action, and effective countermeasures for them. For example, in implementing your decision what supportive resources would you gather for yourself? What supportive resources could benefit your client as their decision is implemented?

Future Research

Future research in the area of rehabilitation counselors assisting clients in end-of-life decision making should focus on identifying if rehabilitation counselors are imposing their values in the decision-making process, whether counselor values are impacting how materials are presented to clients who are making end-of-life decisions, and how to increase competencies and comfortableness of rehabilitation counselors in assisting clients who have to make these decisions. Rehabilitation counselors may not feel comfortable assisting this population because they perceive themselves as not having the necessary knowledge needed to be an asset to the client.

Conclusion

Standard A.9 of the revised the *Code of Professional Ethics for Rehabilitation* Counselors (CRCC, 2010) provides an important framework for rehabilitation counselors working with clients who are terminally ill or their families. While the CRCC 2010) *Code* does not solve all of the problems inherent in such work, it provides some standardization of response and some much-needed clarification. Rehabilitation counselors involved in such work would do well to expand their competencies and gain experience with death and dying, grief and loss, and different spiritual value systems. It is also incumbent upon the counselor to develop a best practice framework in the application of Standard A.9. In aspiring to best practice the rehabilitation counselor will possess a comprehensive grasp of the entire *Code* and also be skilled in the application of pertinent ethical decision-making models. Finally, in the small number of potential cases where client wishes for P-AS are encountered, rehabilitation counselors should engage in exploration of their own values and then seek legal and ethical consultation before proceeding.

Two additional issues also help frame an initial appreciation for the complexities of end-of-life counseling. First, persons with disability have a right to live independently; they have as strong a right to die independently. Yet the healthcare system with its "medical model" of disability can fail such people. For example, the "medical model" of disability emphasizes two dimensions, "normal" and pathological (Smart, 2012). Disability is generally viewed as being pathological, and people without disabilities are viewed as normal. The stigma attached to disability can result in the belief that there is "no point to live because I can never be normal." This may naturally lead to the presumption that P-AS is a better alternative than attempting to focus on strengths and abilities, and not what a person is "unable" to do when someone acquires a disability.

Second, a wide-ranging philosophical and moral debate continues on the topic of P-AS. Doctors are divided between those who see it as their duty to preserve life at all costs and those who see a doctor's primary fimction as working for the beneficence of the patient where beneficence includes happiness even over life (Smart, 2012). Furthermore, the public is divided on the issue as well, often forming lines highly correlated with religious preference or moral stance. The present article is not primarily concerned with this subject; to the extent that it is taken up, it is treated as simply another facet of the end-of-life decision-making process.

Finally, rehabilitation counselors must continuously self-assess themselves to determine what their values are related to end-of-life decisions, and P-AS and disability. As working with in any context related to rehabilitation counseling, the values of the rehabilitation counselor may not be consistent with the values of the client. The rehabilitation counselor should note that they are not making the decision that the client should end their life but rather guiding him or her throughout the decision-making process.

References

Allen, H. A. & Miller, D. M. (1988). Client death: A national survey of the experiences of certified rehabilitation counselors. *Rehabilitation Counseling Bulletin, 32,* 58–64.

Allen, H. A. & Jaet, D. N. (1982). The rehabilitation counselor's experience of client death. *Journal of Applied Rehabilitation Counseling 13(2),* 17–21.

Anastasi, A. (1982). Psychological testing (5th ed.). New York, NY: Macmillan.

Barone, E. (2014, November 3). See which states allow assisted suicide. *Time Magazine.* Retrieved from http:// time.com/3551560/brittany-maynard-right-to-die- laws/

Blevins, D. & Papadatou, D. (2005). Effects of culture on end-of-life situations. In Werth, J.L. & Blevins, D. (APA), *Psychosocial issues near the end of life: A resource for professional care providers* (1st ed., pp,27–55). Washington DC: American Psychological Association.

Blackwell, T. L., & Patterson, J. B. (2003). Ethical and legal implications of informed consent in rehabilitation counseling. *Journal of Applied Rehabilitation Counseling, 34(1),* 3–9.

Barroso, L. R. (2012). Here, there, and everywhere: Human dignity in contemporary law and in the transla- tional discourse. *Boston College International and Comparative Law Review, 35(2),* 331–393.

Botsford, A. L. & King, A. (2005). End-of-life care policies for people with an intellectual disability. *Journal of Disability Policy Studies, 16(1),* 22–30.

Braun, K. L., Pietsch, J. H., & Blanchette, P. L. (2000). An introduction to cuture and its influence on end-of-life decision making. In K. L. Braun, J.H. Pietsch, & P. L. Blanchette (Eds.). *Cultural issues in end of life decision making,* (pp. 1–11). Thousand Oaks, California: Sage.

Caldwell, C.D. & Freeman, S.J. (2009). End-of-life decision making: A slippery slope. *Journal of Professional Counseling Practice, Theory, and Research, 37,* 21–33.

Cates, K. A., Gunderson, C., & Keim, M. A. (2012). The ethical frontier: Ethical considerations for frontier counselors. *The Professional Counselor, 2(1),* 22–32.

Commission on Rehabilitation Counselor Certification. (2010). *Code of professional ethics for rehabilitation counselors.* Schaumburg, IL: Author.

CRCC Desk Reference. (2010). The CRCC desk reference on professional ethics: A guide of rehabilitation counselors. Athens, GA: Elliot & Fitzpatrick.

Daitz, B. (2011, January 24). With poem, broaching the topic of death. *The New York Dimes.* Retrieved from http:// www.nytimes.com/2011/01 /25/health/25navajo.ht-ml?pagewanted=all&_r=0

Greisinger, A. J., Lorimor, R. J., Aday, L. A., Winn, R. J., & Baile, W. F. (1997). Terminally ill cancer patients. Their most important concerns. *Cancer Practice,* 5(3), 147–154.

Hunt, B. & Rosenthal, D. A. (2000). Rehabilitation counselors' experience with client death and death anxiety. *Journal of Rehabilitation, 66* (4), 44–50.

Hunt, B., & Rosenthal, D. (1997). Rehabilitation counsel- ors-in-training: A study for level of death anxiety and perceptions about client death. *Rehabilitation Education, 11,* 323–335.

Kaut, K.P. (2006). End-of-Life assessment within a holistic bio-psycho-social-spiritual framework. In Werth, J. L. & Blevins, D. (APA), *Psychosocial issues near the end of life: A resource for professional care providers* (1st ed., pp. 111–132). Washington DC: American Psychological Association.

Kocet, M. M. (2006) Ethical Challenges in a Complex World: Highlights of the 2005 ACA Code of Ethics. *Journal of Counseling & Development, 84(2),* 228–234.

Lang, F. & Quill, T. (2004). Making decisions with families at the end of life. *American Family Physician, 70(4),* 719–723.

Longmore, P. K. (2005). Policy, prejudice, and reality: Two case studies of physician assisted suicide. *Journal of Disability Policy Study, 16(1),* 38–45.

Manis, A. A., & Bodenhom, N. (2006). Preparation for counseling adults with terminal illness: Personal and professional parallels. *Counseling and Values, 60,* 197–207.

Millington, M. J., & Marini, I. (2014). *Families in rehabilitation counseling: A community-based rehabilitation approach.* New York, NY: Springer Publishing Company.

Muller, J. H., & Desmond, B. (1992). Ethical dilemmas in a cross-cultural context. A Chinese example. *Western Journal of Medicine, 157(3),* 323–327.

National Hospice and Palliative Care Organization. (2009). Chinese-American outreach guide. Retrieved from http://www.nhpco.org/sites/default/files/public/Access/Chinese_American_Outreach_Guide.pdf

NCHS (National Center for Health Statistics. (2009). *Health, United States, 2009.* Retrieved December 20, 2010, from http://www.cdc.gov/nchs/vitalstats.htm.

Olkin, R. (1999). What psychotherapists should know about disability? New York, NY: The Guilford Press

Oregon Death with Dignity Act. (1995). Or. Rev. Stat § 127.800–127.995.

Papalia, D. E., & Martorell, G. (2014). Experience human development. Columbus, OH: McGraw-Hill.

Parker, R. M., Szymanski, E. M. & Patterson, J. B. (2005). Rehabilitation counseling: Basics and beyond. (4th ed., pp. 2–3). Austin, TX: Pro-Ed.

Robinson, E. M., Phipps, M., Purtilo, R. B., Tsoumas, A., & Hamel-Nardozzi, M. (2006). Complexities in decision making for persons with disabilities nearing end of life. *Topics in Stroke Rehabilitation, 13,* 54–67.

Rogers, J. R., Gueulette, C. M., Abbey-Hines, J., Carney, J. V., & Werth, J. L., Jr. (2011). Rational suicide: An empirical investigation of counselor attitudes. *Journal of Counseling & Development, 79(3),* 365–372. doi: 10.1002/j.1556-6676.2001.tbO 1982.x

Smart, J. F. (2009). The power of models of disability. *Journal of Rehabilitation, 75,* 3–11.

Smart, J. (2012). Disability across the developmental life span: For the rehabilitation counselor. New York, NY: Spring Publishing Company.

Sprong, M. E., Dallas. B., Upton, T. D., & Bordieri, J. (2015). The influence of race, causal attribution, and ingroup favoritism on recommendations for rehabilitation services. *Rehabilitation Counseling Bulletin, 58(4),* 227–239. doi: 10.1177/0034355214562071

Tajfel, H., Billig, M. G., Bundy, R. P, & Flament, C. (1971). Social categorization and intergroup behaviors. *European Journal of Social Psychology, 1,* 149–178.

Tajfel, H., & Turner, J. C. (1986). The social identity of inter-group behavior. In S. Worchel & L. W. Austin (Eds.), Psychology of intergroup relations (pp. 7–24). Chicago, IL: Nelson-Hall.

Tarvydas, V. M. (1998). Ethical decision making processes. In R. R. Cottone & V.M. Tarvydas (Eds.), Ethical and professional issues in counseling (pp. 144–158). Upper Saddle River, NJ: Prentice-Hall.

The Patient Self Determination Act, Omnibus Budget Reconciliation Act, Bill Text 101st Congress (1989–1990) H.R.4449.IH

Wadsworth, J., Harley, D., Smith, S.M., & Kampfe, C. (2008). Infusing end-of-life issues into the rehabilitation counselor education curriculum. *Rehabilitation Education, 22,* 113–124

Waldmann, A. K., & Blackwell, T. L., (2010). Advocacy and accessibility standards in the new code of professional ethics for rehabilitation counselors. *Journal of Applied Rehabilitation Counseling, 41* (2), 37–40.

Werth, J. L., Jr., Hastings, S. L., & Riding-Malon, R. (2010). Ethical challenges of practicing in rural areas. Journal of Clinical Psychology, 66, 537–548.

Werth, J. L., Jr., & Rogers, J. R. (2005). Assessing for impaired judgment as a means of meeting the "duty to protect" when a client is a potential harm-to-self: Implications for clients making end-of-life decisions. *Mortality, 10,* 7–21.

Werth, J. L. & Crow, L. (2009). End-of-life care: An overview for professional counselors. *Journal of Counseling & Development, 87(2),* 194–203.

Person-Centered Care and Resident Choice

Jennifer Brush and Margaret Calkins

One perception often interfering with the adoption and implementation of person-centered care practices in nursing homes is apprehension by staff, administrators, and governing boards about potential legal liability and regulatory exposure if residents suffer injuries. This is primarily because a number of person-centered practices, such as offering residents meaningful choices and honoring their decisions, represent significant deviations from prior accepted more paternalistic institution-centered practice. Person-centered care comes from a fundamentally different perspective, which puts considerable value on an individual's right to make decisions concerning every aspect of her or his life. People are not required to follow their healthcare provider's advice, and this right does not change just because care is i being delivered in a care community instead of at home.

Often providers and clinicians want to honor resident choice, but are afraid to do so. The key is finding the balance between providing quality care and keeping clients safe, and allowing choices that may involve risk but will enhance quality of life—both of which are requirements of Medicare- and Medicaid-certified nursing homes.

So how does the care community accommodate resident preferences when the action/activity/behavior is seen as having some potential risk for a negative outcome?

A Process for Care Planning for Resident Choice

The Rothschild Person-Centered Care Planning Task Force, sponsored by the Hulda B. and Maurice L. Rothschild Foundation, worked for a year to create A Proposed Process for Care Planning for Resident Choice (Calkins, Schoeneman, Brush & Mayer, 2014). This process is specifically aimed at care planning when the choice carries sufficient risk that the community is considering not honoring the resident's wishes. Following the Rothschild Person-Centered Care Planning process below will help the community work with the resident (and sometimes the family or representative) to understand and respect choices to the greatest extent possible, in line with Centers for Medicare & Medicaid Services (CMS) regulations.

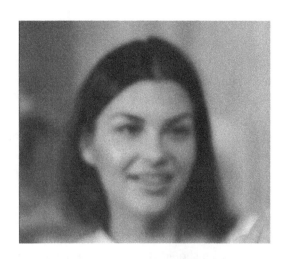

1 Identify and clarify the resident's choice

Interview and observe the resident. Review the resident's history to obtain detailed information about the nature and extent of the choice that the resident wishes to make. Repeat back to the resident your understanding of what she or he desires to choose or refuse, to confirm both parties understand each other. While the decision defaults to the individual, it can be helpful to discuss it with the representative (if one is appointed) in order to better understand some of the context for this individual preference, particularly if the resident is unable to offer a satisfactory explanation.

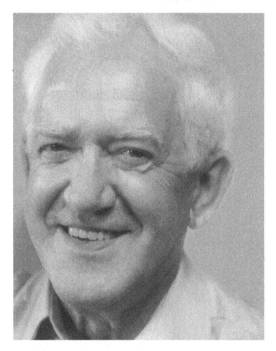

2 Discuss the choice and options with the resident

Discuss with/educate the resident about the potential outcomes of respecting and aiding the resident in the pursuit of her or his choices, as well as the potential outcomes of preventing the person from acting on his or her choices. Consider potential positive outcomes as well as potential negative consequences. Staff should explain that the resident still has the (regulatory) right to make choices and to refuse treatment.

After learning of and considering the potential consequences, the resident may decide not to take his or her initial requested action, to curtail its frequency, or to select an alternative with fewer potential adverse consequences, or may continue to desire the original choice. The team should offer ways in which they can accommodate the choice and also mitigate potential negative consequences as much as possible.

3   Determine how to honor the choice

While some resident requests are potentially too harmful to other people to honor ("I want to drive a car again"), many other requests can and should be honored by virtue of the team creating a plan to mitigate known potential negative consequences or offering a similar activity which has fewer potential adverse consequences (for example, riding in a car to a desired location, but allowing someone else to drive).

The team should compare the resident's choice to the resident's condition to determine the nature of potential risks. If the resident's requested action poses significant danger to others, the team should clearly explain to the resident why they cannot honor that particular choice.

Discuss with/educate the resident about the potential outcomes of respecting and aiding the resident in the pursuit of her or his choices, as well as the potential outcomes of preventing the person from acting on his or her choices. Consider potential positive outcomes as well as potential negative consequences.

4   Care planning the choice

While it is important that all members of the interdisciplinary team be involved in care planning, it is recognized that not every representative can always participate in a face-to-face meeting. It is very important to have the participation and input of the direct care staff as they have the most contact with the resident. Therefore, alternative means of communication should be made available for providing input and review of the plan. On occasion it may be a resident's or representative's choice to meet with a smaller group of people rather than the entire team, and that preference should be accommodated.

5   Monitoring and making revisions to the plan

The interdisciplinary team will monitor the progress of the plan and its effects on the resident's well-being and ongoing desire to continue with the choice. The team will work with the resident to revise the plan as needed and desired by the resident. A person's needs and preferences change over time and so will their expression of them. Care plans and staff should be flexible, as people have the right to change their minds.

6   Quality Assurance and Performance Improvement (QAPI)

The QAPI team should review trends related to resident choice and safety, particularly when residents are routinely denied requests, or when the QAPI team identifies patterns of community care practices that might be improved by performance improvement action plans.

For so long, the focus in long-term care has been on doing what is "in the best interest of the person" as defined by the healthcare professional staff, rather than as defined by the person. The whole process has been based on a historical medical model that assumes the "patient" is the passive and "compliant" recipient of care directed and provided by professionals. In contrast, this care planning process has been developed to help give the person a voice in directing his or her own care. Rather than viewing a person as non-compliant if he or she does not agree with your recommendations, the authors suggest viewing the resident as a member of the care team, participating in the discussion options and potential risks and outcomes.

In cases where a resident expresses a choice that is considered risky, use the described care planning process to discuss the potential outcomes of both respecting and aiding the resident in the pursuit of her or his choices, and review the potential outcomes of preventing the resident from acting on his or her choices. This will demonstrate to residents, state surveyors, family members, and others that a care community has done due diligence with the resident and his or her representative. LTL

The full Process for Care Planning for Resident Choice, which includes blank forms and case studies, can be found at www.IdeasInstitute.com and www. BrushDeveloment.com.

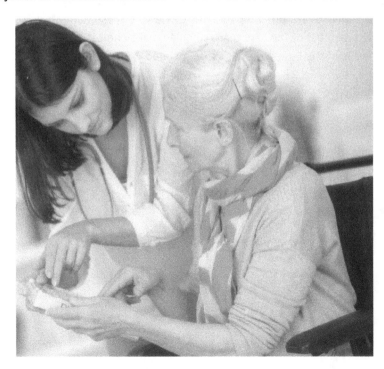

Chapter 5: **Discussion Questions**

1   Describe the challenges facing the development of a sufficient long-term care workforce to meet the needs of the growing elderly population.

   a. How can we increase efficiency by aligning health policies governing elder care?

2   What is a geriatric care manager?

   a. Why, or why not, is this a useful addition to the elder care workforce?

3   How does compensation of the elder care workers affect care?

   a. Do you agree with the author that this is the biggest impediment to improving elder care?

4   Describe the complexities of end-of-life care counseling.

   a. Should families play a role in end-of-life care decisions? Why or why not?

5   How can providers practice person-centered care and provide residents with autonomy and freedom of choice based on their personal priorities?

   a. Explain the difference between clinicians who view patients engaging in risky behavior as non-compliant verses viewing these patients as a valued member of the care team who can make choices based on knowledge of the benefits and risks associated with them.

CHAPTER 6

EVIDENCE-BASED MANAGEMENT AND ECONOMIC HEALTH POLICY

ACOs and the Quest to Reduce Costs

Ken Perez

Accountable care organizations have done reasonably well at curtailing wasteful spending while promoting the sort of innovation that can help organizations succeed in a value-oriented healthcare environment.

The United States will spend more than $3 trillion on health care in 3014, according to the Centers for Medicare & Medicaid Services (CMS), with much of this spending being unnecessary and wasteful. When Donald M. Berwick, MD, was preparing to leave his post as CMS administrator in late 2011, he noted that 20 to 30 percent of healthcare spending yields no benefit to patients.[a]

Accountable care organizations (ACOs) are key components of the Obama administration's strategy to stem the high cost and waste of health care. ACOs address both quality and cost, employing economic carrots and sticks to change the way providers deliver care. The headline of one news article described ACOs as "Obamacare's Secret Weapon in the War on Exorbitant Healthcare Costs."[b] Berwick tied ACOs to the triple aim of sought-after improvements in U.S. health care: "The creation of ACOs is one of the first delivery-reform initiatives that will be implemented under the [Affordable Care Act]. Its purpose is to foster change in patient care so as to accelerate progress toward a three-part aim: better care for individuals, better health for populations, and slower growth in costs through improvements in care.[c]

---

a   Pear, R., "Health Official Takes Parting Shot at 'Waste'," *The New York Times*, Dec. 3, 2011.

b   Lopez, G., "Meet Obamacare's Secret Weapon in the War on Exorbitant Healthcare Costs," Vox, May 17, 2014.

c   Berwick, D. M., "Launching Accountable Care Organizations—The Proposed Rule for the Medicare Shared Savings Program," *New England Journal of Medicine*, March 31, 2011.

How ACOs Have Fared

In December 2008, the Congressional Budget Office estimated that ACOs could save Medicare $5.3 billion between 2010 and 2019. According to the Medicare ACO business model, the member organizations—usually including physicians and hospitals—share in the savings if they meet certain quality-reporting or performance requirements and a cost-savings target.

If an ACO falls short of the target, members receive no rewards, which could make them less motivated to continue their participation. Cost savings are critical to sustaining the ACO model.

Physician Group Practice (PGP) demonstration. The PGP demonstration, which took place in 2005–10, was Medicare's first pay-for-performance initiative for physicians.

Under terms of the PGP demonstration, 10 large, multispecialty physician groups were eligible to earn performance payments of up to 80 percent of the savings they generated. By the third and fourth years, five of the 10 groups shared in savings by meeting cost-reduction goals and hitting targets on key quality measures, according to a CMS fact sheet released in July 2011. The overall performance improved during the first four years of the demonstration, with incentive payments totaling $7.3 million in year one, $13.8 million in year two, $25.3 million in year three, and $31.7 million in year four. The average payments in year four alone—$6.3 million per physician group—represented a sizable return on the average up-front investment of $1.7 million. (Overall performance dipped slightly in year five, with four of the 10 groups qualifying for performance payments totaling $29.4 million.)

Although reaching the cost-savings targets certainly was not a slam dunk for the participating organizations, the targets became more attainable with practice. This trend has remained apparent in subsequent ACO models.

Medicare Shared Savings Program (MSSP). On Jan. 3o, CMS released interim financial results for the MSSP ACOs that began operating in 2012. In their first 12 months, 54 of 114 MSSP ACOs (47 percent) had lower expenses than projected, exceeding their cost-savings benchmarks, according to a U.S. Department of Health and Human Services (HHS) news release announcing the results. Of those 54 ACOs, 29 achieved levels at which they were eligible for shared savings, which totaled more than $126 million.

AT A GLANCE

- Accountable care organizations (ACOs) have been described as a "secret weapon" in the effort to slow the exponential growth of healthcare costs while improving the quality of care.

- Short-term cost savings are crucial to sustaining the ACO model because without revenue from shared- savings incentives, participating organizations might not be motivated to continue their involvement.

- ACOs of various types have achieved cost savings in recent years while improving care for their patients, and opportunities lie ahead for ACOs to become even more effective.

Provider organizations in Medicare ACOs are free to use various technologies and explore innovative approaches that will reduce the utilization of services.

These ACOs generated $128 million in net savings for the Medicare trust funds. HHS also notes that most of the program's impact is expected to be seen in subsequent years.

Pioneer ACOs. Announced in December 2011, the Pioneer ACO model, a CMS Innovation Center program, features higher levels of potential reward and risk than does the MSSP model.

At the launch of the Pioneer ACO model, CMS noted that the initiative, which at the time had 32 participating Pioneer ACOs, would generate $1.1 billion in savings over five years. Although the projection has been met with criticism, given that Medicare's annual budget is more than $500 billion, the critics do not recognize the pilot nature of the Pioneer program, which represents an experiment in bending the cost curve that could provide valuable lessons for the healthcare industry.

In July 2013, CMS shared first-year results of the Pioneer program, disclosing that all 32 Pioneer ACOs successfully reported the required quality measures. Eighteen of the 32 delivered savings, with 13 achieving levels at which they were eligible for shared savings.

Of the 19 Pioneers that failed to qualify for shared savings, seven opted to step down to the less-risky MSSP and two decided to cease operating as Medicare ACOs altogether. The 10 others chose to remain in the Pioneer program, suggesting they planned to take a "wait-and-see" attitude regarding the viability of the model.

Costs grew by 0.3 percent in 2012 for the approximately 669,000 Medicare beneficiaries in Pioneer ACOs, compared with 0.8 percent for comparable beneficiaries outside the ACOs, according to CMS. As noted by HHS in its Jan. 30 news release, an independent evaluation concluded that the Pioneer ACO program saved $147 million in the first year. That total was $60 million higher than the savings initially reported by CMS.

Pioneer and MSSP ACOs had yielded combined savings of more than $380 million as of January, according to the HHS release. Expenditures were below projections for almost half—72 of 146—of the participating ACOs.

In a separate release issued the same day, Blair Childs, senior vice president of public affairs for Charlotte, N.C.-based Premier, Inc., notes the "significant early progress" that was evident in the savings figures. "We hope these results will prove the potential of accountable care, and incent other payers and providers to join the growing movement away from today's broken fee-for-service system, and toward a more value- based, cost-effective future," Childs says.

Medicaid ACOs. More than 20 states have launched ACOs that cover Medicaid and Children's Health Insurance Program populations, according to the National Academy for State Health Policy. The largest such ACO, Colorado's Accountable Care Collaborative (ACC), has been operational since 2011 and manages care for more than 350,000 members, or 47 percent of the state's Medicaid population. The ACC has focused on connecting members with their primary care physicians, deploying care coordinators, and using analytics extensively.

The ACC generated gross savings of $44 million in its fiscal year ending in June 2013, according to the Colorado Department of Health Care Policy and Financing, returning $6 million to the state after expenses. It also slowed the growth of emergency department (ED) utilization and reduced hospital réadmissions (by 15 to 20 percent), use of high-cost imaging services (by 25 percent), and hospital admissions for patients with chronic obstructive pulmonary disease (by 22 percent). Most important, key health metrics (e.g., rates of chronic conditions, such as hypertension and diabetes) improved for ACC members relative to Medicaid enrollees who were not in the ACC.

> ACOs are an aggressive, innovative means of shifting the business of health care from the well-entrenched fee-for-service model to a fee-for-value approach.

Neighboring Utah's four Medicaid ACOs, which went live on Jan. 1, 2013, and encompass 85 percent of the state's Medicaid population, have been less publicized, but may turn out to be even more successful: They are on track to save the state's taxpayers more than $2.5 billion during the next seven years.[d]

Commercial ACOs. More than 300 ACOs are led by commercial health plans, with the largest plans each orchestrating dozens of these arrangements. Relatively little has been disclosed about their performance, in part because many commercial ACOs only recently have become operational and also because of their status as private entities.

In 2010, Blue Shield of California launched an innovative shared-savings model involving a purchaser (the California Public Employees Retirement System [CalPERS]), a physician group (Hill Physicians Medical Group), and a hospital system (Dignity Health). The ACO serves approximately 42,000 CalPERS employees and their families who are covered by Blue Shield. It has generated gross savings of $105 million, with net savings of $95 million to CalPERS members.[e]

In 2011, Advocate Health Care and Blue Cross & Blue Shield of Illinois started an ACO called AdvocateCare. It provides financial incentives for physicians and hospitals to meet quality, patient-satisfaction and cost-reduction goals for a defined population of about 380,000 members.

Between 2011 and 2012, Advocate and its network of 4,000 physicians improved key care metrics for the approximately 200,000 members in the ACO's preferred provider organization (PPO):

- The hospital admission rate decreased 1.4 percent, compared with an increase of 2.2 percent at other hospitals in the Blue Cross broad PPO network.
- Average length of stay increased 1.7 percent, compared with 2.7 percent for the rest of the network.
- Inpatient days increased 0.3 percent, compared with 4.7 percent for the rest of the network.

Factoring in positive outpatient metrics, Advocate-Care's costs were trending 2.5 percent below the other hospitals in the Blue Cross PPO network.[f]

d   Liljenquist, D., "Utah's Medicaid Reform Has Been a Quiet Success," *Deseret News*, April 10, 2014.

e   Melnick, G., and Green, L., "Four Years Into a Commercial ACO for CalPERS: Substantial Savings and Lessons Learned," *Health Affairs* blog, April 17, 2014.

f   Wang, A.L., "Advocate-Blue Cross ACO Sees improvement in Utilization, Costs," *Crain's Chicago Business*, Jan. 21, 2014.

FUTURE ACO OPPORTUNITIES

Many areas of opportunity exist for ACO expansion or development, including:

- Medication adherence initiatives
- Renal-specific ACOs
- Oncology ACOs
- Post-acute care integration
- Retail pharmacy utilization
- Wellness programs
- Mobile health

Areas of Opportunity

CMS's final rules for the MSSP and Pioneer ACO models explain in great detail how per capita expenditures are set. But they are silent as to how ACOs should go about achieving the cost-reduction targets.

Provider organizations in Medicare ACOs are free to use various technologies and explore innovative approaches that will reduce the utilization of services. A review shows that high-performing ACOs employ a data-driven approach and use analytics extensively, including to carry out risk stratification, identify gaps in care, improve care coordination, and enhance patient engagement.

The pursuit of cost savings by ACOs has spurred interest in management of high-cost and chronic diseases, and of areas where the care delivery chain somehow breaks down. Promising approaches include renal-specific ACOs, advocated by DaVita Inc., the nation's second-largest dialysis provider; oncology ACOs, piloted by Aetna and Florida Blue; and medication adherence initiatives, which have been shown to lower hospitalization rates and ED use, resulting in a significant net reduction in healthcare costs.

Taking the 'Long View'

ACOs are an aggressive, innovative means of shifting the business of health care from the well-entrenched fee-for-service model to a fee-for-value approach. They are an example of practicing the art of the possible, effecting fundamental change in a large, capitalist society where the healthcare system is a complex web of public- and private-sector involvement.

Some view the mixed results of ACOs regarding cost reduction as proof that the basic concept is flawed. But surely unaccountable care is not the answer.

We should refine the existing ACO programs and launch new ones, sharpen our strategies and tactics, and improve population health management. "We have to take the long view, and be focused on iterating, evolving, and improving the concept, rather than seeking summary judgment," says Farzad Mostashari, a visiting fellow at the Brookings Institution and former national coordinator for health information technology.[g] If we take that approach, we will see greater successes in our effort to solve the problems of unacceptably high healthcare costs and poor quality.

---

g   Stuckey, M., "Poised for Growth, Commercial ACOs Also Face Considerable Challenges," *California Healthline*, May 21, 2014.

Clinical Integration

A Cornerstone for Population Health Management

Kenneth W. Kizer

The primary business of healthcare today is managing chronic conditions such as diabetes, asthma, heart disease, and arthritis. Approximately three fourths of all healthcare expenditures are for the care of chronic conditions, and about one half of Medicare patients are treated for five or more chronic conditions and see, on average, seven to 11 physicians annually (Pham, Schrag, O'Malley, Wu, & Bach, 2007).

The diffusion of responsibility for a patient's care over multiple caregivers too often results in fragmented care that is uncoordinated, unsafe, unsatisfying, and unnecessarily expensive. Recognizing that fee-for-service payment has fueled fragmented care, healthcare payers are increasingly moving to value-based payment models that incentivize improved coordination of care, quality, and efficiency.

The movement to value-based payment is accelerating, as demonstrated by, among other things, the recent Centers for Medicare & Medicaid Services announcement that one half of Medicare spending outside of managed care will be paid for via value-based models by 2018 (Burwell, 2015) and by the creation of the Health Care Transformation Task Force (a group of large employers, payers, and health systems), which intends to shift 75 percent of its member business to value-based contracts by 2020 (Health Care Transformation Task Force, 2015).

In the emerging value-based healthcare economy, it will be necessary for health systems to rigorously manage the health of populations, whether the population is defined by chronic condition, age, geography, gender, or other characteristics. Indeed, population health management will be a requisite core competency for health system success in the future.

Clinically Integrated Services

Successful population health management will require that health systems integrate clinical services across providers, settings of care, conditions, and time. Toward this end, many healthcare organizations are pursuing alliances, partnerships, or structural changes aimed at facilitating clinical integration. Prominent among these are efforts to consolidate providers into vertically *integrated delivery systems* (IDSs). Many health systems are purchasing physician practices and employing the formerly independent physicians, believing that employment will better align physician interests with the goals of improving quality and lowering costs.

Proponents of vertically integrated consolidation strategies argue that full administrative and financial integration is necessary for clinical integration. They say that the IDS organizational structure leads to more coordinated care across the continuum of services, less unnecessary or duplicative care, lower administrative and transactional costs, better use of expensive medical technology, and more resources for health promotion and other community needs. Despite the enthusiasm with which IDS proponents make their case, there is scant evidence to support the claimed efficiency benefits, or quality performance advantages of vertically integrated health systems (Baker, Bundorf, & Kessler, 2014; Blossom & Wan, 1999; Burns, Goldsmith, & Sen, 2013; Goldsmith, Burns, Sen, & Goldsmith, 2015; Hwang, Chang, LaClair, & Paz, 2013).

It is important to point out that *integrated delivery system* and *integrated patient care* are not the same and should not be equated. Integrated patient care (which results from clinical integration) is about the patient and how patient care services are provided in a coordinated manner, whereas an IDS is about the structure of the organization and how its parts fit together. The latter is not a priori linked to the former. This distinction was well illustrated by the Veterans Affairs Healthcare System in the early 1990s, during which time the VA was unquestionably an IDS but was not providing integrated patient care (Kizer & Dudley, 2009).

Notwithstanding that some IDSs have achieved a high degree of clinical integration, the preponderance of evidence simply does not show that integration achieved through common ownership is superior to other models of clinical integration (Baker et al., 2014; Blossom & Wan, 1999; Burns et al., 2013; Goldsmith et al., 2015; Hwang et al., 2013). Both experiential and empirical evidence make clear that it is not organizational structure or size that is necessary to achieve clinical integration and integrated patient care. Instead, it is the organization's culture, commitment to continuous quality improvement, and possession of key functional abilities that link most closely to better care quality, financial performance, and patient satisfaction (Shortell et al., 2005). The fact that some IDSs possess these attributes should not be taken to mean that it is the IDS structure that is responsible for them.

A close examination of clinically integrated health systems reveals that the following seven key functional abilities and characteristics are necessary to achieve integrated patient care regardless of organizational structure.

1   **A Values-Based Shared Vision of Healthcare Delivery That Is Patient Centric and Population Health Focused.** An organization's vision succinctly articulates what it aspires to be and what it broadly hopes to accomplish. The vision should be rooted in explicitly stated core values that signify the manner in which the organization will conduct itself in achieving its vision; these values are the cornerstone for its culture.

A patient-centric vision embodies the view that services will be provided in a culturally sensitive manner respectful of individual preferences, needs, and values, and that these considerations will be used to inform all clinical decision making. Patients and caregivers are understood to have a shared responsibility for health outcomes, and this mutuality is valued. Care and information are made accessible by multiple means, and the "access dose" is determined by patient needs. The vision is population focused in that service delivery resources are matched to the needs of the population being served, with the important roles of social and environmental determinants of health being recognized and factored into service delivery.

2   **A Governance Structure That Establishes Clear Clinical Goals and Oversees Implementation of Policies and Procedures for Coordinating Care Across the Continuum of Services.** Governance refers broadly to the mechanisms and processes by which an organization is directed and controlled so that it is able to purposefully set goals and implement the means to achieve them. In a clinically integrated health system, clinical goals and associated policies and procedures about care coordination and communication across providers, settings of care, conditions, and time are established to promote a seamless continuum of services that are provided in the most cost-effective, clinically appropriate setting. Services are arranged to minimize overutilization and underutilization, facilitate information flow, and maximize the likelihood that all needed services are delivered safely and effectively in a timely manner. Transitions between care settings and handoffs between providers are managed to avoid disruption of care. Clearly specified clinical aims facilitate meaningful assessment of performance and sharing of performance data.

3   **Strong Clinical Leadership That Drives Integrated Care and Engages Frontline Caregivers.** The most frequently observed success factor for achieving clinical integration is strong clinical leadership that builds trust in the organization and promotes a culture of teamwork and collaboration, transparency, continuous quality improvement, and accountability. Clinical leaders define and communicate priorities to frontline caregivers, serve as the critical bridge between the boardroom and the bedside, ensure that core values are incorporated into operational policies and practices, and align and harmonize competing agendas. Clinical leadership is critical for creating an environment that supports innovation and learning, identifying and communicating stories that highlight what is valued, and ensuring that appropriate recognition is given to reinforce and reward desired behaviors and outcomes.

4   **Information Management Tools and Other Supporting Infrastructure.** A robust infrastructure is needed to support clinical integration. This infrastructure includes information technology (IT) resources (e.g., an electronic health record, health information exchange, clinical decision support, and data analysis tools), human resources, physical space, financial and contractual management, and knowledge management resources. Among the specific tools and systems needed to support clinical integration are utilization and demand management programs; patient scheduling and registration systems; evidence-based clinical guidelines and care pathways; performance measurement and other quality improvement systems; care management programs; clinical service lines; and disease registries.

    In recent years, much attention has been appropriately directed toward developing information management capacity, and especially to support population health management, but it is important to keep in mind that the value of the data provided by IT will not be realized if the human capital and administrative support systems are not in place to operationalize needed interventions.

5   **Team-Based Care.** For all but trivial maladies, multidisciplinary teams of caregivers are needed to provide high-quality and accessible care. However, effective teams do not just happen. Team-based care must be nurtured by the health system and grounded on the principles and practices of effective team-based care (American Hospital Association, 2012; Goldberg, Beeson, Kuzel, Love, & Carver, 2013; Mitchell et al., 2012).

6   **Methods of Accountability, Including a Performance Management System That Consistently Measures and Monitors Clinical Performance.** Among the various methods of accountability needed to support clinical integration, perhaps the most important is a performance management system. As has been noted often, measurement is a requisite for improvement. When establishing performance management systems, healthcare leaders need to remember that performance measurement can produce both intended positive consequences and unintended negative consequences (Kizer & Kirsh, 2012). Whether positive or negative effects predominate depends on the organization's culture and how performance measurement results are used (Kizer & Kirsh, 2012; Kizer & Jha, 2014). Successful performance measurement systems strive to clearly define performance goals, measure results that matter, ensure stakeholder involvement at every level of the performance measurement process, couple top-down or externally imposed measurements with flexibility to address local circumstances, and use performance measurement results to support learning and continuous improvement.

7   **Shared Financial Risks and Rewards for Clinical Outcomes.** Health systems can use various shared financial risk and reward mechanisms to support care coordination across providers. Typically, these involve a risk-adjusted per capita payment model wherein provider payments include a significant incentive bonus for achieving quality and efficiency goals. For the risk and reward system to be successful, however, providers

must understand how the system works and their individual roles and responsibilities for achieving the outcomes that will be rewarded or penalized.

Conclusion

Effective population health management requires that patient care services be clinically integrated. This can be achieved through various organizational models involving different degrees and forms of administrative and financial integration. No one integration model has proven to be clearly superior to others, and the ability of an organization to achieve tangible improvements in cost and quality depends more on strong clinical leadership and the organization's culture and commitment to improvement than it does on any particular structural model.

References

American Hospital Association's Physician Leadership Forum. (2012). *Team-based health care delivery: Lessons from the field*. Chicago, IL: American Hospital Association. Retrieved from http://www.ahaphysicianforum.org

Baker, L. C., Bundorf, M. K., & Kessler, D. P. (2014). Vertical integration: Hospital ownership of physician practices is associated with higher prices and spending. *Health Affairs, 33(5)*, 756–763.

Blossom, Y. J., & Wan, T. T. H. (1999). Analysis of integrated healthcare networks' performance: A contingency-strategic management perspective. *Journal of Medical Sciences*, 22(6), 467–485.

Burns, L. R„ Goldsmith, J. C., & Sen, A. (2013). Horizontal and vertical integration of physicians: A tale of two tails. In J. Goes, G. T. Savage, & L. Friedman (Eds.), *Annual review of health care management: Revisiting the evolution of health systems organization, 15,* (pp. 39–117). West Yorkshire, England: Emerald Publishing Group.

Burwell, S. M. (2015, January 26). Progress towards achieving better care, smarter spending, healthier people [U.S. Department of Health and Human Services Web log post]. Retrieved from http://www.hhs.gov/blog/2015/01/26/progress-towards-better-care-smarter-spending-healthier-people.html

Goldberg, D. G., Beeson, T., Kuzel, A. J., Love, L. E., & Carver, M. C. (2013). Team-based care: A critical element of primary care practice transformation. *Population Health Management, 16(3)*, 150–156.

Goldsmith, J., Burns, L. R., Sen, A., & Goldsmith, T. (2015). *Integrated delivery networks: In search of benefits and market effects*. Washington, DC: National Academy of Social Insurance.

Health Care Transformation Task Force. (2015). Major health care players unite to accelerate transformation of U.S. health care system. Retrieved from http://www.hcttf.org/releases/2015/1/28/major-health-care-players-unite-to-accelerate-transformation-of-us-health-care-system

Hwang, W., Chang, J., LaClair, M., & Paz, H. (2013). Effects of integrated delivery system on cost and quality. *American Journal of Managed Care*, 19(5), el75–el84.

Kizer, K. W., & Dudley, R. A. (2009). Extreme makeover: Transformation of the Veterans Health Care System. *Annual Review of Public Health, 30,* 313–339.

Kizer, K. W., & Jha, A. K. (2014). Restoring trust in VA health care. *New England Journal of Medicine, 371*(4), 295–297.

Kizer, K. W., & Kirsh, S. R. (2012). The double edged sword of performance measurement. *Journal of General Internal Medicine, 27*(4), 315–317.

Mitchell, P., Wynia, M., Golden, R., McNellis, B., Okun, S., Webb, C. E., ... & Von Kohorn, I. (2012). *Core principles & values of effective team-based health care.* Discussion paper, Washington, DC: Institute of Medicine. Retrieved from http://www.iom.edu/tbc

Pham, H. H., Schrag, D., O'Malley, A. S., Wu, B., & Bach, P. B. (2007). Care patterns in Medicare and their implications for pay for performance. *New England Journal of Medicine, 356*(11), 1130–1139.

Shortell, S. M., Schmittdiel, J., Wang, M. C., Li, R., Gillies, R.R., Casolino, L. P., ... & Rundall, T. G. (2005). An empirical assessment of high-performing medical groups: Results from a national study. Medical Care Research Review, 62(4), 407–434.

The Ethics of Evidence-Based Management

Best Practices will Produce Better Outcomes for all Healthcare Stakeholders

Paul B. Hofmann

The advantages of evidence-based medicine have been demonstrated repeatedly. Indisputably, the adoption of clinical guidelines, pathways and protocols has contributed to improved clinical outcomes. Could the development and application of evidence-based management practices have a comparable benefit for patients, staff and, ultimately, healthcare organizations and their communities?

The succinct answer is yes, absolutely. Unfortunately, the slow and uneven adoption of best management practices is not recognized as an ethical issue. When economic resources are insufficient to acquire new technology, employ additional staff and expand or even maintain existing programs, the importance of using evidence-based management cannot be over-emphasized.

Failing to adopt documented best practices is ethically indefensible. We have an inherent fiduciary and moral responsibility to energetically pursue and implement improved management tools and techniques.

Reasons for Slow Adoption of Best-Demonstrated Practices

There are a variety of reasons why leaders may not move quickly to replicate highly successful management practices. Four come to mind.

First, some executives believe they are well experienced, know how to manage properly and do not need to invest time and effort to examine how others may be more successful in managing their organizations. They would not consider themselves to be egotistical or arrogant but, rather, confident that internal resources are sufficient to maintain continued improvement.

When economic resources are insufficient to acquire new technology, employ additional staff and expand or even maintain existing programs, the importance of using evidence-based management cannot be over-emphasized.

Second, other leaders not only are convinced they know most of the keys to effective management, but they also contend that, unlike medicine, which is primarily based on objective scientific findings, management is more of an art. Therefore, these executives view evidence-based management as an attractive academic concept but one whose value is relatively unproven.

Third, another group of executives do not feel compelled to make adoption of evidence-based management practices a high priority because the incentives for doing so are not obvious. The governing body has not expressed any concern about current practices, medical staff members continue to support the executive team and the organization is well respected by its community.

Fourth, many executives believe they simply do not have time to acquire and review potentially useful information concerning best- demonstrated management practices. These executives acknowledge the benefits of replicating best practices, but they feel overextended by confronting a seemingly unending number of crises and instead decide to delay action.

Taking a Pragmatic Approach

The case for evidence-based management must be made more persuasively. We need to think systematically and creatively about how management best practices can be more rapidly and effectively promoted, disseminated and implemented. For example, we know many institutions have won significant stare and national awards for superior performance in a wide variety of areas, including:

- Improving patient safety
- Preventing and minimizing never events
- Decreasing healthcare-acquired infections
- Making care more timely and patient centered
- Increasing patient satisfaction
- Minimizing employee turnover and absenteeism
- Reducing the cost of services
- Maximizing the value of information technology
- Promoting accountability and transparency
- Creating a learning culture

- Improving community health status
- Reducing healthcare disparities
- Demonstrating community benefit

We also know there will be more hospitals recognized for their success in:

- Lowering re-admission rates within 30 days of discharge
- Adopting electronic health records
- Expanding the cost-effective use of telemedicine
- Reducing energy consumption

Undoubtedly, many of the institutions that have won the Malcolm Baldrige National Quality Award, the American Hospital Association-McKesson Quest for Quality Prize, the Thomson Reuters 100 Top Hospitals Performance Improvement Leaders award and similar honors are led by CEOs who learned from their peers. Consequently, these same executives are almost always interested in sharing their lessons with others. The key point is that right now in each of the above areas there are reliable management policies, programs and practices that are contributing to irrefutable improvements in organizational outcomes.

Timely and Informative Resources

In addition to learning from successful organizations, a growing number of recent publications contain valuable insights regarding verified means and methods for achieving exceptional progress. Five of these are particularly noteworthy.

- *Evidence-Based Management in Healthcare* by Anthony R. Kovner, PhD, David J. Fine, PhD, FACHE, and Richard D'Aquila, FACHE (Health Administration Press, 2009). The book explains how healthcare leaders can move from making educated guesses to using the best available information to make decisions.
- *Journey to Excellence: How Baldrige Health Care Leaders Succeed* by Kathleen J. Goonan, MD, Joseph A. Muzikowski and Patricia K. Stoltz (ASQ Quality Press, 2009). The book describes how nine Baldrige Award healthcare winners approached their Baldrige journey and what other healthcare leaders should do to accomplish similar benefits.
- *What Top-Performing Healthcare Organizations Know: 7 Proven Steps for Accelerating and Achieving Change* by Greg Butler and Chip

We have an inherent fiduciary and moral responsibility to energetically pursue and implement improved management tools and techniques.

Caldwell, FACHE (Health Administration Press, 2008). The authors researched more than 220 healthcare organizations to determine what differentiates high performers from organizations that fail to achieve lasting operational success.

- *Hospitals in Pursuit of Excellence [HPOE]: A Guide to Superior Performance Improvement* (American Hospital Association, 2009). This guide comprises 28 case studies of hospitals that have made significant strides in one of AHA's four initial HPOE focus areas: health-care-acquired infections, medication management, patient throughput and patient safety. The guide is available on CD, and the print version was mailed to every hospital in the United States in 2009.

- *Better: A Surgeon's Notes on Performance* (Metropolitan Books, 2007). Written by the remarkable surgeon and acclaimed author Atul Gawande, MD, this book is both eloquent and inspiring. Gawande notes, "Better is possible. It does not take genius. It takes diligence. It takes moral clarity. It takes ingenuity. And above all, it takes a willingness to try."

Accelerating the Adoption of Evidence-Based Management

Hospitals and other healthcare organizations have a solid track record regarding the implementation of clinical pathways, guidelines and protocols. Similarly, our most effective executives have been successful in replicating exemplary management practices through learning collaboratives and by developing innovative programs on their own. Nonetheless, we still can and should do more to close the too-large gap between the best performing institutions and those that rationalize they don't have the intellectual or financial resources to make more rapid progress.

As the public becomes better informed about the number and magnitude of problems afflicting the healthcare field, citizens legitimately will question why healthcare providers have not implemented well-documented management best practices as quickly as clinical best practices. It will be difficult to defend the status quo on an ethical basis because it cannot and should not be done.

But discomfort about being criticized is not a sufficient or compelling reason to employ evidence-based management. The motivation should be to create and sustain more effective organizations that are better able to serve our communities.

Chapter 6: **Discussion Questions**

1   How might accountable care organizations help reduce health care waste?

   a.   Do you think these organizations will improve health care quality? Why or why not?

2   How do ACOs shift health care from a fee-for-service model to a value-based approach?

   a.   What cost savings have resulted from the ACO model?

3   Describe value-based payment models in contrast to past fee-for-service payments.

   a.   What changes are health organizations making to provide clinically integrated services?

4   List three types of administrative tools/infrastructure that aid health care organizations in providing value-based health care.

   a.   Why is team-based care more effective for chronic conditions?

5   Is it unethical for a healthcare organization to fail to adopt evidence-based management practices? Why or why not?

   a.   Evidence-based management practices lead institutions to win awards based on several different categories and improvements; however, many institutions fail to employ these practices based on lack of finances. What motivations other than awards should inspire institutions to adopt these best practices?

CHAPTER 7

ORGANIZATIONAL CULTURE IN HEALTH CARE

Diagnosing the Patient Experience

Ellen Lanser May

Identifying Pain Points in the Patient Experience

Seven years ago, Cleveland Clinic ranked lowest among 15 peer institutions in patient satisfaction when it came to patient-physician communication.

Although the academic medical center was well known for the quality of care it provided, it ranked well below average on individual measures of the patient experience, such as staff responsiveness, communication with nurses, noise levels and room cleanliness, on its first HCAHPS survey in 2008. Later, an employee engagement survey indicated staff felt unappreciated.

The surveys were a wakeup call for Cleveland Clinic leaders, who sought to change the organization's culture and formalize its commitment to improving the patient experience.

In 2009, the clinic became the first major academic medical center to appoint a chief patient experience officer, and it was one of the first to create an office of patient experience. Using "Patients first" as its guiding principle, the office of patient experience collaborates with departments throughout the organization to ensure consistent delivery of patient-centered care, monitors national and local trends to identify how topperforming hospitals attain success on HCAHPS measures, studies clinical care data and observes patient care in action to identify and promote best practices.

"To influence the organizational culture and improve the patient experience, you have to recognize that you can't come in with a 'smile campaign' or a coach or trainer and expect to make a significant, lasting change," says James Merlino, MD, an ACHE Member who formerly served as chief patient experience officer for Cleveland

Ellen Lanser May, "Diagnosing the Patient Experience," *Healthcare Executive*, vol. 30, no. 4, pp. 22, 24-28, 30. Copyright © 2015 by Health Administration Press. Reprinted with permission. Provided by ProQuest LLC. All rights reserved.

> "You can't come in with a 'smile campaign' or a coach or trainer and expect to make a significant, lasting change. You must deliberately and strategically create a culture of engaged and satisfied caregivers who come to work knowing they're part of something bigger than their job description."
>
> **—James Merlino, MD**
> Press Ganey

Clinic and is now chief medical officer for Press Ganey. "You must deliberately and strategically create a culture of engaged and satisfied caregivers who come to work knowing they're part of something bigger than their job description."

One way Cleveland Clinic strengthens clinician communication is building a narrative of patient-provider experiences around inpatient and outpatient data as well as data gathered through other feedback channels, such as comments, letters and phone calls. Information about each caregiver for the organization is compiled and shared in a nonblinded fashion with the organization's physicians, nurses and other clinical team members.

This level of transparency initially drove some modifications to physician and clinician behavior; however, Cleveland Clinic's leaders believed they needed to do more to support physicians and nurses in better navigating emotionally complex patient issues.

In 2010, Cleveland Clinic established the Center for Excellence in Healthcare Communication. Using evidence-based communication skills, more than 50 specially trained physicians and advanced care providers facilitate courses for physicians and nurses on topics such as delivering bad news, demonstrating empathy, managing difficult communication scenarios, encouraging changes to patients' health behavior and asking "What else?" until all of a patient's questions have been answered.

"We use a model of communication that isn't physician centered or patient centered but rather, relationship centered," says Adrienne Boissy, MD, chief patient experience officer for Cleveland Clinic. "Beyond teaching specific skills, we're hoping to nudge our physicians and clinicians toward thinking about their roles differently. This means not just listening more effectively, but also thinking about what it takes to build a relationship with a patient in a way that has meaning for both parties. If we can do that, we'll improve the patient experience, the caregiver experience and our outcomes."

> "Whether it's seeing a patient for five minutes before surgery or providing support as a patient learns to manage a chronic illness, we are responsible for the relationships we forge. Having a framework for meaningful conversations with patients has been empowering for our care team."
>
> **—Adrienne Boissy, MD**
> Cleveland Clinic

Cleveland Clinic's Center for Excellence in Healthcare Communication recruited and trained 42 physician facilitators from more than 25 different specialties, many of whom were surgeons. Sixteen advanced clinical care providers also were trained to present programs, including physician assistants, nurse practitioners, nurse managers, social workers and others with significant patient contact.

Today, more than 2,000 staff physicians, more than 1,000 clinical trainees and more than 500 advanced clinical care providers have completed the program, which is now mandatory for all on-boarding staff and clinical trainees. In 2013, Cleveland Clinic's executive leaders also took part in the program.

"We chose to focus on communication skills for our providers not only because it is easily within caregivers' power to influence and change these skills, but also because we know patient loyalty, confidence, trust and engagement depend on it," Boissy says.

Through the efforts of medical center leaders, physicians and staff, Cleveland Clinic has improved its HCAHPS scores across the board. Today, patient satisfaction with physician communication has risen from the 10th percentile in 2008 to nearly the 70th percentile in 2014.

Physicians also have benefitted from improved communication with patients: Diagnostic accuracy, efficiency, self-confidence, job satisfaction and engagement all have improved significantly as a result of the training, while professional burnout, malpractice claims and costs of care have decreased.

"Whether it's seeing a patient for five minutes before surgery or providing support as a patient learns to manage a chronic illness, we are responsible for the relationships we forge," Boissy says. "Having a framework for meaningful conversations with patients has been empowering for our care team."

A Prescription for Change

In 2001, leaders at Sharp HealthCare, based in San Diego, began a sweeping performance improvement initiative to make the organization the best place to work, the best place to practice medicine and the best place to receive care.

This initiative became known as "The Sharp Experience," with a focus on transforming the healthcare experience for caregivers, patients and families. As Sharp's chief experience officer Lynn Skoczelas sees it, The Sharp Experience isn't about any one thing the organization does; it's about everything the health system's physicians, clinicians, leaders and staff do each day.

"We are committed to delivering high-quality care and service with dignity, compassion and respect," Skoczelas says. "We've successfully engaged people from the C-suite to the front lines and allowed our people to be the architects of change within our organization. That's what has made us so successful."

From the beginning of its performance improvement journey, leaders for Sharp—which was honored with the Malcolm Baldrige National Quality Award in 2007—determined staff engagement would be critical to enhancing the patient experience. Sharp's Standards Action Team—which comprises employees from across the system—developed 12 behavior standards upon which staff are to model their daily actions and interactions with patients. These standards include:

- Creating a lasting impression through positive attitudes
- Communicating with courtesy, clarity and care in both verbal and nonverbal messages
- Building relationships and fostering teamwork

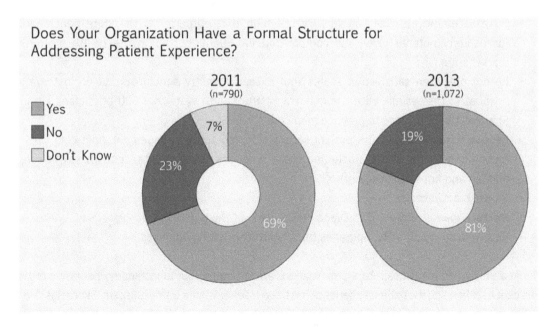

Does Your Organization Have a Formal Structure for Addressing Patient Experience?

Source: The Beryl Institute and Catalyst Healthcare Research

All employees at Sharp Healthcare—including executives—are held accountable to the health system's behavior standards in their annual performance reviews. Each month, the health system focuses on improving performance around one of the 12 standards.

"It may seem like a basic approach to modifying behavior, but holding team members accountable to these standards has been an incredibly effective way to shape our culture," Skoczelas says. "Now that these standards have been in place for more than a decade, we have the right people working here—people who want to be part of this culture. Those who have not found our culture to be a good fit have self-selected out of the organization."

Staff attitude has a clear impact on how patients view the quality of care and service provided by hospitals and health systems. In the customer service industry, experts often refer to positive moments of truth—experiences that create a positive impression for customers or a negative one that stays in their subconscious. Sharp developed "signature moments" to create positive memories for patients and their families. Staff and volunteers design and deliver these signature moments daily, from baking cookies in hospital lobbies to offering patients flowers cut from hospital gardens and serving juice and crackers on a silver tray after a patient receives a colonoscopy.

"If you give employees permission to create the environment in which they want to work and to create experiences that reflect why they chose to work in the healthcare field, you'll find that it affects them in profound ways," Skoczelas says. "Our staff come forward with ideas on how to create a better experience for patients, and they're rewarded with patients' gratitude. The feedback they receive fires them up to do even more for patients and their families."

The positive impact of The Sharp Experience is indisputable. From its inception in 2001 through 2014, Sharp's initiative has helped the organization:

- Increase employee retention to a record high that outperforms the state benchmark (particularly notable given the competition for qualified staff in the health system's market area)
- Record physician satisfaction scores that exceed industry benchmarks at almost every hospital in the system, with the majority of the health systems 2,600 physicians citing Sharp as the best place to practice medicine
- Receive national awards for patient satisfaction, employee engagement, physician satisfaction and quality of care (including in the areas of critical care, cancer care, stroke care and hip and knee replacement)
- Increase net revenue
- Increase market share in San Diego during each of the past 14 years
- Receive a string of rating upgrades from healthcare rating agencies

"At a time when many healthcare organizations are struggling, our longstanding, pervasive commitment to enhancing the patient experience has been essential to our overall success," Skoczelas says.

Should Your Organization Invest in a Patient Experience Officer? 7 Things to Consider

The role of the patient experience officer in healthcare is an evolving one, and its scope and responsibilities vary based on the needs of the organization.

At its core, the chief patient experience officer is more than a symbolic post. "Establishing a senior-level position for transforming the patient experience makes an unwavering statement that your organization recognizes that healthcare is really about the experience of patients and families," says Jason Wolf, PhD, president, The Beryl Institute, Nashville, Tenn. "Healthcare organizations that have committed the resources to having a dedicated executive who drives patient experience strategy are outperforming other hospitals and health systems in this area."

According to Wolf, there are seven critical factors for a chief patient experience officer's success.'

Commitment. The chief patient experience officer should be able to focus 100 percent of his or her time on improving the patient experience. Healthcare leaders should assess their organization's readiness and willingness to support and sustain such an effort, which should be a strategic initiative for the organization.

Authority. The patient experience executive should report to the organization's CEO, just as most central roles in the C-suite do, and should have authority equivalent to his or her peers. This reinforces the importance of the patient experience to the organization's strategy.

Diverse experience. Chief patient experience officers do not necessarily need to be physicians or nurses, although this may be the best option in some settings such as academic medical centers. Candidates for chief patient experience officer also may have experience in the service or retail industry.

Broad scope. The chief patient experience officer guides and actively influences—but not always directly manages—macro strategies across quality, safety and service. Various patient-related departments could be placed under the chief patient experience officer's leadership such as patient relations, complaints, surveying and analytics, and volunteer staff.

Support. The chief patient experience officer must have adequate resources within the context of the organization such as budget, staff or other types of support. This may be the greatest opportunity in the experience equation. It is one thing to identify a patient experience officer; it is another to support that person's efforts to provide the best experience possible for all who are in your organization's care.

Strategic focus. Healthcare leaders should consider the critical nature of this role in building and guiding the organizational culture. The chief patient experience officer should guide key people strategies focused on culture, consistency and accountability.

Flexibility. Recognize that this role is still relatively new and will continue to evolve. Be willing to experiment with what works for your organization—and be willing to fail. But also be ready to get back up and continue patient experience initiatives with unwavering intent.

*Adapted with permission from The Chief Experience Officer—An Emerging & Critical Role, The Beryl Institute, November 2014.

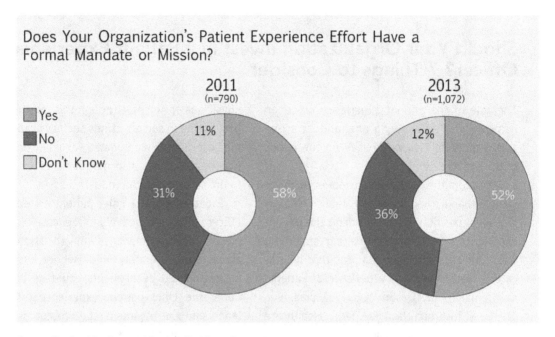

Does Your Organization's Patient Experience Effort Have a Formal Mandate or Mission?

Source: The Beryl Institute and Catalyst Healthcare Research

Keeping a Pulse on the Patient Experience

In 2012, Riverside Health System in Newport News, Va., rewrote its mission statement to reflect a philosophical shift across the organization: *To care for others as we would care for those we love—to enhance their well-being and improve their health.*

"The healthcare industry today has been more focused on the transaction," says Nancy Littlefield, FACHE, DNP, senior vice president and CNO at Riverside. "But our organization wanted to refocus our culture on the relationships we create with our patients and our caregivers. Every action, process and function at Riverside is meant to amplify our mission and our commitment to relationship building."

More recently, Riverside has examined ways to enhance the patient experience and drive patient satisfaction in the context of relationship building. Transparency is an integral component of this effort. For example, to give a more visible platform to the voice of the patient, Riverside has created two family engagement councils; by the end of 2015, six such councils will provide feedback around the health system's five acute care hospitals, 11 nursing homes and various specialty facilities situated throughout northeastern Virginia.

"Through these councils, our patients and families talk to us at the advisory board level and advise us on operational priorities," Littlefield says.

Last summer, Riverside leaders participated in a monthly roundtable discussion convened by the president of the Virginia Hospital & Healthcare Association, which was concerned that

Virginia ranked 30th among the nation's 50 states in HCAHPS scores. Through these sessions, Riverside learned higher survey return rates are often correlated with higher rankings.

Through their work with the Virginia Hospital & Healthcare Association, Riverside's leaders identified three critical patient experience initiatives for the health system:

- Purposeful rounding (a structured, hourly rounding routine)
- Phone calls to patients after discharge
- Daily huddles on units

Riverside experienced an immediate bump in its HCAHPS scores in the first quarter after implementing purposeful rounding. "Our purposeful rounding isn't simply task-focused," Littlefield says. "It is a way to communicate with the patient to make sure the patient is pain-free, safe and responding as expected to treatment. When our patients leave the hospital, our nurses continue to build on that relationship by calling and saying, 'I cared for you when you were in the hospital, and I want to make sure you're okay—that you were able to make a follow-up appointment and fill your prescriptions.'"

Riverside's leaders also believed the organization could improve the way it told its story to better engage its team members. The health system implemented Champions of Caring, a program in which patients, their families and Riverside staff recognize team members who go above and beyond in their care and the service they provide.

In 2013, 1,700 Champions of Caring nominations were received; in 2014, more than 7,000 nominations were submitted.

"For our team, experiencing such a tangible expression of patients' gratitude helps them to feel valued and to recognize just how critical they are to the care of our patients," Littlefield says. "In the simplest of terms, focusing on the relationships we form with patients and their families aligns our heads with our hearts. It pushes us to reconnect with the reason most of us chose healthcare as a career."

Continual Follow-Up is the Key to Success

Efforts to enhance the patient experience cannot be viewed as "one and done." Although strategies and tactics are part of the journey, The Beryl Institute's Wolf notes an organization's ability to execute those strategies and weave them into its culture is a predictor of its longterm success.

"It's about taking a macro-level approach to the patient experience," he says. "We can't say we've fixed the patient experience and move on. It's a forever issue."

Maximum Medicine: In Lubbock, Texas, A Weak Heart Gets the Full Treatment

Its Doctors Like Angioplasty, and Who is to Say the Patient Doesn't Need It? Cities and Their Specialties

George Anders

Lubbock, Texas—No one relocates here because of the scenery or the weather. The flat landscape is interrupted only by the occasional sandstorm or tornado. But in the late 1980s, when heart doctor Robert Wey needed another partner in his seven-physician group, he ran a tiny classified ad in the New England Journal of Medicine that captivated doctors across the U.S.

"Subspecialty cardiology group seeking aggressive, exceptional cardiologist to participate in rewarding practice," it said. Potential yearly earnings: more than $1 million.

The phone started ringing. "Are you really making that much money?" an excited doctor in California asked. "I said yes," Dr. Wey recalls. "The next thing he wanted to know was, 'When can I move out and join you?'"

This West Texas city of 200,000 has become the heart-care industry's El Dorado. Cardiologists here are rich enough to buy Cessna jets and breed Arabian horses. Pacemaker salesmen covet the territory. Although Lubbock is too small for any more than a minor-league baseball team, its main hospital is among the 20 busiest heart centers in the U.S.

Local Tastes

Such showcase cities are becoming famous—or notorious—in the treatment of many major ills. People with weak hearts, sore backs or breast cancer may think their symptoms alone decide their care. Not so. A patient's odds of getting a major, invasive procedure can be swayed by something else: his or her zip code.

A study by Dartmouth Medical School and the American Hospital Association found huge regional fluctuations in the way medicine is practiced. Boulder, Colo., leads the nation in prostate-cancer surgery per 1,000 residents. In Rapid City, S.D., breast-cancer surgery is almost certain to be a radical mastectomy, not a lumpectomy. Provo, Utah, is the back-surgery capital. And in Lubbock, cardiologists perform two major heart procedures about twice as often as the national average.

To public-health experts, such treatment patterns constitute something close to a medical scandal. "These high rates aren't just of interest to insurance companies," says Dartmouth investigator John Wennberg in Hanover, N.H. "This matters to patients as well. They may be getting treatments where the risks exceed the benefits."

Regulatory files in Texas are packed with accusations that patients got unneeded pacemakers, back surgeries and other procedures. But such charges "are very difficult cases to prove," says Tim Weitz, chief counsel at the Texas State Board of Medical Examiners. "Maybe nine out of 10 doctors will disagree with what the physician did. Maybe in hindsight he shouldn't have done the procedure." But if doctors can produce expert witnesses justifying a procedure, regulators will be hard-pressed to prevail in a disciplinary case.

Cardiac Costs

The stakes are highest in the treatment of heart disease, the nation's costliest illness and its No. 1 killer. Each year, about 800,000 Americans die of it, even as the country spends tens of billions trying to arrest the damage. Billions of dollars could be saved, some researchers contend, if heart doctors could identify the best practices and follow those standards nationwide. Instead, each medical community has its own norms.

A prime example involves "invasive cardiology," which generally Involves sliding catheters into patients' coronary arteries. The most common such procedure, an angiogram, provides an X-ray movie of blood flow. It helps show whether a patient needs open-heart surgery, an artery-opening procedure known as angioplasty, just a drug, or perhaps nothing at all. Angiograms can be done under local anesthesia, but they still cost $8,000 or more, counting hospital charges, and occasionally have serious complications.

Both angiograms and angioplasty are done at an unusually high rate in Lubbock, according to the Dartmouth study. And last. year, the New England Journal of Medicine reported that Texas doctors did angiograms on 45% of Medicare patients following heart attacks, while New York doctors did them in only 30% of cases. The greater frequency in Texas didn't, on the whole, save lives or improve patients' well-being, says Edward Guadagnoli, a Harvard Medical School professor who led the study. (Bypass operations aren't performed at an unusually high rate in Lubbock; they can be done only by surgeons, not by cardiologists.)

Lubbock Style

So how do these pockets of maximum medicine arise? And who wins or loses when one part of the U.S. practices medicine so differently?

In Lubbock, aggressive treatment of heart disease began in the 1970s as a personal mission of a few local doctors. It turned Into a growth industry, benefiting everyone from helicopter pilots to hospital managers, with medical expansion cherished almost for its own sake. A Lubbock style of medicine took hold—aided by the arrival of out-of-state cardiologists angling for the big money.

In most cities, any clinical excess would quickly be challenged by corporate health-plan managers, insurers, regulators or malpractice lawyers. But in Lubbock, such restraints are scarce. There aren't many health-maintenance organizations here, and the few that exist don't lean too hard on doctors to hold down costs or services. Most efforts to prevent medical overuse in Texas are concentrated on the big population centers, Dallas and Houston.

Lubbock's leading cardiologists defend their practice style. "We're a strong role model in appropriateness of procedures," says Paul Waller, president of Cardiology Associates of Lubbock. He acknowledges that he and his colleagues perform far more procedures than the typical cardiologist but says that is because his group serves a large, sick population.

Even so, some families here seethe about what they see as excess doctoring. Karen Vardy won a six-figure settlement from some Cardiology Associates doctors last year after an angiogram on her husband led to severe bleeding. He died 10 weeks later. Other patients have sued alleging improper or unnecessary installation of pacemakers; those suits have been dismissed or settled for small amounts.

Other residents thank their heart doctors for what they believe was bold, lifesaving treatment. "People in West Texas are extremely trusting of doctors," observes M. Wayne Cooper, a cardiologist who practiced in Lubbock in the 1980s, when he moved to the East Texas city of Tyler. "They think of physicians as deities. That power can be misused."

For all its current sweep, heart medicine in Lubbock started small. Old-timers remember the city's first cardiologist, Harvard-trained William Gordon, who settled here in 1946 because the dry air allayed his wife's asthma. Patient care then was done mostly by stethoscope and prescription. Dr. Gordon bought an electrocardiograph, put it in his car and drove to small towns so he could analyze patients' heartbeats.

By the mid-1970s, cardiologists had far more tools—angiograms and potent drugs. Dr. Gordon's practice grew into Cardiology Associates, with a new partner recruited every few years from the University of Colorado, a training ground for angiogram enthusiasts. Their high-tech style became part of the Lubbock way.

They found patients galore. More than 500,000 people lived within a 100-mile radius. Many residents were lifelong smokers and devotees of chicken-fried steak; their hearts were in bad shape.

"The first weekend I got here in 1975, I had 20 cases," Dr. Wey recalls. "That was more than I'd had for an entire month in training in Colorado. I thought I'd died and gone to heaven."

Soon, the two biggest hospitals in town were vying for the cardiologists' business, courting them with an intensity hospitals more typically extend only to surgeons. St. Mary of the Plains built two catheterization labs. Methodist Hospital struck back with a six-story Heart Center, with six "cath labs" and $9 million of equipment.

Local leaders were pleased. "One of the few driving forces in the Lubbock economy was medicine," Dr. Wey says, "The driving force of medicine was cardiology."

Doctors whom Cardiology Associates hired from the East and West Coasts brought skills Lubbock hadn't seen before. They also arrived with a swagger that didn't always sit well. One new doctor annoyed his neighbors by turning his huge backyard into a pasture for six Arabian horses. Another decorated his office with full-length mirrors. A third became a collector of Mont Blanc pens.

Dr. Wey, who headed Cardiology Associates in the early 1990s, urged colleagues to share not just in the "gravy"—procedures that could pay $1,000) for an hour's work—but also in the "scut work"—office visits and lab tests at awkward times. His appeals didn't always work. One physician was overheard muttering, "Treadmill tests are the crabgrass of cardiology."

Internal pay records show that in 1990, when the group had nine doctors, eight earned at least $1 million. Last year, 11 of the group's 14 doctors cleared the $1 million barrier—figures that astound cardiologists elsewhere.

Paul Overlie earned nearly S1.3 million last year. He did 454 angiograms and 133 angioplasties at Methodist and scores more procedures at St. Mary. Some nurses and doctors call him Dr. Overplasty.

"I don't overplasty," Dr. Overlie responds. He says that if a single artery is 60% closed, he won't open it, though he will intervene if it is 90% closed. He acknowledges that not all cardiologists would do angioplasty even then, but he thinks the cautious ones may be making a mistake. "I get their patients at night," after heart attacks, he says.

Pilot Project

In the late 1980s, two Lubbock cardiologists leased helicopters to bring emergency cases from outlying farm towns. Of course, many of those burgs lacked helipads. "We hired contractors to pour concrete in at least 20 towns," says one of the doctors, Howard Hurd.

Once again, West Texas developed its own practice style. In most of the U.S., tiny rural hospitals treated heart-attack patients on site, giving clot-busting drugs. But Lubbock cardiologists told rural doctors that patients ought to be flown to a cath lab for emergency angiograms and angioplasties. Result: a $3,000 helicopter bill per case, a $2,000 cardiologist fee and $12,000 or more for a Lubbock hospital.

Lubbock cardiologists went all-out to make angioplasty seem like the wise choice. Doctors who relied on drugs, known as thrombolytics, were belittled as "thrombolunatics." Studies were circulated showing better survival rates for angioplasty. In some cases, Lubbock physicians jumped in the helicopter themselves, rather than rely on an air nurse and technicians to get the case started.

Dr. Wey became a hero in Muleshoe, Texas, for flying out to rescue the father of town doctor Robert Purdy after a heart attack. The payoff was substantial: Dr. Purdy became a huge fan of the helicopter service and now sends at least 30 heart-attack cases a year to Lubbock.

Emergency angioplasty isn't always a lifesaver. According to the Center for Health Industry Performance Studies in Columbus, Ohio, Lubbock's Methodist Hospital in 1994 had a 4.1% death rate for Medicare patients getting single-vessel angioplasty. That was nearly double the national average. Cardiology Associates, the main heart group practicing at Methodist, disputes the data and says most of its angioplasty deaths occurred in extremely grave heart-attack cases where other doctors might not have tried the procedure.

Lasers and Stents

New techniques found favor in Lubbock. Delivery trucks in the early 1990s pulled into Methodist and St. Mary with cargoes of lasers, ultrasound probes, highspeed "ablading" devices and wire-mesh stents to prop open arteries after angioplasty. Lubbock's heart doctors became co-investigators in many nationwide research trials, testing new treatments.

"It was a heady time," Dr, Walter says. "There was this incredible enthusiasm that we could solve all sorts of problems that otherwise would have required surgery. With just a half-hour treatment, we could open an artery—and then have someone ready to go back to work the next week."

Some new techniques lived up to their promise. Dr. Overlie inserted more than 100 stents a year, with impressive results. "He's shown slides of my arteries at conferences around the world," boasts stent patient Hubert Setliff, 82.

Other ideas flopped. Lubbock doctors for a while tried using lasers to burn away arterial plaque. They billed as much as $5,000 for a half-hour procedure, triple the rate for conventional balloon angioplasty. But one doctor who tried this 10 times abandoned it after deaths or complications in four cases.

Norma Wines, age 70, underwent laser angioplasty in Lubbock. Her husband and daughters were so confident they went home after the procedure started to make a big pot of soup and wait for her to come home. She never did. Medical records show that Mrs. Wines sank into critical condition after the procedure, needed emergency surgery, and died.

Three years later, her widower, Weldon, sits in his darkened kitchen and talks about the case. "I know how to build houses, and I know how to grow tomatoes," he says, "but I don't understand heart medicine. When they recommended this laser treatment, we just signed the papers." Mr. Wines has sued one of the doctors, Fawwaz Shoukfeh, in state court, alleging negligence and unwarranted treatment. Dr. Shoukfeh denies the charges. A trial is set for the fall.

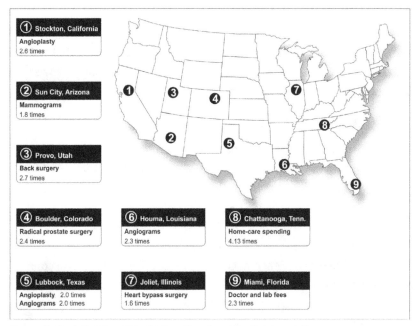

Source: Dartmouth Atlas of Health Care/American Hospital Association

Second Thoughts

Dartmouth didn't measure pacemaker use, but Mark Riley, a salesman for Intermedies, a pacemaker firm, says, "I've been in medical-equipment sales for a long lime, and I've never seen a town like this." He says Methodist Hospital buys as much of some common heart devices as the biggest hospital in Dallas, though Dallas has five times as big a population.

Lately, a schism has developed between Lubbock's older heart doctors and new arrivals. Most of the veterans are native Texans who identify with the farmers, oilmen and ministers they serve and say they don't mind spending time on simple preventive counseling. They question whether some newer colleagues share those values. "I got tired of apologizing for my colleagues' behavior," says Dr. Hurd, 52, who left Cardiology Associates to set up his own practice.

Another alumnus, 64-year-old Sam King, says he is uneasy about other heart doctors' fondness for angioplasty. "It's very lucrative," he remarks. "As far as the patients' well-being, it's not always the best thing." Frequently, he notes, arteries rapidly close again. "And every time you do one, there's myocardial loss. By the time patients are considered candidates for surgery, the heart ventricle isn't that good any more. You convert someone from a good surgical risk to a poor risk."

So far, Lubbock has lagged far behind the rest of the U.S. in feeling pressure from employers and managed-care companies to use health resources more frugally. The biggest private-sector employer here, Texas Instruments Inc., says it is too busy overseeing medical costs in its larger Houston and Dallas sites to focus much on Lubbock.

What Diet?

In the past few months, Lubbock's heart doctors have become worried that managed care will soon make inroads here. Cardiology Associates retained Ernst & Young to advise on ways to cut costs and be better positioned for managed care.

Capitals of High-Intensity Medicine

Cities that lead in frequency of procedures or in spending level per 1,000 residents. Figures are a multiple of the national average and are based on an analysis of Medicare data for 1992 and 1993.

How Reseachers Figured Regional Medical Norms

Researchers at Dartmouth Medical School and the American Hospital Association divided the U.S. into 306 hospital-referral regions, each anchored by a city. They tallied procedures for Medicare patients living in each region in 1992 and 1993 and divided the totals by the region's, Medicare population Rates were adjusted to even out different mixes in age, sex or race. The method omits out-of-area I Patients who may be attracted to a renowned medical center.

Mostly, however, the city's heart-care juggernaut keeps rolling along. Elsewhere, health plans are trying to nudge heart patients into intensive diet and exercise programs; in Lubbock, patients keep queuing up at the cath labs. Waiting rooms are packed with anxious men and women, mostly 50 and over, wanting to know how bad off their hearts are.

"These patients don't know much about hearts," says Frank Harmon, a former medical manager in Lubbock. "They're pretty much at the mercy of their doctors. And the doctors know that."

Among Lubbock's grateful patients is 59-year-old Buddy Sexton, a retired school principal. Over 13 years, he has been a steady cardiology customer, undergoing 10 procedures, including five angioplasties. His arteries periodically renarrow; doctors respond with another angioplasty.

Doctors have told Mr. Sexton that he is a poor risk for heart surgery. He is overweight, and his current cardiologist, Dr. Overlie, has told him to diet, but the advice hasn't been very practical. At one point, Dr. Overlie said: "I want you to eat nothing but salad until you turn into a salad." Mr. Sexton hasn't had much luck holding to a healthy diet and blames himself. Meanwhile, he praises Dr. Overlie for "prolonging my life."

On a recent visit to the hospital, Mr. Sexton sheepishly asked a nurse, "Am I the only slob who can't stick to his diet?" The reply, he says, was as follows: "No. We have file cabinets of people like you. We wouldn't have a practice if everyone did what they were told."

Chapter 7: Discussion Questions

1   What does HCAHPS stand for?

  a. How did the survey data impact and change Cleveland Clinic's organizational culture?

2   What methods can health care organizations employ to adapt their culture to improve quality of care for the patients?

  a. How does the staff's attitude impact health care outcomes?

3   What is the role of a patient experience officer?

  a. How does data impact improvement efforts?

4   What is Lubbock style medicine?

  a. List three organizations that profited from the over-prescription of health care services in Lubbock, Texas.

5   Would you want to receive cardiovascular care in Lubbock, Texas in the 1980s? Explain.

  a. According to the author, how did Lubbock's low health literacy and the providers' attitudes affect population health in the city?

CHAPTER 8

HEALTH DISPARITIES AND HEALTH POLICY

Health Justice and the Future of Public Health Law

Lawrence O. Gostin and Lindsay F. Wiley

A community's health is as much the result of institutional policies and practice as it is personal choice. Which communities have fresh, nutritious food? Where do governments allow dumping? Who is more often targeted by advertisers with unhealthy products? Which communities have state-of-the-art medical facilities? Which ones don't?

All of these factors (or social determinants) are symptoms of the bias and privilege that shape virtually every aspect of our lives. It is no secret that across nearly every indicator of health status, poor people and people of color are more likely to be sick, injured, or die prematurely.... It will take organizing from the ground up; social change that transforms the current systems of neglect, bias, and privilege into systems—policies, practices, institutions—that truly support healthy communities for all. That's health justice.

—The Praxis Project, 2014

Public health is typically regarded as a positivistic pursuit, and undoubtedly our understanding of the etiology and response to disease and injury is heavily influenced by scientific inquiry. [...] Law creates a mission for public health agencies, assigns their functions, and specifies the manner in which they may exercise their authority. In public health work, the law is a tool that is used to identify and respond to health threats, set and enforce health and safety standards, and influence norms for healthy behavior.

Social justice is at the heart of this work. Although protecting and promoting overall population health is vitally important, justice also demands action to reduce disparities in health. Gains in average life expectancy belie stagnant or worsening health outcomes for the poor and socially marginalized. A social justice approach to public health demands that society embed fairness into the environment in which people live and that it allocate services equitably, with particular attention to the needs of the most disadvantaged.

The essential job of public health agencies is to identify what makes people healthy and what makes them sick, and then take the steps necessary to ensure that the population encounters a maximum of the former and a minimum of the latter. At first glance, this task would seem to be uncontroversial, but protecting the public's health and reducing health disparities create fundamental social and political disputes almost by definition. Public health is rooted in the biomedical and social sciences, but from the moment of asserting some collective responsibility for the population's health, officials have to manage a complex political process and operate with finite resources. Public health agencies, in particular, confront well-financed political opposition and face inherent problems of legitimacy and trust. These are not barriers to good public health that somehow can be overcome by law. They are, rather, unavoidable conditions of public health, conditions with which agencies must find ways to cope.

Public health has always been politically controversial. And public health law—which concerns the extent of government authority to intervene to protect the public's health—lives in the thick of this controversy. In recent decades, as public health science, practice, and law have expanded to tackle noncommunicable disease threats, injuries, the social determinants of health, and health disparities, the political controversy over public health has grown. This chapter offers brief concluding reflections on the public health field and its inescapable connection to politics and government in a constitutional democracy.

Health Disparities

> Health and the social distribution of health function as a kind of social accountant. So intimate is the connection between our set of social arrangements and health that we can use the degree of health inequalities to tell us about social progress in meeting basic human needs.
>
> —Michael Marmot, foreword to Sridhar Venkatapuram, *Health Justice,* 2011

Deep and enduring socioeconomic inequalities form the backdrop to any public health policy, and these disparities help explain why social justice is a core value of public health. Poverty, inferior educational opportunities, unhygienic and polluted environments, social disintegration, and other causes lead to systematic hardships in health and in nearly every other aspect of social, economic, and political life. Prevailing inequalities beget other inequalities, which is one major reason that those who are already disadvantaged suffer disproportionately from health hazards.

Over the last few decades, life expectancy has increased dramatically among people in the top half of the income distribution while remaining nearly flat among those in the bottom half,[1] and even declining among women in many parts of the United States.[2] Average life expectancy can vary by as much as twenty-five years between neighborhoods just a few miles apart. African-Americans are eight times more likely to be diagnosed with HIV, twice as likely to die within the first year of life, and 50 percent more likely to die prematurely of heart disease or stroke than their non-Hispanic white peers.[3] Black children are about 1.6 times as likely to be diagnosed with asthma than their peers, and they are six to seven times as likely to die of resulting complications.[4] Hispanic women are 1.6 times as likely as non-Hispanic white women, and people living in poverty are about twice as likely as those with higher incomes, to be diagnosed with diabetes.[5]

Some of these disparities are caused by unequal access to health care. Explicit, implicit, and structural biases continue to shape the health care experiences of racial and ethnic minorities and other socially and economically disadvantaged people. People of color, people with disabilities, and people with limited means are less likely to have health insurance coverage and less likely to receive needed medical care even if they do have coverage. The quality of care that they receive tends to be lower, they are subject to higher rates of medical error, and their health outcomes suffer as a result.[6] Recent efforts to make reduction of health disparities a priority for federal agencies,[7] which include development of the National Partnership for Action to End Health Disparities,[8] its National Stakeholder Strategy for Achieving Health Equity,[9] and the HHS Action Plan to Reduce Racial and Ethnic Health Disparities,[10] focus largely on addressing disparities in access to and quality of health care.

But significant health disparities persist even in places where there is universal access to health care. Safe working conditions, safe housing free from community violence and toxins like lead and radon, clean air and water, healthy food, and improved sanitation are more powerful drivers of health than access to health care. Many of the "causes of the causes" of poor health and premature death are linked to household income, formal education, race and ethnicity, and neighborhood.[11] The population perspective of public health and the "health in all policies" approach to action on the social determinants of health are more responsive to social justice concerns than a narrow view focusing on health care access and quality.

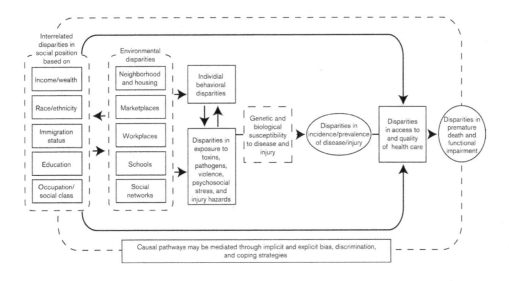

Figure 8.1.1 A conceptual model of health disparities.

Social Justice as a Core Value of Public Health Law

Public health must go "back to the future" and integrate power and agency into our models for promoting the public's health. History sensitizes us to the interplay of the varied social, political, and economic forces that positioned public health at different moments in time, regardless of the areas of responsibility the field claimed. History demands that we understand not only the forces that shaped public health action in the past but also the current forces that will shape the potential and limits of what we can do as professionals committed both to science and to its application.

—Amy L. Fairchild, David Rosner, James Colgrove, Ronald Bayer,
and Linda P. Fried, "The Exodus of Public Health," 2010

The ideal of social justice is a core value of public health and is foundational to our conception of public health law. We define social justice as a communitarian approach to ensuring the essential conditions for human well-being, including redistribution of social and economic goods and recognition of all people as equal participants in social and political life. Like public health practice, social justice is, by its nature, politically charged.[12]

The Community Orientation

The choice of the term *social* justice reflects "the idea that all developments relating to justice occur in society" and "the related desire to restore the comprehensive, overarching concept of the term 'social,' which in recent times has been relegated to the status of an appendix of the economic sphere."[13] It is inherently communitarian in its "attention to what is often ignored in contemporary policy debates: the social side of human nature; the responsibilities that must be borne by citizens, individually and collectively, in a regime of rights; the fragile ecology of families and their supporting communities; the ripple effects and long-term consequences of present decisions."[14] Social justice firmly rejects the libertarian view of society as "an aggregation of individuals for whom the meaning of freedom is choice within the scarcity of each person's 'own' resources."[15] In contrast, social justice views assurance of the essential conditions for human well-being as the legitimating purpose of government.

Civic Participation

Among the most basic and commonly understood meanings of *justice* is fairness or reasonableness, especially in the ways people are treated and decisions affecting them are made. Justice stresses fair disbursement of common advantages and the sharing of common burdens. But it also goes further by demanding equal respect for and recognition of all members of the community as full and equal participants in social interaction and political life.[16] Experience has shown that community engagement at every stage of public interventions—from the initial assessment of health needs to the ultimate evaluation of an intervention's impact—promotes effective public health practice.[17]

The dual goals of redistribution (which emphasizes material outcomes) and recognition (which emphasizes process, participation, respect, and identity) threaten to pull public health in opposing directions. But they can and should function as complementary strains of the social justice approach, allowing for advocacy strategies that combine a "cultural politics of identity" with a "social politics of equality," promoting just distribution of economic and social goods rooted in participatory parity.[18] Social justice requires action to preserve human dignity for all, particularly for those who suffer from systematic disadvantage.[19]

Social Justice and Health Disparities in Three Recent Movements

> Reproductive Justice analyzes how the ability of any woman to determine her own reproductive destiny is linked directly to the conditions in her community—and these conditions are not just a matter of individual choice and access.... Moving beyond a demand for privacy and respect for individual decision making to include the social supports necessary for our

individual decisions to be optimally realized, this framework also includes obligations from our government for protecting women's human rights.

> —Sistersong Collaborative, "Why Is Reproductive Justice
> Important for Women of Color?," 2015

Three recent social movements—environmental justice, reproductive justice, and food justice—have adopted health disparities as a central focus. Each has emerged as a critique from within a progressive project. The environmental justice movement originated as a civil rights–based critique of the process and outcomes of environmental protection. The reproductive justice movement began as a critique by women of color within the prochoice movement. And the food justice movement emerged in response to concerns about elitism in the alternative food movement, which seeks to reform industrial food production. In each case, the response has involved particular attention to the wide-ranging impacts of income inequality and white privilege, with eventual expansion to address other issues of bias and structural advantage such as ableism,[20] privileged gender expression,[21] heteronormativity,[22] and nativism.[23]

Environmental Justice

Galvanized by controversy over the location of waste and industrial sites in predominantly black communities, the environmental justice movement emerged in the 1980s as a response to environmental racism.[24] Its focus is more expansive than that of the environmental protection movement. Posing crucial questions about "how individual events reflect broader historical and societal inequities,"[25] the movement emphasizes just distribution of environmental risks and benefits and recognition of socially marginalized groups in related decision-making processes.[26] Together, the sustainability and environmental justice movements "guard against the risk of 'tunnel vision': one-dimensional environmental policymaking that fixates on a single goal ... without considering or addressing broader implications."[27]

The relationship between environmentalism and environmental justice is not entirely harmonious. "Since at least the early 1990s, activists from the environmental justice movement consistently have criticized what they consider the 'mainstream' environmental movement's racism, classism, and limited activist agenda."[28] In their efforts to probe the influence of elitism on mainstream environmentalism, environmental justice advocates raise difficult questions about the appropriate role for lawyers and other experts in defining the movement's priorities and strategies.[29] They have also grappled at length with the tension between the distributive and participatory commitments of social justice.[30] Especially in cases where Native American tribal governments have opted to allow environmentally hazardous operations within their jurisdictions, legal scholars have struggled to conceptualize and implement the environmental justice movement's commitment to procedural justice and self-determination for socially disadvantaged communities.[31]

The environmental justice framework has had significant influence at the federal level. A 1994 executive order from President Bill Clinton directed all federal agencies, not merely the EPA, to incorporate the achievement of environmental justice into their missions by "identifying and addressing ... disproportionately high and adverse human health or environmental effects of [their] programs, policies, and activities on minority populations and low income populations."[32]

The articulation of environmental justice in terms of disproportionate "human health *or* environmental effects" would arguably encompass all health disparities.[33] Indeed, the Interagency Working Group created by Clinton's executive order and reconvened by the Obama Administration in 2010[34] has, at times, interpreted the "environmental" part of environmental justice quite broadly to encompass "greater access to health care, clean air and water, healthy and affordable food, community capacity building through grants and technical assistance, and training to educate the health workforce about environmentally associated health conditions."[35]

DHHS strategies developed pursuant to Executive Order 12898 frequently reference the agency's broader efforts to increase access to health care, healthy food, and healthy living conditions, but with an emphasis on how those efforts are particularly relevant to the narrower environmental justice project of "reducing the health disparities that may result from disproportionate exposures to environmental hazards in minority and low income populations and Indian Tribes."[36] For example, DHHS officials emphasize national objectives in traditional environmental protection areas like air and water quality and hazardous waste disposal. EPA officials recognize that "addressing environmental health disparities through the lens of EPA is touching the tip of the iceberg[;] populations that experience health disparities related to other social determinants of health, such as access to health care and access to healthy foods, tend to be the same populations that live in communities overburdened with environmental pollution."[37] The fact that the environmental justice work of federal agencies is broad-based and cross-cutting is fortuitous for the future of public health law.

Reproductive Justice

The reproductive justice movement represents a transformation of the prochoice agenda into a much broader effort to protect and promote "the right to have children, not have children, and to parent the children we have in safe and healthy environments."[38] Loretta Ross, a key figure in the reproductive justice movement, traces its roots to the 1994 International Conference on Population and Development in Cairo,[39] which "was explicitly given a broader mandate on development issues than previous population conferences, reflecting the growing awareness that population, poverty, patterns of production and consumption and the environment are so closely interconnected that none of them can be considered in isolation."[40] The program of action that arose out of the Cairo meeting recognized reproductive health as a human right and recognized gender equality, women's empowerment, and equal access to education for girls as priorities for sustainable development.

Access to health care—not merely as a matter of ensuring women's right to choose contraception or abortion, but as a matter of providing access to a wide range of affordable, culturally appropriate health services for women and families—is a priority issue for the reproductive justice movement. Additionally, reproductive justice advocates' emphasis on "safe and healthy environments" for raising children encompasses access to clean air and water and safe and healthy food as well as health care, housing, education, employment, and other essential needs.

Food Justice

The food justice movement arose out of the confluence of environmental justice and the alternative food movement.[41] The influential food writer Michael Pollan has said that the alternative food movement is "unified as yet by little more than the recognition that industrial food production is in need of reform because its social/environmental/public health/animal welfare/gastronomic costs are too high."[42] Critics soon noted, however, that "with its focus on farmers' markets and a do-it-yourself avoidance of processed food ... many of the [alternative] food movement's goals ... seem aimed at those with disposable income and disposable time."[43] In contrast, the food justice movement "focuses on the barriers that low income or otherwise marginalized groups face in realizing the goals of the broader food movement, such as access to fresh, unprocessed food."[44]

Noting that "communities of color have long faced disproportionate rates of cancer, diabetes, and illnesses associated with lack of access to nutritious food and other forms of environmental racism," many food-justice advocates put health disparities front and center, describing the movement as arising from "a deepening community health crisis."[45] Similarly, Just Food (a nonprofit organization devoted to "building a just and sustainable food system" for New York City) defines food justice in terms of "communities exercising their right to grow, sell, and eat healthy food."[46] The group goes on to define healthy food in a way that extends beyond a narrow conception of physical human health: "Healthy food is fresh, nutritious, affordable, culturally appropriate, and grown locally with care for the well-being of the land, workers, and animals." The group also emphasizes the benefits of "people practicing food justice" in terms of "a strong local food system, self-reliant communities, and a healthy environment." On the other hand, food justice advocates "almost never speak in terms of obesity, though some commentators see that as one underlying motivator. They speak instead about rights, equality, community empowerment, cultural appropriateness, and, of course, justice."[47]

An Emerging Movement: Health Justice

> The question of health-care reform in America, including politically acceptable and fair health-care rationing, is ideologically leveraged. If we find, after all the fuss, that politically we can't do much to make the distribution of medical care more just, in spite of the apparent present opportunities to do so, then a pessimistic conclusion may be irresistible: we may abandon hope for any more widespread or general democratic concern for social justice. But if we do now make substantial and recognizable political progress in this one urgent matter, we may learn more, from the experience, about what justice itself is like, and we might find it to our taste, so that we can steadily, bit by bit, incrementally, fight the same battle in other areas.... Health might not be more important than anything else—but the fight for justice in health might well be.
>
> —Ronald Dworkin, "Justice in the Distribution of Health Care," 1993

Political philosophers and ethicists have begun a productive discussion of the multifaceted relationship between health and social justice, which ranges far beyond individual patient rights and allocation of health care resources to focus on collective needs and problem solving with respect to the social determinants of health.[48] At the same time, a growing number of nonprofit organizations are pursuing ambitious and wide-ranging aims within an emerging health justice framework. For example, the Praxis Project, a nonprofit company that supports community organizers, situates its work with environmental and food justice groups and those committed to health care access under the label of health justice. Praxis defines health justice broadly, with an emphasis on the social determinants of health, fighting cultural bias, and promoting health at the community level.

The health justice framework unites the science and politics of public health. It cuts across long-standing divisions in public policy, integrating health care and population health priorities to meet the needs of the public and reduce health disparities. It emphasizes social, economic, cultural, and political inequalities not to despair over them, but rather to attack them with the power and agency that emerge when science, law, and politics are recognized as inextricably intertwined. Health justice demands an examination of the influence of social bias and structural advantage on interventions aimed at reducing health disparities, particularly measures that adopt an individualistic, victim-blaming approach. Interventions to reduce health disparities should maximize community engagement and empowerment. Scientific expertise, community knowledge, and shared values can and must be united as advocates and experts face the many political, legal, and cultural challenges that stand in the way of health justice.

The Challenges: Public Health, Politics, and Money

> From my perspective, as a White House official watching the budgetary process, and subsequently as head first of a health care financing agency and then of a public health agency, I was continually amazed to watch as billions of dollars were allocated to financing medical care with little discussion, whereas endless arguments ensued over a few millions for community prevention programs. The sums that were the basis for prolonged, and often futile, budget fights in public health were treated as rounding errors in the Medicare budget.

—William Roper, "Why the Problem of Leadership in Public Health?," 1994

While few dispute the basic goal of reducing health disparities, lawmakers, judges, scholars, and the general public are deeply divided over the most appropriate means for doing so. Sharp disagreement over our increasingly collective approach to health care financing is spilling over into a national conversation about personal versus public responsibility for health, in which political ideology and cultural biases threaten to overwhelm scientific inquiry and commitments to social justice.[49]

The ability of public health authorities to attract support is essential to their success, for, as its daily practice reminds us, public health operates in a world of choices in the allocation of limited resources. The great sanitarian Herman Biggs famously remarked that "public health is purchasable," but because there will always be limits on how much we are willing to buy, public health will always turn on allocational decisions.[50] Under these conditions, apathy toward the needs of the least advantaged threatens to widen existing health disparities. Thus the field of public health is as inherently political (i.e., concerned with the distribution of resources in society and addressing the social determinants of health disparities) as it is technological (concerned with the deployment of scientific knowledge).

One might assume that attracting public and financial support would not be difficult given the undoubted communal benefits of health. But the condition of public health is one of paradox. Although most people support a high level of public health, fewer are eager to pay for it. Public health officials have enormous legal power, yet they often cannot exercise it for political, cultural, or practical reasons. The public cares passionately about health threats, but that passion is often not proportional to the magnitude of the risk. The measures that will provide the most societal benefit often provide little or no discernible benefit to any one person, and vice versa. Although there is a virtually bottomless purse for the medical treatment of illness, it appears there is little in the budget to prevent it or, more generally, to ensure the conditions in which people can be healthy.

Even within the relatively modest budgets devoted to public health, there remain hard choices. Public health officials are inevitably faced with the need to divide a small pie among many worthy competitors for resources. Injuries, HIV, emerging infectious diseases, bioterrorism, chronic diseases, child and maternal health, and many other priorities are, in some sense, in competition for prevention resources. Difficult decisions must be made about the most effective allocation of funds. Thus, rationing—a controversial notion in medicine—is, in public health, a "moral imperative ... in the face of scarce resources."[51]

Additionally, public health officials increasingly face opposition from well-financed and politically powerful interests. Criticism of modern public health law is to some extent inevitable: as Roger Magnusson observes, "The use of law as a policy tool to respond comprehensively to environmental exposures, unhealthy lifestyles, and accidental injuries threatens to impinge on the interests of a wide variety of industries, and to significantly expand sites for state intervention."[52] By extending the reach of public health law beyond the traditional domain of infectious disease to the social and economic influences of infectious and noncommunicable disease and injuries, social epidemiologists have inquired into causal connections between ill health and such powerful institutions as tobacco companies, industrial polluters, firearm manufacturers, industrial agriculture, beverage companies, and fast food chains.

Legitimacy and Trust at Risk

> In democratic social orders, the formation of science policy is an ethical and political process.... Policy formation ... include[s] contestable judgments, the search for credibility and legitimation, the marshalling and critique of evidence, and often rhetorical appeals to the public good.
>
> —Leigh Turner, "Politics, Bioethics, and Science Policy," 2005

Social justice demands more than fair distributions of benefits and burdens. Failure to engage community groups with diverse needs and interests harms the whole community by eroding public trust and undermining social cohesion. Public health agencies rely heavily on voluntary cooperation by those at risk of harm and the support of the population at large. Consequently, they must appear credible in the advice they render and trustworthy in their practices. Despite its importance, agencies face considerable challenges in maintaining public confidence both because they are organs of government and because, by necessity, they are engaged in a highly political process.

Public health agencies are fixtures of public administration, part of the structure of government since the earliest times of the Republic. As such, they face the daunting task of ensuring the conditions required for people to be healthy while bearing the burden of antigovernment sentiment: generalized mistrust, doubts about efficiency and efficacy, and fear of oppression. If the public perceives health officials simply as the tool of an overreaching government captured by special interests, their ability to engage collaboratively with communities and earn their support is compromised. Likewise, public health measures are subject to general legal limitations on government activity and to prevailing attitudes about the sorts of things government ought to do. This dynamic can be seen in multiple public health activities characterized as interference by the "nanny state"—e.g., laws mandating the use of seat belts and motorcycle helmets, fluoridation of public water supplies, smoking bans in public places, and healthy eating initiatives. Many disputes in public health turn less on its goal, which everyone professes to support, and more on the proper scope of government intervention to achieve it.

Health officials and experts must maintain scientific rigor while engaging effectively in the political process, and these aims sometimes appear to conflict. To maintain legitimacy and public trust, public health authorities rely on expert scientific knowledge. Scientific decisions are thought to be more objective and systematic and less captive to political ideology. Health officials know that this expertise gives them the authority and the ability to convince. Yet to be effective, health officials must also be willing to embrace and excel in the political process. Many fear that this political involvement risks weakening the impression of professional neutrality and expertise from which health officials draw their public credibility.

Are the science and politics of public health in conflict? Can the public's trust be ensured only if health agencies and experts remain within the cramped confines of the "basic six" public health functions—collecting vital statistics; controlling communicable disease; sanitation; laboratory services; maternal, infant, and child health services; and health education?[53] If so, then public health must resign itself to ineffectiveness and irrelevance.

While health officials fret over the effect of politicization on the authority derived from their scientific expertise,[54] that authority is already waning among those who distrust mainstream science. Critics across the political spectrum call the validity of scientific evidence into question. Counterintuitively, distrust of science with regard to some issues—especially vaccination, fluoridation, and genetic engineering of foods and medicines—is highest among those who have higher household incomes and more formal education.

Frustrated by the lack of individual control over such hazards as air, water, and soil pollution, many people become irrationally concerned with ensuring the "naturalness" of the products they can control. The fetishization of "natural" foods, household products, and medical therapies and rejection of seemingly "unnatural" interventions like water fluoridation, vaccination, antimicrobial drugs, and sunscreen is linked to justifiable fears about toxic exposures but reflects irrational thinking about priorities and scientific evidence.

The public's trust in scientific expertise is undermined by perceived conflicts of interest. Antivaccination crusaders accuse provaccination experts of being shills for the pharmaceutical industry and ignore volumes of scientific evidence on the grounds that it is all biased. Similar accusations are made against proponents of sunscreen use, water fluoridation, and the potential for genetic engineering to generate solutions to pressing health problems. As Michael Specter has observed, "Denialism couldn't exist without the common belief that scientists are linked, often with the government, in an intricate web of lies. When evidence becomes too powerful to challenge, collusion provides a perfect explanation."[55] Health justice demands recognition of public values and concerns, even—perhaps especially—when they conflict with orthodox expertise.

Health justice also requires recognition, participatory engagement, and voice for historically underrepresented groups. This insistence on participatory parity may generate tension over the appropriate role for lawyers, scientists, and other formally educated experts, as it has in the environmental and reproductive justice movements. In some cases, law and policy interventions to serve the interests of the poor and disenfranchised may conflict with the autonomy of those groups to choose other approaches that might be disfavored by experts.[56] Striking the balance between the substantive and procedural commitments of social justice is challenging, but it is crucial to successful public health strategies.

Efforts to ensure access to health care and healthy living conditions must be firmly rooted in community engagement and participatory parity. The processes of "public participation and deliberation in political decisions and social choice [are] a constitutive part of public policy."[57] They "are crucial to the formation of values and priorities, and we cannot, in general, take preferences as given independently of public discussion."[58]

Many of the most effective public health measures are pioneered at the local level. Although local government is typically associated with greater democratic accountability and civic engagement, in the case of many recent healthy eating and tobacco control measures, there has been a deliberate attempt to eschew political accountability in favor of decisions by insulated experts. Mayor Michael Bloomberg explicitly framed New York City's pioneering public health law interventions as efforts to reduce health disparities. These measures threaten the interests of politically powerful industries, and for that reason it is perhaps entirely understandable that Bloomberg pursued them through the New York City Board of Health, which is far more insulated from political pressure than the directly elected city council. On the other hand, public health, local government, and administrative law scholars have been critical of the antidemocratic nature of Bloomberg's strategy.[59] For example, Wendy Parmet has recently suggested that popular backlash against Bloomberg-style interventions might be better understood as resistance to expert opinion in favor of the democratic process, rather than opposition to paternalism.[60]

Pursuing substantive reforms believed to be in the interests of the poor without recognizing affected community members as full participants in a collaborative problem-solving process may remedy distributive injustices, but it perpetuates and exacerbates failures of respect and recognition.[61] Bloomberg's public health legacy raises important and difficult questions about how best to reconcile the substantive and procedural aims of social justice.

The Problem of Framing

> People must take responsibility for their own lives. They must recognize that the pose of helplessness is not just detrimental to their individual dignity, it also saps them and their communities of the spirit of enterprise that makes a healthy and vibrant society. The real epidemics threatening Britain today are not smoking or obesity; they are passivity, the culture of victimhood and stifling government paternalism.
>
> — *The Times* (London), 2004

Under the Affordable Care Act, the health care system is shifting away from "actuarial fairness" (whereby each individual pays according to the likelihood that he or she will require services) toward a "mutual aid" approach (all individuals pay rates determined at the community level, contributing toward a common pool of resources to provide care for those who need it).[62] This shift toward a more collective approach to health care financing has generated increased public interest in the root causes of poor health. When health care costs affect society as a whole, we share a common interest in prevention.

There is major disagreement, however, over whether the root causes of poor health are a matter of collective responsibility or personal responsibility.[63] On the one hand, social epidemiology suggests that social, economic, and environmental factors are the true "causes of the causes" of death, disease, and disability, demanding collective action to regulate commercial activities that are harmful to the public's health and ensure social support for basic human needs. On the other hand, measures that put the onus on individuals to change their behaviors, without necessarily making it more feasible for them to do so, are far more politically palatable. Many of the most important drivers of death and disability—cancer, heart disease, injuries, diabetes, and stroke attributable to tobacco use, alcohol and drug abuse, unhealthy eating, and physical inactivity—are constructed as matters of individual choice and personal responsibility. In the popular imagination, these behaviors are divorced from their social bases.[64]

Our collective inability to overcome the stubborn persistence of health inequalities reflects deep ambivalence about efforts to reduce disparities.[65] The cultural and political resonance of arguments against the "nanny state" and in favor of personal responsibility is readily apparent. These arguments are fueling political opposition to law and policy interventions (such as soda taxes); legal challenges aimed at striking down newly enacted public health laws (such as tobacco and portion-control regulations); the failure of public health litigation (such as lawsuits against the firearms and fast food industries); and efforts to roll back long-standing public health interventions (such as water fluoridation).

The attribution of ill health to personal responsibility is intimately connected to deep-seated cultural biases. Viewing the another person's poor health as the consequence of internal, controllable causes—rather than sheer chance—is comforting.[66] Attribution of illness to individual failings "serves a symbolic, or value expressive function ..., reinforcing a world view consistent with a belief in a just world, self determination, the Protestant work ethic, self-contained individualism, and the notion that people get what they deserve."[67] People like to think of themselves and others as autonomous agents making fully informed, independent judgments. Blaming other people for their own problems makes it easier to make sense of the world, justifying complacency in the face of overwhelming human needs.

Health justice demands collective responsibility for health rather than individualistic, behavior-based interventions. "Victim-blaming misdefines structural and collective problems of the entire society as individual problems, seeing these problems as caused by the behavioral failures or deficiencies of the victims. These behavioral explanations for public problems tend to protect the larger society and powerful interests from the burdens of collective action, and instead encourage attempts to change the 'faulty' behavior of victims."[68] Personal responsibility interventions to discourage unhealthy behaviors through individually targeted incentives and penalties are counter to the communitarian commitment of social justice. The health justice framework demands more rigorous attention to these issues. Scholars and lawyers have an obligation to probe proposed interventions ostensibly aimed at reducing health disparities for evidence of social and structural biases. Even well-intentioned public health officials may sometimes neglect the disadvantaged and propose interventions that exacerbate underlying inequalities.

Moving forward in the face of the backlash against the "nanny state" and apathy toward the plight of the socially disadvantaged will require a reframing of public health action in controversial areas. Public health has a proud tradition of promoting equity and justice. It should not surrender the moral high ground to industry groups casting themselves as defenders of individual liberty. What is needed is a salient, culturally resonant vision of communities coming together to create healthier living conditions.[69] Government is not an external force: it is how "we the people" achieve collectively what we cannot achieve individually. Some interventions may ultimately prove to be unwise from a policy standpoint, but to kill innovative local government experiments in their infancy, to block the will of the people expressed through the democratic process based on a counter-majoritarian protection of commercial interests, would be a tragic loss for the health of the republic.

We are undoubtedly making gains, especially on access to health care. Many of the interventions being proposed and deployed in the name of reducing health disparities are encouraging from a social justice standpoint. But as the public health ethicist Dan Beauchamp has cautioned, "As long as these actions are seen as merely minor exceptions to the rule of individual responsibility, the goals of public health will remain beyond our reach."[70] The health justice framework offers a powerful critique of the ways in which dominant norms about fairness, emphasizing "just deserts," shore up a narrow vision of health that is dominated by the health care industry, an impoverished vision of community as the aggregation of quasi-contractual relationships between autonomous and atomized individuals and their exogenous social environment, and a lopsided vision of reform as driven by privileged experts who fail to engage meaningfully with the communities they purport to serve.

The Future of Public Health Law

> Either the social epidemiologists' contention that socioeconomic dispari-
> ties are a primary factor in causing good public health is accurate, or it is
> not.... [I]f socioeconomic disparities are truly productive of public health,
> policies consistent with the narrow model [of old public health], which
> by definition do nothing to ameliorate social conditions, will do little to
> actually improve health in the aggregate.... If public health practice is
> not intended to facilitate the public's health, it is unclear what use such a
> practice has and why public monies should be forthcoming to support it.
>
> —Daniel S. Goldberg, "In Support of a Broad Model of
> Public Health," 2009

[...] [W]e have sought to provide a fuller understanding of the varied roles of law in advancing the public's health. The field of public health is purposive and interventionist. It does not settle for existing conditions of health but actively seeks effective techniques for identifying and reducing health threats. Law is a very important, and increasingly recognized, tool in furthering the public's health. Public health law should not be seen as an arcane, indecipherable set of technical rules buried deep within state health codes. Rather, it should be seen broadly as the authority and responsibility of government to assure the conditions for the population's health. As such, public health law has transcending importance in how we think about government, politics, and policy.

Critics of public health efforts to address noncommunicable diseases and the social determinants of health begin from the proposition that, regardless of the validity of social epidemiology as a scientific matter, it does not necessarily follow that state authority to intervene "under the banner of public health" should be expansive.[71] They stress the need "to more clearly differentiate between public health *analysis* and public health *authority*," arguing that "public health law is much more limited than public health science."[72]

In a subtle but fundamental way, the division between science and law championed by these critics would also disconnect public health from the social justice mission that has been integral to its disciplinary identity for centuries. We agree that scientific inquiry to describe the causes and patterns of health conditions at a population level should aim for neutrality. But eliminating threats to public health involves multiple activities that are far from being exclusively within the domain of either law or science. The demarcations among science, practice, policy, and law are inherently blurry. It is not possible for the science of public health to exist in a vacuum. The questions it seeks to answer (and the answers it eventually provides) are informed by practice, policy, and law. The identification of causal pathways is intimately tied to developing and evaluating potential interventions within them. The practice of public health is useless unless it is informed by science and guided by policy. And public health policy easily blends into the law, which is its expression.

Law is a vitally important determinant of population health. The interplay among law, social norms, cultural beliefs, health behaviors, and healthy living conditions is complex. To limit the scope of public health law to the control of proximal determinants of infectious diseases, to cut off the law and policy of public health from the advances of health science and practice, would be utterly unjustifiable in the face of so much preventable death, disability, and disparity. The push to limit public health law's scope is deeply counter-majoritarian and undemocratic, threatening to disable communities from undertaking measures to improve their own wellbeing.

We reject the critics' contention that public health science should (or even could) be cut off from its social justice mission, but we do believe their fundamental concern is a valid one. Designating a concern as a public health threat has important legal consequences. To the extent that the public interest is invoked as a liberty-limiting principle, it should be thoughtfully defined and theorized. While government has responsibility to assure the conditions for health, at times, public health has overreached, failing to consider the full range of concerns and interests of the public it seeks to protect.

Communities may rightly weigh ends and values other than health differently than public health experts would. In this regard public health advocates could take a page from the environmentalists' book. As Douglas Kysar puts it: "Environmental law must form part of the social glue that binds a political community together in pursuit of long-term and uncertain goals. To serve that function, in turn, laws must have continuity with the concepts, values, and discourses expressed by real people."[73] Public health law, likewise, should strive to reflect community engagement.

This objective leads to one of the most complicated problems in the field, which is how to balance the collective good achieved by public health regulation with the resulting infringements of individual rights and freedoms. The difficult trade-offs between collective goods and individual rights form a major part of the study of public health law. Civil liberties, including free speech, have intrinsic value for libertarians and progressives alike—and they play an important role in promoting public health.

Public health, like the law itself, is highly political, influenced by strong social, cultural, and economic forces. As these forces shift over the years, as different political ideologies and economic conditions take hold, the field of public health will change and adapt, as it has always done. It will continue to provide intellectually enticing and socially important terrain for scholars and practitioners to explore.

John Ruskin, a nineteenth-century British scholar whose work ranged from art history, literary criticism, and mythology to the pervasive health hazards of the industrial economy, captured better than most the essential message of this book: "I desire, in closing the series of introductory papers, to have this one great fact clearly stated. There is no wealth but life. Life, including all its powers of love, of joy, and of admiration. That country is the richest which nourishes the greatest number of noble and happy human beings; that man is richest, who, having perfected the functions of his own life to the utmost, has also the widest helpful influence, both personal, and by means of his possessions, over the lives of others."[74]

Notes

Substantial portions of this chapter are reproduced from Lindsay F. Wiley, "Health Law as Social Justice," *Cornell Journal of Law and Public Policy,* 24, no. 1 (2014): 47–105.

1 Peter G. Peterson Foundation, "Increases in Longevity Have Been Greater for High Earners," November 21, 2014, http://pgpf.org/Chart-Archive/0015_life-expectancy, discussing data from a 2007 Social Security Administration report.

2 See, for example, David A. Kindig and Erika R. Cheng, "Even as Mortality Fell in Most U.S. Counties, Female Mortality Nonetheless Rose in 42.8 Percent of Counties from 1992 to 2006," *Health Affairs*, 32, no. 3 (2013): 451–58, 53; Haidong Wang, Austin E. Schumacher, Carly E. Levitz, Ali H. Mokdad, and Christopher J. L. Murray, "Left Behind: Widening Disparities for Males and Females in US County Life Expectancy, 1985–2010" *Population Health Metrics,* 11, no. 8, (2013): 3.

3 Gloria L. Beckles and Benedict I. Truman, "Education and Income: United States, 2009 and 2011," *Morbidity and Mortality Weekly Report,* 62, no. S3 (2013): 9–19, 13.

4 Lara J. Akinbami, Jeanne E. Moorman, Paul L. Garbe, and Edward J. Sondik, "Status of Childhood Asthma in the United States, 1980–2007," *Pediatrics*, 123, no. S3 (2009): S131–S145. Notably, Puerto Rican children have the highest rates of asthma: they are about 1.5 times as likely as non-His-panic black children, 2.5 times as likely as non-Hispanic white children, and about three times as likely as Mexican-American children to be diagnosed.

5 Gloria L. Beckles and Chiu-Fang Chou, "Diabetes: United States, 2006 and 2010," *Morbidity and Mortality Weekly Report,* 62, no. S3 (2013): 99–104, 101.

6 Pamela A. Meyer, Paula W. Yoon, and Rachel B. Kaufmann, "Introduction: CDC Health Disparities and Inequalities Report—United States, 2013," *Morbidity and Mortality Weekly Report,* 62, no. S3 (2013): 3–5, 3.

7 See Gwendolyn Roberts Majette, "Global Health Law Norms and the PPACA Framework to Eliminate Health Disparities," *Howard Law Journal,* 55, no. 3 (2012): 887–936, 926–27.

8 U.S. Department of Health and Human Services, "Learn about the NPA," National Partnership for Action to End Health Disparities, April 4, 2011, http://minorityhealth.hhs.gov/npa/templates/browse.aspx?lvl=1&lvlid=11.

9 U.S. Department of Health and Human Services, "National Stakeholder Strategy for Achieving Health Equity," National Partnership for Action to End Health Disparities, September 19, 2011, http://minorityhealth.hhs.gov/npa/templates/content.aspx?lvl=1&lvlid=33&ID=286.

10 U.S. Department of Health and Human Services, *Action Plan to Reduce Racial and Ethnic Health Disparities: A Nation Free of Disparities in Health and Health Care* (Washington, DC: Department of Health and Human Services, 2011) http://minorityhealth.hhs.gov/npa/files/Plans/HHS/HHS_Plan_complete.pdf.

11 Michael Marmot and Richard G. Wilkinson, eds., *Social Determinants of Health,* 2nd ed. (New York: Oxford University Press, 2006).

12 International Forum for Social Development, *Social Justice in an Open World: The Role of the United Nations,* U.N. Doc. ST/ESA/305 (New York: United Nations, 2006), 11.

13 Ibid., 3.

14 Communitarian Network, "The Responsive Communitarian Platform," Institute for Communitarian Policy Studies, George Washington University, www.gwu.edu/~ccps/platformtext.html, accessed October 15, 2014.

15 Rand E. Rosenblatt, "The Four Ages of Health Law," *Health Matrix: Journal of Law-Medicine,* 14, no. 1 (2004): 155–96, 96.

16 Nancy Fraser, "Rethinking Recognition," *New Left Review,* 3 (2000): 107–20.

17 See, for example, Barbara A. Israel, Amy J. Schulz, Edith A. Parker, and Adam B. Becker, "Review of Community-Based Research: Assessing Partnership Approaches to Improve Public Health," *Annual Review of Public Health,* 19 (1998): 173–202.

18 Nancy Fraser, "From Redistribution to Recognition?: Dilemmas of Justice in a 'Post-socialist' Age," *New Left Review,* 212 (1995): 68–93, 69; see also Nancy Fraser, "Social Justice in the Age of Identity Politics: Redistribution, Recognition, and Participation," in *Redistribution or Recognition? A Political-Philosophical Exchange,* ed. Nancy Fraser and Axel Honneth (New York: Verso, 2003): 7–109.

19 Dignity is a multifaceted concept, with scholars disagreeing on its status as the foundation or the content of human rights. See, for example, Jeremy Waldron, "Dignity and Rank," *European Journal of Sociology,* 48, no. 2 (2007) 201–37; Christopher McCrudden, "Human Dignity and Judicial Interpretation of Human Rights," *European Journal of International Law,* 19, no. 4 (2008): 655–724; George Kateb, *Human Dignity* (Cambridge, MA: Harvard University Press, 2011); Michael Rosen, *Dignity: Its History and Meaning* (Cambridge, MA: Harvard University Press, 2012); Jeremy Waldron, "Is Dignity the Foundation of Human Rights?," in *Philosophical Foundations of Human Rights,* ed. Rowan Cruft, S. Matthew Liao, and Massimo Renzo (Oxford: Oxford University Press, 2015), 117–137.

20 See, for example, Valerie Ann Johnson, *Bringing Together Feminist Disability Studies and Environmental Justice* (Washington, DC: Center For Women Policy Studies, 2011); Mia Mingus, "Disabled Women and

Reproductive Justice," Pro-choice Public Education Project, http://protectchoice.org/article.php?id=140, accessed February 10, 2015.

21 See, for example, Rachel Stein ed., *New Perspectives on Environmental Justice: Gender, Sexuality, and Activism* (New Brunswick, NJ: Rutgers University Press, 2004); Laura Nixon, "The Right to (Trans) Parent: A Reproductive Justice Approach to Reproductive Rights, Fertility, and Family-Building Issues Facing Transgender People," *William and Mary Journal of Women and the Law*, 20 (2013): 73–103.

22 See, for example, Alisa Wellek and Miriam Yeung, "Reproductive Justice and Lesbian, Gay, Bisexual and Transgender Liberation," The Pro-choice Public Education Project, http://protectchoice.org/article.php?id=135, accessed October 15, 2014.

23 See, for example, Chinese Progressive Association, "Immigrant Power for Environmental Health and Justice," www.cpasf.org/node/12, accessed October 15, 2014;, "Health Equity is a Matter of Reproductive Justice," *National Latina Institute for Reproductive Health* blog, April 25, 2012, http://latinainstitute.org/en/2012/04/25/health-equity-is-a-matter-of-reproductive-justice; Jessica Gonzales-Rojas and Aishia Glasford, "Immigrant Rights and Reproductive Justice," Pro-choice Public Education Project, http://protectchoice.org/article.php?id=136, accessed October 15, 2014.

24 See Gerald Torres, "Environmental Justice: The Legal Meaning of a Social Movement," *Journal of Law and Commerce*, 15, no. 2 (1996): 597–622, 598–607, describing the origins of the environmental justice movement as a response to "environmental racism" while also critiquing its framing in terms of racism as opposed to white supremacy or white advantage; Alice Kaswan, "Environmental Justice and Environmental Law," *Fordham Environmental Law Review*, 24, no. 2 (2013): 149–79, 50–51, noting that a siting dispute over a polychlorinated biphenyl (PCB) disposal facility in a predominantly African American community in North Carolina in the 1980s "was a nationally galvanizing event, sparking widespread attention to distributional, participatory, and social environmental justice."

25 Kaswan, "Environmental Justice," 151.

26 See Gordon Walker, *Environmental Justice: Concepts, Evidence and Politics* (New York: Routledge, 2012), I, defining environmental justice very broadly to encompass

> the intertwining of environment and social difference—how for some people and some social groups the environment is an intrinsic part of living a "good life" of prosperity, health and well-being, while for others the environment is a source of threat and risk, and access to resources such as energy, water, and greenspace is limited or curtailed ... how some of us consume key environmental resources as the expense of others, often in distant places, and about how the power to effect change and influence environmental decision-making is unequally distributed.... the way that people should be treated, the way the world should be.

27 Ibid., 171.

28 Ronald Sandler and Phaedra C. Pezzullo, eds., *Environmental Justice and Environmentalism: The Social Justice Challenge to the Environmental Movement* (Cambridge, MA: MIT Press, 2007), 2.

29 See, for example, Luke W. Cole, "Empowerment as the Key to Environmental Protection: The Need for Environmental Poverty Law," *Ecology Law Quarterly*, 19, no. 4 (1992): 619–83, 49: "Solutions to poor peoples' environmental problems should be found by the victims of those problems, not by environmental lawyers"; Eleanor N. Metzger, "Driving the Environmental Justice Movement Forward: The Need for a Paternalistic Approach," *Case Western Reserve Law Review*, 45, no. 1 (1994): 379–98.

30 See Kevin Gover and Jana L. Walker, "Escaping Environmental Paternalism: One Tribe's Approach to Developing a Commercial Waste Disposal Project in Indian Country," *University of Colorado Law Review*, 63, no. 4 (1992): 933–43, 42; Giancarlo Panagia, "Tota Capita Tot Sententiae: An Extension or Misapplication of Rawlsian Justice," *Penn State Law Review*, 110, no. 2 (2005): 283–343, 305; Yves Le Bouthillier, Miriam Alfie Cohen, Jose Juan Gonzalez Marquez, Albert Mumma, and Susan Smith, eds., *Poverty Alleviation and Environmental Law* (Cheltenham, UK: Edward Elgar, 2012), exploring apparent tensions between the goals of poverty alleviation and environmental protection.

31 See, for example, Ezra Rosser, "Ahistorical Indians and Reservation Resources," *Environmental Law*, 40, no. 2 (2010): 437–550, 472–74, arguing that these scenarios necessitate a reconceptualization of environmental justice.

32 Exec. Order 12898, 59 Fed. Reg. 7629 (1994).

33 Ibid. (emphasis added).

34 See Kaswan, "Environmental Justice," 153–55.

35 J. Nadine Gracia and Howard K. Koh, "Promoting Environmental Justice," *American Journal of Public Health*, 101, no. S1 (2011): S14–S16, S15.

36 U.S. Department of Health and Human Services, *2012 Environmental Justice Strategy and Implementation Plan* (Washington, DC: U.S. Department of Health and Human Services, 2012), 6.

37 Onyemaechi C. Nweke and Charles Lee, "Achieving Environmental Justice: Perspectives on the Path Forward through Collective Action to Eliminate Health Disparities," *American Journal of Public Health*, 101, no. S1 (2011): S6–S8.

38 SisterSong Women of Color Reproductive Justice Collective, "Why Is Reproductive Justice Important for Women of Color?," www.sistersong.net, accessed October 15, 2014; Loretta Ross, "Understanding Reproductive Justice: Transforming the Pro-choice Movement," *Off Our Backs*, 36, no. 4 (2006): 14–19.

39 Ross, "Understanding Reproductive Justice." See also Joan C. Chrisler, "Introduction: A Global Approach to Reproductive Justice; Psychosocial, and Legal Aspects and Implications," *William and Mary Journal of Women and the Law*, 20, no. 1 (2013): 1–24.

40 United Nations, *Report of the International Conference on Population and Development, Cairo, 5–13 September 1994*, U.N. Doc. No. A/CONF.171/13 (New York: United Nations, 1995).

41 Rebecca L. Goldberg, "No Such Thing as a Free Lunch: Paternalism, Poverty, and Food Justice," *Stanford Law and Policy Review*, 24 (2013): 35–98, 48–49.

42 Michael Pollan, "The Food Movement, Rising," *New York Review of Books*, June 10, 2010, quoted in Daniel S. Goldberg, "In Support of a Broad Model of Public Health: Disparities, Social Epidemiology and Public Health Causation," *Public Health Ethics*, 2, no. 1 (2009): 70–83, 73.

43 Michael Pollan, quoted in Goldberg, "No Such Thing as a Free Lunch," 49.

44 Ibid.

45 Ibid. Others have similarly pointed to the ways in which "food oppression" is a form of structural racism. See, for example, Andrea Freeman, "Fast Food: Oppression through Poor Nutrition," *California Law Review*, 95, no. 6 (2007): 2221–59; Kate Meals, "Nurturing the Seeds of Food Justice: Unearthing the Impact of Institutionalized Racism on Access to Healthy Food in Urban African-American Communities," *Scholar: St. Mary's Law Review on Race and Social Justice*, 15, no. 1 (2012): 97–138.

46 Just Food, "About Us," and "Food Justice," http://justfood.org, accessed October 15, 2014.

47 Just Food, "Food Justice," 50–51.

48 See, for example, Sridhar Venkatapuram, *Health Justice: An Argument from the Capabilities Approach* (Cambridge: Polity Press, 2011); Shlomi Segall, *Health, Luck, and Justice* (Princeton, NJ: Princeton University Press, 2010); Jennifer Prah Ruger, *Health and Social Justice* (New York: Oxford University Press, 2009); Norman Daniels, *Just Health: Meeting Health Needs Fairly* (New York: Cambridge University Press, 2008); Madison Powers and Ruth Faden, *Social Justice: The Moral Foundations of Public Health and Health Policy* (Oxford: Oxford University Press, 2006).

49 See Janet L. Dolgin and Katherine R. Dieterich, "Weighing Status: Obesity, Class, and Health Reform," *Oregon Law Review*, 89, no. 4 (2011): 1113–77; Dayna Bowen Matthew, "The Social Psychology of Limiting Healthcare Benefits for Undocumented Immigrants: Moving beyond Race, Class, and Nativism," *Houston Journal of Health Law and Policy*, 10, no. 2 (2010): 201–26; Lindsay F. Wiley, "Access to Health Care as an Incentive for Healthy Behav-ior? An Assessment of the Affordable Care Act's Personal Responsibility for Wellness Reforms," *Indiana Health Law Review*, 11, no. 2 (2014): 635–709, 641.

50 New York City Health Department, *Monthly Bull*, October 1911, quoted in Barbara Gutmann Rosenkrantz, *Public Health and the State: Changing Views in Massachusetts, 1842–1936* (Cambridge, MA: Harvard University, 1972), 5.

51 Richard H. Morrow and John H. Bryant, "Health Policy Approaches to Measuring and Valuing Human Life: Conceptual and Ethical Issues," *American Journal of Public Health*, 85, no. 10 (1995): 1356–60.

52 Roger S. Magnusson, "Mapping the Scope and Opportunities for Public Health Law in Liberal Democracies," *Journal of Law, Medicine and Ethics*, 35, no. 4 (2007): 571–87, 72.

53 Amy L. Fairchild, David Rosner, James Colgrove, Ronald Bayer, and Linda P. Fried, "The Exodus of Public Health: What History Can Tell Us about the Future," *American Journal of Public Health*, 100, no. 1 (2010): 54–63, 56: "In 1940, the American Public Health Association passed a resolution codifying the standard repertoire of services that local health departments should provide, what became known as the 'basic 6.' … Thus, at the same moment that it prioritized objective science over social reform and alliances with relatively powerful progressive constituencies such as labor, charity, social welfare organizations, and housing reformers, the field was marginalized and left with no political base."

54 Daniel S. Goldberg, "Against the Very Idea of the Politicization of Public Health Policy," *American Journal of Public Health*, 102, no. 1 (2012): 44–49.

55 Michael Specter, *Denialism: How Irrational Thinking Hinders Scientific Progress, Harms the Planet, and Threatens Our Lives* (New York: Penguin, 2009), 5.

56 Artika R. Tyner, "Planting People, Growing Justice: The Three Pillars of New Social Justice Lawyering," *Hastings Race and Poverty Law Journal*, 10, no. 2 (2013): 219–63, 19–20. Some, social justice advocates, like Ascanio Piomelli, have gone so far as to suggest a shift in "what we mean by and count as social justice and social change": a shift away from substantive law reform to better serve the interests of low income and otherwise marginalized communities and toward a process-based conception of social justice lawyering as a democratic, participatory, collaborative project to ensure recognition of and self-determination for marginalized individuals. Ascanio Piomelli, "Sensibilities for Social Justice Lawyers," *Hastings Race and Poverty Law Journal,* 10, no. 2 (2013): 177–90, 82–83.

57 Ruger, *Health and Social Justice,* 55.

58 Amartya Sen, *Development as Freedom* (New York: Alfred A. Knopf, 1999), 153.

59 But see Paul A. Diller, "Local Health Agencies, the Bloomberg Soda Rule, and the Ghost of Woodrow Wilson," *Fordham Urban Law Journal*, 40, no. 5 (2013): 1859–901, arguing that the New York City Board of Health could have better insulated the portion rule from a separation-of-powers challenge by relying more explicitly on its health sciences expertise.

60 Wendy E. Parmet, "Beyond Paternalism: Rethinking the Limits of Public Health Law," *Connecticut Law Review,* 46, no. 5 (2014): 1771–94.

61 Fraser and Honneth, *Redistribution or Recognition?,* 86–87.

62 Deborah A. Stone, "The Struggle for the Soul of Health Insurance," *Journal of Health Politics, Policy and Law,* 18, no. 2 (1993): 287–317.

63 Howard M. Leichter, "'Evil Habits' and 'Personal Choices': Assigning Responsibility for Health in the 20th Century," *Milbank Quarterly,* 81, no. 4 (2003): 603–26.

64 Venkatapuram, *Health Justice,* 11.

65 Dolgin and Dieterich, "Weighing Status," 1139.

66 See, for example, Claudia Sikorski, Melanie Luppa, Marie Kaiser, Heide Glaesmer, Georg Schomerus, Hans-Helmut König, and Steffi G. Riedel-Heller, "The Stigma of Obesity in the General Public and Its Implications for Public Health: A Systematic Review," *BMC Public Health*, 11 (2009): 661, describing the role of attribution theory in obesity stigma.

67 Christian S. Crandall and Rebecca Martinez, "Culture, Ideology, and Antifat Attitudes," *Personality and Social Psychology Bulletin,* 22, no. 11 (1996): 1165–76, 66.

68 Ibid., 104; see also Venkatapuram, *Health Justice,* 77 n. 58, arguing that outdated models of disease "misclassif[y] causes as beyond social action."

69 Lindsay F. Wiley, Micah L. Berman, and Doug Blanke, "Who's Your Nanny? Choice, Paternalism and Public Health in the Age of Personal Responsibility," *Journal of Law, Medicine and Ethics*, 41, no. S1 (2013): S88.

70 Dan E. Beauchamp, "Public Health as Social Justice," *Inquiry,* 13, no. 1 (1976): 3–14, 6.

71 Richard A. Epstein, "Let the Shoemaker Stick to His Last: A Defense of the 'Old' Public Health," *Perspectives on Biology and Medicine,* 46, no. S3 (2003): S138–S159, S154.

72 Mark A. Hall, "The Scope and Limits of Public Health Law," *Perspectives on Biology and Medicine,* 46, no. S3 (2003): S199–S209, S202; Epstein, "Let the Shoemaker Stick to His Last," S138, attempting to draw a distinction between "the conception of public health that is internal to the public health discipline, and the conception of public health as it has been understood outside the public health field by historians and lawyers who are interested in defining the appropriate use and limitations of the state power of coercion."

73 Douglas A. Kysar, *Regulating from Nowhere: Environmental Law and the Search for Objectivity* (New Haven, CT: Yale University Press, 2010).

74 John Ruskin, *"Unto This Last": Four Essays on the First Principles of Political Economy* (New York: Wiley & Son, 1872), 125–26.

Working against Racial Injustice

Bringing the Message to Community Mental Health Providers

Judith Shola Willison and Rebecca Jackson Garcia

Abstract: This narrative offers the experiences and reflections of two colleagues and friends in their efforts to work for racial justice including the use of Community Circles. This pair acts as a bi-racial training dyad to address implicit racial bias, racial microaggressions, and cross-racial dialogue in community mental health settings. Challenges in acting as a white ally are presented, as well as the toll being a facilitator takes on people of color.

Keywords: mental health; anti-racism

Introduction

Our national conversation about both interpersonal and institutional racism has moved this past year in response to the surfacing in mainstream media of police brutality toward black men. Some of us knew this painful legacy continued, but I can't tell you how many white folks have said to me "isn't this happening more?!" We live in predominantly racially and economically segregated communities in the U.S. and those of us with the privileges that come with being white in this racialized society have the luxury of not having to know this violence is happening. These stories are not historically covered on mainstream news media but thanks to community mobilization in places like Ferguson, MO and Baltimore, MD, the nation has been faced with issues of racial injustice. My friend and colleague Rebecca Garcia and I began talking about what we can do at a community mental health level to forward racial justice and support others who are doing so. This essay outlines some of the efforts we made to contribute to the national movement against racism, our experiences, and our reflections on what we learned.

Racial injustice in all its forms is relevant for mental health providers. We know that perceived racism is one of the stressors that research has identified as contributing to psychological distress, depression, anxiety, and poor overall mental health (Kwate & Goodman, 2015; Soto, Dawson-Andoh, & BeLue, 2011) as well as chronic and serious medical conditions and early death (Goosby & Heidbrink, 2013). We also know that "color-blindness" in white mental health clinicians can lead to a lack of empathy for clients of color (Burkard & Knox, 2004), and that racial bias is associated with misdiagnosis, and the criminalization of mental illness (Pottick, Kirk, Hsieh, & Tian, 2007). Therapeutic relationships as well as dispositional decisions are profoundly impacted by a white mental health providers' level of racial implicit bias and whether they have the capacity to engage in reflection around racism.

The brutality visited upon black men figures into the way in which our clients of color live their lives. Our clients want and need to talk about this, and many white mental health clinicians are at a loss for how to have these conversations. Even worse, our clients may not talk to us about these issues because they can pick up on our discomfort with the topic of race and racism by what we don't say, or the conversations that we don't initiate. We are also sometimes at a loss for how to connect with our colleagues around racial justice issues. We as mental health clinicians need to know how to respond to concerns of those in communities of color who are impacted by racism on a daily basis.

The Co-Authors Response to the Killing of Black Men by Police

Rebecca: I completed my MSW six years ago, I am an African American woman, and many of the clients I have worked with are people of color, of all ages. In particular, I have a strong inclination toward working with young men of color. This is partly a result of my own experience with community violence in my previous career as a pastor, when I lost a member of my church. He was shot in the head outside of a bar and died a month later. This experience gave me a deep seated passion for working with men of color. During my time working at an agency that places social workers at police stations, I was able to work even more with young men of color, mostly ranging in age from 16–25. These men were coming into contact with the criminal justice system, either as a result of their own activities as gang members, or their association with friends who were involved in some type of criminal activity. I consider this work to be a privilege, because the lived experiences of these young men are not fully understood in our society. To be able to sit with a young man who has lost a sibling to violence and talk to him about the depth of his pain, or to talk to another young man about what it's like to be regularly profiled by the police, and assumed to be guilty of crimes that he didn't commit, is an honor that not many clinicians get to experience. Part of this is their level of comfort talking about the issues of race, which is much harder for white clinicians, in general, than clinicians of color.

I always talk about race with my clients. In response to the murders of young Black men over the past few years, beginning with Trayvon Martin, I organized a community circle. The goal of the circle was to create space for those of us who work with young people, especially young Black men, to talk about the impact of systemic racism on their lives, and as a result on our work. The community circle is based upon Native American circle practices, in which there is a talking piece and every person sitting in the circle has the opportunity to speak (or not). There is usually an opening and closing by the circle keeper, and questions asked in the circle to prompt thought. I decided to use this format because I wanted to provide a forum that would allow people to speak freely and that would be containing at the same time. It is my belief that we do not take enough time to pause and talk about the lived experience of our clients who battle being stereotyped and targeted by the police, and are therefore at risk of being killed by a police officer or vigilante every moment of their lives. If we as clinicians are not processing this, how do we have the space in our minds and hearts to be able to talk about it with our clients? Since our initial community circle in response to George Zimmerman's not guilty verdict, we have held other circles in response to Ferguson and Baltimore. Another way that I have been working for social and racial justice is by co-facilitating anti-racism workshops with Judith Willison, a former professor turned colleague, friend, and mentor. We have co-facilitated two workshops for mental health providers in community mental health centers, geared toward people who are doing clinical work with low income people in the inner city, mostly people of color.

Judith: As a white educator at a public university in a School of Social Work, and a social work practitioner for over twenty years in the criminal and juvenile justice systems, I am committed to remaining involved in community-level work in order to link my scholarship to advocacy, consciousness raising, and systemic change. Although I was involved in numerous initiatives on campus this past year focused on racial justice and the success of students of color, I felt compelled to do more in the community. Fortunately, a number of my friends of color who work in urban community-based mental health centers felt similarly. The clients served by these centers are primarily impoverished people of color. My friends knew that we needed to create forums for community mental health workers to grapple with how racism impacts the lives of our clients and our interactions with those clients.

Part of the reason my friends asked me to facilitate these workshops was that they believe, and I agree, that having a white ally speak to white folks about implicit racial bias, racial microaggressions, and racial justice can be powerful. And of course, white supremacy is a problem that we white people need to fix. I can talk to other white clinicians about white privilege, how to overcome our fears of reaching across the racial divide, our mistakes and how to recover from them, and the responsibility we have to dismantle the systems of racial injustice that exist. I can talk about how moving past white guilt through understanding how the Cycle of Socialization (Harro, 2008) indoctrinates us to the laws of white supremacy is the only road to taking action to change that cycle.

However, I felt strongly that the workshops I was asked to facilitate should be done in partnership with a colleague/friend of color, and so Rebecca Garcia and I decided to partner in these endeavors. Rebecca and I talked about why using a bi-racial dyad for these forums would be important: Rebecca would legitimize my role for folks of color in the workshops; she would act as a cultural liaison of sorts, we would offer a model of cross-racial dialogue and connection, as well as provide a picture of what cross-racial cooperation can accomplish. We wanted to bring hope to folks who felt worn down and discouraged by racial injustice and the lethal violence visited upon men of color every day. We aimed to engage in dialogue with each other in order to spark dialogue with the workshop participants.

Rebecca: As a woman of color who teaches graduate social work students part time and lives in the racialized United States full time, with a Black husband, the reality of racism and oppression is also a part of my everyday life. When I stand up in front of a mostly white audience and reveal my personal experiences, this includes the emotional weight of sharing my life with a Black man who I am fully aware is a target, I am exposing a vulnerable part of my life for the purpose of educating others. There is an emotional price that I pay to do that. I'm not always clear on what it is, but it costs me something. When I prepare to engage a class discussion about the uprising in Ferguson or Baltimore and I think about the young men that I work with, I have to be willing to share that emotion with my students. My hope is that in sharing my experience, a student in the classroom, or a mental health professional in the audience will be moved to the point of a different level of understanding and action. Perhaps that action will be having a conversation with a client that they wouldn't have had before. Perhaps it will be seeking out more knowledge about systemic racism and police brutality. Perhaps it will be getting involved in some community action and eventually leading others to do the same.

I have been teaching for four years, and have experienced multiple microaggressions as an African-American woman teaching mostly white students about systemic racism. I have also conducted multiple workshops with various audiences in which I, as the facilitator, am the target of microaggressions and misplaced anger. Co-facilitating with Judith, a white anti-racist educator, makes this experience markedly different. When Judith talks about white supremacy and systemic racism, the reaction and receptivity of a white audience is different. They're much more open to hearing about that from another white person. Working with Judith lightens the burden on me, which makes it easier for me to share my personal experiences and talk about facts without feeling as though the weight of the workshop rests entirely on me, a Black woman. It also allows me the freedom to connect more with the people of color in the audience, who generally seem to feel relief from having a Black co-facilitator.

The Community Mental Health Anti-Racism Workshops

Both workshops that we co-facilitated were attended by a range of mental health professionals including social workers, psychologists, psychiatrists, supervisors, and administrators. The first workshop of about 25 people was small enough so we could engage the participants in dialogue right away. We asked them to tell us who they were and why they were attending the workshop, what we might address that would be helpful for them in their work. We covered concepts such as racial implicit bias, racial microaggressions, and cross-racial communication. The workshop evolved into a very interactive dialogue whereby the participants shared their personal and professional experiences with interpersonal and institutional racism, and we brainstormed about possible avenues for addressing issues of racial injustice is their work with clients and colleagues. The second workshop was a more formal Grand Rounds with a larger audience of about 50 people.

Judith: In the second workshop one of my opening remarks was intended to not alienate participants who had police people in their close social circles. Rebecca and I had talked about how to address this, and Rebecca's experiences working closely with male policemen of color was on our agenda as well. I said something like "Our national conversation has been informed by the black men who have died over the past year at the hands of police people. Police people are our heroes, but their actions are shaped by the militarization of the police by the federal government, subsequent to the war on drugs, which is in reality a war on impoverished people of color." Rebecca and I immediately saw a Black woman in the front row begin shaking her head "no" vigorously. We will call her Simone. I thought to myself "She may have lost a son, or a husband to police violence, and I just called them heroes, what have I said?!" It was a stressful moment for me, but I realized that I had to address Simone's response if she wanted to discuss it.

I talked about how cross-racial dialogue about racism is difficult and often avoided by us white folks because we are afraid we will say the wrong thing and offend a person of color. In fact, I continued, I may have already done that this afternoon...I asked "Have I offended anyone so far?" And much to her credit, Simone answered my question and made it clear, with emotional passion, that police officers are not considered heroes in communities of color, but rather an extension of the criminal justice system which targets men of color... she made excellent points about the role of the police as enforcers of the laws of white supremacy which oppress people of color. All the points Simone made are points I have made in the past...I thought, "Yes, I agree! Didn't I mention Michelle Alexander's book The New Jim Crow? I am a white ally, I agree! But I had to temper my message in order to reach the white folks in the room and not alienate anyone!" I felt like my values and commitment were in question. But then I realized that this was not about me, it was about her, and the other people of color in the room. I had made a terrible mistake through my use of language about police as "heroes" and that in fact, first and foremost I needed to connect with her, to validate her, to reach across the racial divide and to demonstrate cultural humility in that moment, to really act like an ally. And so instead of defending myself, which is what I was compelled to do, I listened, I moved toward Simone, I looked her in the eye respectfully and nodded, and I agreed with her, and then I apologized and said I would never use that word again to describe police people, that I had misspoken, made a mistake, and that I appreciated her perspective and feedback. After the workshop, both Rebecca and I approached Simone and spoke with her more about her views and she thanked us for making space for her experiences in the workshop.

Rebecca: When I saw Simone, who was sitting right in the front row, vigorously shaking her head in response to Judith's statement. I smiled and nodded at her because I thought I knew what she was thinking: "the police aren't our/my heroes." Having worked with police officers, this conversation is one that challenges me. I know from personal experience that not all police officers are bad, and not all police officers are heroes. But some are. I've talked to some of my police officer friends about the killing of Mike Brown in particular, and their perspective is much different from a civilian perspective. I have to respect that, and hold the complexity of multiple perspectives while maintaining my own personal lens, which is informed by diverse stories that I've been privileged to know. When Judith responded to Simone by genuinely agreeing with her, it freed up the space for me to share my nuanced perspective on the police. As a Black woman, I can say that I know police officers who are making a positive difference, and I also have had clients who've been abused by police officers in the very station where I worked. This type of nuance is not easy to express in such a diverse audience, but having Judith and Simone openly share allowed me to do that.

Judith: Later in the workshop, a white participant discussed her attempts to connect with clients of color and characterized her attempts as 'lame.' She asked what our advice was about making a cross-cultural connection with clients. We validated her attempts, and I discussed my opinion that as white clinicians we need to demonstrate to our clients early on that we are open to talking about race and racism, and that we see racism exists in order to establish a safe place to talk with us. I offered specific ways to talk about current events with clients to indicate our values and our position on racism. But the most helpful comment came from Simone who told the white participant that simply acknowledging that we are trying to communicate across culture and are open to learning from our clients of color is a truly powerful way to connect. It seemed to me that this was also a moment of meaningful cross-cultural dialogue between colleagues.

Rebecca: It has been my experience that clients are often relieved to have their clinician name racism as a factor in their lives. However, this if often very difficult, particularly for White clinicians. Perhaps because of white guilt, perhaps because they don't know where to take the conversation, or perhaps because they don't know how to hold the conversation and simply sit with the despair and hopelessness that often accompanies these discussions.

Reflections on Our Learning

Judith: As Rebecca and I reflected on the presentation afterwards with the friend who had invited us, they pointed out to me that I had used a potentially conflictual interaction as an opportunity to act as a white ally who was open to hearing when I was wrong, or when I had offended someone of color. I reflected that it is only after 25 years of this work that I could gain that sort of perspective and respond the way I did. I also thought about how important it is that we white folks can bear witness to the pain and anger that some people of color experience, without responding out of guilt or defensiveness, but rather, truly validating that person and accepting that a legacy of racial injustice and violence has led them to the point they are at today.

Later, in talking with Rebecca further, I expressed that one of the reasons I had been able to make an attempt to connect with the participant was that Rebecca was there by my side. I knew that Rebecca understood my commitment to racial justice, and I knew she would support me in my efforts to connect with Simone. I felt truly grateful to be in partnership with Rebecca.

Rebecca: I shared with Judith that I did not feel any anxiety during her encounter with Simone. This mostly comes from my thorough trust of Judith, which I hope our audiences see and can provide some hopeful modeling of cross-cultural relationships. I knew that Judith would handle this situation gracefully, and I also wasn't left with the pressure of handling it by myself. I think the open way in which we addressed this disagreement, allowing space for multiple perspectives, is what needs to happen more in order for social justice to become a reality, which will require people from diverse backgrounds and different life experiences to come together in a common cause. This unity cannot happen without the open airing of grievances, disagreements and the exchange of different stories.

Rebecca: Lately I have been struggling with the feeling that talking, creating space to talk, is not enough. As a co-worker of mine said 'we need to do something.' I agree. But as another colleague often points out, we can rush to action without spending enough time in the relationship building. Without this, we don't even know what to do or where to do. If we don't understand what the problem is, what another person's story or experience is, how can we 'do something?' We cannot 'do' without first having knowledge and understanding. This is not just a goal, it is a process. The more we have space to share our stories with those who are different from ourselves, the more equipped we are to bridge gaps and help create lasting change. We must be committed to communicating our hurts and hearing the hurts of others so that we can work together to fight for social and racial justice.

References

Burkard, A.W., & Knox, S. (2004). Effect of therapist color-blindness on empathy and attributions in cross-cultural counseling. *Journal of Counseling Psychology, (51)*, 387–397. doi: 10.1037/0022-0167.51.4.387

Goosby, B. J., & Heidbrink, C. (2013). The transgenerational consequences of discrimination on African-American health outcomes. *Sociology Compass, 7/8*, 630-643. doi: 10.1111/soc4.12054

Harro, B. (2008). Updated version of the cycle of socialization (2000). In M. Adams, W. J. Blumenfeld, R. Castaneda, H. W. Hackman, M.L. Peters, X. Zuniga (eds.), *Readings for Diversity and Social Justice* (pp. 15–21). New York: Routledge.

Kwate, N. O., & Goodman, M. S. (2015). Cross-sectional and longitudinal effects of racism on mental health among residents of black neighborhoods in New York City. *American Journal of Public Health, 105*, 711–718.

Pottick, K. J., Kirk, S. A., Hsieh, D. K., & Tian, X. (2007). Judging mental disorders in youths: Effects of client, clinician, and contextual differences. *Journal of Consulting and Clinical Psychology, 75*, 1–8. doi: 10.1037/0022-006X.75.1.1

Soto J. A., Dawson-Andoh N. A., & BeLue, R. (2011).The relationship between perceived discrimination and generalized anxiety disorder among African Americans, Afro Caribbeans, and non-Hispanic Whites. *Journal of Anxiety Disorders, 25*, 258–265.

Transparency for Food Consumers

Nutrition Labeling and Food Oppression

Andrea Freeman

I. Introduction

Transparency for consumers through nutrition labeling should be the last, not the first, step in a transformative food policy that would reduce dramatic health disparities and raise the United States to the health standards of other nations with similar resources. Nonetheless, transparency in the food system is a key focal point of efforts to improve health by providing consumers with necessary information to make good nutritional choices, as well as to achieve sustainable food chains and ensure food safety and quality.[1] In fact, nutrition labeling on packaging and in restaurants is the centerpiece of policy designed to decrease obesity, a condition many health advocates consider to be the most urgent public health crisis of the twenty-first century.[2] The resulting increased transparency about food ingredients has led to some changes in industry practices and allowed many middle- and upper-income consumers to make informed choices about the products they purchase and consume. Unfortunately, however, research reveals that increased nutritional information does not improve health.

Most consumers do not use nutrition labeling to ameliorate their food choices, and those who do are already in good health. Further, low-income consumers who must select foods based entirely on availability and affordability derive few, if any, benefits from transparency. This is because their choices reflect structural conditions, not lack of information. Instead, transparency primarily benefits health-conscious, wealthier constituents as well as food corporations, which incur minimal costs from labeling in comparison to the expense that other, more impactful reforms would impose.

To eliminate or decrease socioeconomic and racial health disparities, structural changes that expand access to healthy food, regulate harmful food ingredients, and create opportunities for more active lifestyles are necessary. Therefore, to the extent that it replaces more meaningful structural reform, transparency's primacy in food policy deepens the health divide between wealthy and poor individuals, and between whites and other racial groups.[3] The immediate goal of transparency in the food system should accordingly not be to provide consumers with information about food ingredients and processes, but to expose the partnerships between the food industry and the government that lead food policy to prioritize private profit over public health.

This paper begins by describing nutrition labeling requirements and the research on their effectiveness. It then explores the obstacles that prevent information provision from effecting positive change. It interrogates how alliances between the government and corporations lead to food oppression, which arises from facially neutral laws and policies that disproportionately harm socially subordinated groups, and examines how racial stereotypes and popular perspectives on health exacerbate these harms. It concludes by proposing new directions in food policy that would render transparency more useful for all consumers and reduce health disparities.

II. Nutrition Labeling

Americans consume one third of their calories and spend half of their food budgets on food prepared outside the home.[4] This practice of eating pre-packaged and restaurant food, particularly from fast food establishments, correlates with obesity and other indicators of poor health.[5] In an attempt to improve the health outcomes associated with eating food cooked outside the home, Congress enacted Section 4205 of the Patient Protection and Affordable Care Act. This provision requires chain restaurants to list the calorie content of their standard food and drink items on menus and menu boards,[6] thereby ensuring that restaurant patrons receive information about menu items that overlaps with what manufacturers must display on packaged food products.[7]

Food manufacturers, under the Nutrition Labeling and Education Act (NLEA), must include a label titled "Nutrition Facts," displaying the amount of calories, sugars, fat, saturated fat, vitamins A and C, calcium, iron, fiber, and carbohydrates contained in a packaged food product.[8] Manufacturers may also voluntarily post other nutritional content.[9] In 2014, the Food and Drug Administration (FDA) proposed amendments to the NLEA that would create a new line on the label for added sugars (previous labels did not distinguish between added and natural sugars, such as those that come from fruit); adjust the serving size to reflect realistic portions; and make the calorie count more visible.[10] Many food and health advocates view these amendments as an important victory for consumers.[11]

Research reveals, however, that nutrition labels and restaurant calorie counts have little or no impact on consumer choice and health.[12] Both teenagers and adults notice calorie counts when restaurants provide them, but neither group alters their food selection in response.[13] Similarly, behavioral economic strategies designed to encourage healthy selections by making certain products more accessible and prominent in lunchrooms or restaurants do not appear to reduce overall caloric consumption, and instead may, in some instances, increase it.[14] For example, one study demonstrated that consumers did, in fact, make healthier selections based on the addition of healthy items to a fast food restaurant menu.[15] Nonetheless, they then compensated for making a healthy choice, such as a sandwich instead of a burger, by adding an unhealthy item, such as fries or a milkshake, to their meal.[16] Ironically, the healthy selection served to assuage the consumer's guilt about unhealthy eating, opening the door to further unhealthy choices. Similarly, another study found that adding a healthy option, like a salad, to an otherwise unhealthy fast food menu increases selections of unhealthy products even when the consumer does not purchase and consume the salad.[17] Merely viewing the healthy option on the menu satisfies the eater's need for good health practices.[18]

Nutrition labels on packaged foods sold in stores also do not appear to improve health outcomes by reducing consumers' intake of calories, saturated fats, or sodium.[19] Instead, the evidence suggests that labeling only facilitates better choices for middle and high-income consumers, the Whole Foods shoppers who already engage in healthy eating habits. Consequently, the labels fail to result in an overall change in consumer health.[20] In addition to socioeconomic class, gender can determine the use and effect of labeling. Women are more likely than men to read nutrition labels[21] and, while women usually use nutritional information to attempt to lose weight, men often employ it to increase their caloric intake, or "bulk up."[22]

However, although nutrition label requirements appear to have only a minimal impact on consumer health and behavior, they do influence the conduct of manufacturers, who sometimes reformulate ingredients in anticipation of new rules to gain a competitive advantage. Several large food companies, for example, altered their products in reaction to trans fat labeling requirements[23] and the 2005 Dietary Guidelines' recommendations of a specific daily intake of whole grains.[24] Additionally, changes implemented in response to the guidelines' advice to eat foods lower in fat content significantly increased the market share of fat-modified cheese products and cookies.[25] Chain restaurants similarly reacted to labeling requirements by reducing the calories in many of their non-core menu items.[26] It is not clear, however, that these changes by manufacturers and restaurants result in better health outcomes for consumers, as more nutritious products may only appeal to already health-conscious consumers.[27] Moreover, in a phenomenon branded "the Snackwell's effect," some people binge on foods, such as low-fat Snackwell's cookies, in the mistaken belief that these foods are healthy due to their low-fat content.[28] In fact, the reverse is true, as these types of foods usually contain high amounts of sugar and chemicals that disrupt metabolism and engender other negative health consequences.[29] Increased production of foods labeled low-fat and, by implication, healthy, can therefore lead to poorer health outcomes.

Nutrition labels may similarly contribute to this type of consumer confusion because the information they present is difficult to decipher.[30] To improve consumers' comprehension, an

FDA study recommends that, instead of dividing calories and other nutritional content into servings, labels should post the total number of calories that are in the package.[31] Even with this improvement, however, it is likely that consumers would not fully understand the significance of the numbers that appear on labels cross-listed with calories and other food components. Clearer labeling might, however, lead to significant changes. For example, David Kessler, the former commissioner of the FDA who designed and oversaw the implementation of the first nutrition label, proposes that instead of displaying the required information on the side of packaged foods, manufacturers should prominently feature the three top ingredients, the number of calories per serving, and the amount of additional ingredients on the front of packages.[32] Research demonstrates that this type of plain language can alter consumer behavior. For example, in one study, six Baltimore convenience stores posted large, brightly colored signs on refrigerators containing sweetened beverages that stated how long it would take to walk off the calories in each drink.[33] There was a corresponding drop from 98% of adolescent shoppers choosing sugary beverages to 89%.[34]

Similarly, a study conducted at Massachusetts General Hospital cafeteria labeled foods with red, yellow, and green symbols intended to evoke responses to food items ordinarily associated with traffic symbols.[35] Green (go) signified the healthiest options, including fruits and vegetables; yellow (proceed with caution) indicated a need for moderation in consuming those foods; and red (stop) signaled items containing little or no nutritional value.[36] To boost these symbols' effectiveness, posted signs encouraged customers to choose according to the colors and provided more detailed nutritional information.[37] This experiment led to significant decreases in purchases of red items and corresponding increases in the selection of green items.[38] Despite these promising results, however, nutrition labeling in any form faces a number of serious limitations to its potential to alter behavior and health for most consumers.

III. Obstacles to the Effectiveness of Nutrition Labeling

There are a multitude of factors that contribute to individuals' decisions regarding what foods to buy and consume, of which nutrition labeling is only one. Therefore, even when consumers have the luxury—in terms of time, resources, and choice—to consider nutrition information, external factors may inhibit the usefulness of this information. For example, behavioral economics research indicates that the acquisition of information simply may not have the power to increase self-control, particularly when a person is hungry.[39] Further, individuals tend toward impulsivity in food selection, which allows environmental factors at the point of purchase, such as colors, smells, and product positioning, to exert greater influence over decision-making than rational thinking about diet and health.[40] Finally, people possess a limited capacity to process new information that may be exhausted when the time to make food choices arrives.[41]

Food preferences are also resistant to change because the food industry has invested millions in perfecting the exact measurements and proportion of sugar, salt, and fat that will render a food addictive.[42] This addiction is powerful enough to overcome rational thinking about the health impact of consuming a food perfectly balanced in sugar, salt, and fat, such as McDonald's McGriddles, a breakfast sandwich consisting of egg, bacon, and cheese layered between two sweet pancakes studded with syrup. Further, food corporations devote extensive resources to studying how to motivate consumption once hunger is satiated.[43] They use the results of these studies to develop marketing tactics that successfully increase the desire to eat junk food, such as M&Ms, regardless of the body's lack of need for surplus calories.[44]

Even more importantly, for many consumers, taste, price, and convenience matter more than nutritional content.[45] Moreover, although price and convenience are salient factors in all consumers' food decisions, they are determinative for those who lack access to a range of foods. For example, most individuals living in low-income urban communities have seen their grocery stores relocated to suburbs.[46] These distant locations often do not fall on bus or train lines.[47] In their place, corner stores sell poor quality produce at inflated prices.[45] These establishments usually sell only one brand of each type of food offered, such as soup stock or pasta, making choice based on nutritional content impossible. The fact that these products often contain harmful preservatives that increase shelf life further compounds this harm.[49]

Additionally, the predominance of fast food restaurants in these neighborhoods ensures that residents have no alternatives to the unhealthy, high calorie items on offer.[50] Realistically, fast and cheap junk foods often represent the most prudent choice for individuals who must struggle to stretch thin food budgets to maximize the intake of calories required to fulfill overwhelming work and family responsibilities. Finally, public schools provide students with an array of unhealthy foods in their lunchrooms, often as a result of the USDA's need to support subsidized commodities, such as meat, dairy, wheat, rice, corn, and soybeans, the last two primarily through secondary markets of high fructose corn syrup and oils.[51]

All of these structural factors prevent nutrition labeling from improving food choices and health for individuals living on or near the poverty line. In 2013, more than fourteen million people in the United States lived in poverty, and many others lived in near-poverty.[52] Members of racialized groups, such as Blacks, Latinos, Indians, Native Hawaiians and Pacific Islanders are overrepresented among the poor and in federal nutrition programs.[53] Therefore, to the extent that food policy focuses on nutrition labeling and other strategies targeted at individuals to improve health, instead of structural reform, that policy is a manifestation of food oppression.

IV. Food Oppression

Food oppression is institutional, systemic, food-related action or policy that physically debilitates a socially subordinated group.[54] It is present where there is a facially neutral law, policy, or government action that disproportionately harms a socially marginalized group that experiences health disparities in food and nutrition-related deaths and diseases. To constitute food oppression, the law, policy, or action must result at least in part from corporate influence, and the disproportionate harm that it causes must erroneously appear to arise from cultural or individual, not structural, factors, because of racial stereotypes and mistaken beliefs about what motivates or causes health-related choices and outcomes.[55] Food oppression falls heaviest on individuals who experience marginalization along multiple axes, including race, class, gender, sexuality, ability, age, gender identity, and immigration status.[56]

Facially, The policy choice to showcase nutrition labeling and other strategies directed toward influencing individual behavior, such as education and behavioral economics, is a race-neutral one. Although there is some recognition of racial health disparities in government literature outlining objectives for improving health outcomes, such as Healthy People 2020,[57] laws and regulations that mandate labeling and other information provision do so in a completely race-neutral way, focusing solely on manufacturers' and restaurant owners' duties, not consumers' social identities. Despite this appearance of neutrality, however, the impact of this policy choice falls heaviest on the communities who face the greatest structural obstacles to healthy eating. These communities include residents of low-income, urban Black and Latino neighborhoods and individuals living on lands colonized by the United States, including Hawai'i and Puerto Rico, among others.

The adverse impact of nutrition labeling on marginalized communities manifests itself in several ways. At best, nutrition labeling has no effect on most members of these communities, because they simply are not in a position to exercise choice in food selection based on nutritional content due to the environmental and financial constraints described above. This absence of impact is not, however, an absence of harm, because the harm is located in the focus on nutrition labeling, not the degree to which it influences consumer behavior. Policy designed to improve health by altering consumer conduct effectively obfuscates and negates the primacy of structural determinants of health, and stands in the way of meaningful reform.

Identifying nutrition labeling as an essential pathway to improving health supports the popular misperception that good health reflects a combination of sufficient information, intelligence, and willpower. Society commonly reads robust health as a manifestation of an individual's positive characteristics. However, this widely held belief is wrong on both broad and narrow scales. Social psychology reveals, for example, that personality predicts very few, if any, of the decisions we make.[58] Instead, studies demonstrate, we respond to situations in pre-determined ways unrelated to what we consider to be our own, particularized philosophies and perspectives, or disposition.[59] This insight is especially relevant in the context of food because external factors almost entirely shape access to healthy food and, even where some degree of choice exists, social position and financial conditions created by historical and present discrimination circumscribe those choices.

Some of the historical events and present conditions that relegate certain groups to poverty and ill health are slavery; the invasion, occupation, and colonization of island nations; the theft of land from indigenous and Mexican people; the perpetuation of racial myths and stereotypes through media and popular culture; punitive and restrictive immigration laws; devaluing of Black and Latino/a lives by law enforcement and the criminal justice system; and an inadequate social safety net. Although advocates for both food and social justice often do not draw these connections, all of these powerful forces play a part in determining communities' and individuals' ability to eat in a way that sustains good health. The obfuscation of these links allows for an insistence on nutrition labeling as a solution to poor eating and bad health that perpetuates harmful myths about the importance of information and willpower in relation to food selection.

Further, focusing on individual agency instead of the roles played by corporate and government actors in limiting food choices reduces the likelihood that the government will enact structural reform. The conclusion to this paper proposes a number of steps that the government could take to improve the health of marginalized communities and reduce health disparities. Under the health paradigm exemplified by the promotion of nutrition labeling as a primary solution to poor health, however, these strategies would be ineffective because individuals will continue to make bad food choices arising from their personal deficiencies. Therefore, by reinforcing common understandings of food-related health conditions, information provision serves as a panacea and distraction from the potential for more meaningful change through stricter regulation of food companies and government nutrition programs.

There are significant racial and socioeconomic health disparities that buttress the contention that food policy focused on consumer behavior disproportionately harms socially marginalized communities. Blacks, Latina/os, Indians, Pacific Islanders, Native Hawaiians and other racialized groups[60] experience greater health problems than whites.[61] Specifically, there are pronounced racial disparities in diseases and deaths related to food and nutrition, including obesity diagnoses,[62] high blood pressure,[63] diabetes,[64] high cholesterol,[65] and cancers.[66] Many factors contribute to these disparities, including access to care, racial bias in treatment, environmental harms prevalent in segregated neighborhoods, mass incarceration, medical research priorities, colonialism, and correlation with poverty.[67] Food policy that focuses on consumer behavior is another important factor that is instrumental in creating and widening health disparities.

In the United States, a desire to satisfy the interests of the food and agricultural industries drives much of food policy. These industries derive their influence over policy through campaign contributions,[68] lobbying,[69] and a revolving door between corporate and administrative positions.[70] Their efforts yield impressive results, including control over the wording of the federal Dietary Guidelines;[71] low standards for school lunches, despite considerable public pressure to increase them;[72] subsidization of food commodities that leads to unhealthy eating habits;[73] and the dismantling of pesticide regulations, even where legislatures have voted to maintain them.[74]

Significantly, nutrition labeling imposes relatively small costs on food corporations in terms of printing and posting and, in its present form, appears not to lead to lost sales. Therefore, in comparison with other possible laws and regulations designed to improve health, such as the removal of harmful chemical preservatives from packaged foods, nutrition labeling is a bargain for food corporations. Nonetheless, the industry remains vigilant in its efforts to minimize the reach and impact of food labeling laws. For example, movie theatres, after extensive lobbying by the National Association of Theatre Owners, remain exempt from nutrition labeling require-ments imposed on other food sellers, despite the high content of unhealthy oils in movie theater popcorn.[75] Similarly, food companies have so far successfully lobbied to prevent the adoption of David Kessler's proposal to require clearer and more prominently placed nutrition labels.[76] The content and form of nutrition labeling requirements thus appear to be additional manifestations of corporate influence over government policy.

The success of corporations in achieving their food policy goals, however, relies in part on public acquiescence to the health paradigms underlying government efforts to combat obesity and other health problems. These public perceptions of the proper path to better health arise from popular and pervasive framing of health issues as products of individual decisions.[77] This type of blaming is most apparent in the context of weight and obesity, where it is common to associate excessive weight with poor eating choices,[78] despite evidence that corporations play a significant and deliberate role in causing and perpetuating obesity.[79] Even before the obesity crisis, however, people associated illness with poor choices. For example, the attribution of AIDS transmission to the choice to lead a gay lifestyle and the homophobia this perspective embodied led to tragic consequences, as the government delayed funding for AIDS research while thousands of people died.[80]

In fact, it is rare for the public to associate sickness with environmental and structural factors under any circumstances. For example, even when communities experience the harmful side effects of industrial pollution, they often become marginalized and blamed for their own ill health. This allows corporations to exploit racism and indifference to poverty by deliberately locating their most toxic enterprises in poor neighborhoods of color, where others will associate the resulting harms to health with the residents' social defects instead of the companies' acts.[81] Similarly, support for nutrition labeling stems from an internalized belief that people are re-sponsible for their own health and an optimistic view that sufficient information will transform shopping and eating habits. Unfortunately, however, even the most detailed and prominently placed information cannot alter the structural forces and corporate tactics that determine eating habits.

Popular views about the relationship between eating, weight, and personality traits receive reinforcement from the proliferation of racial stereotypes that portray obesity and related health conditions as endemic to certain groups. For example, most overweight characters on television are Black.[82] one example of a common racial trope in television is the "sassy Black woman."[83] An overweight version of this character first appeared on shows from the 1970s and 1980s, such as *What's Happening!!,*[84] *Good Times,*[85] and *Gimme a Break!.*[86] More recent popular shows, including *How I Met Your Mother,*[87] *The Big C,*[88] and *Glee,*[89] continue to feature her. The negative implications of this sassy Black woman's weight (that she is lazy and unattractive) diminish her positive qualities (that she is outspoken and honest).

Similar stereotypes about Hawaiians and Pacific Islanders lead to discrimination based on weight that can lead to serious health consequences and social neglect.[90] For example, a study of Tongans and Pacific Islanders living in the United States revealed their frustrations in dealing with a Western doctor fixated on their obesity.[91] One participant in the study explained, "In reality, our wellness challenge is not obesity, but to live and work in the U.S. legally, obtain decent paying jobs with safe working conditions, have access to caring legal representation, and to tap into opportunities for education and quality child care for our children so they can go to college instead of being victims of community violence."[92]

Moreover, obesity and related health problems among Native Hawaiians arise from the disruption of their diets after the American overthrow of their monarchy that led to the near obliteration of traditional food practices.[93] After its subsequent occupation of the Hawaiian Islands, the United States sought to increase consumption of American junk foods, such as spam, and eliminate reliance on locally grown, traditional foods.[94] The solution to Native Hawaiians' poor diets thus lies in complex approaches to sovereignty and independence, not consumer education.

Other popular racial stereotypes, such as the welfare queen,[95] also mask the realities faced by individuals with limited or no access to privilege and political process. This stereotype suggests that poor black mothers are greedy, lazy, and indifferent to their children's wellbeing, instead of constrained by racism and poverty. All of the factors outlined above—the facially neutral character of nutrition labeling that belies its disproportionate impact on marginalized communities; significant racial and socioeconomic health disparities; successful efforts by food and agricultural corporations to influence food policy; and pervasive perspectives on health combined with racial stereotypes that create the illusion of personal responsibility for health and discourage structural reform—establish that the primacy of nutrition labeling in federal food policy is a form of food oppression. The conclusion of this Article offers a few proposals to dismantle or mitigate the effects of this oppression.

V. Conclusion

There are a number of directions food policy could take that would reduce health disparities and improve health outcomes generally. All of them involve change relating to corporate or government, not individual, conduct. First, and most importantly, the FDA and the USDA should operate independently of industry influence. Public health should be their top priority. This mandate should guide reforms that include: de-subsidization of commodities that fuel the markets for non-nutritious foods such as fast food, sweetened beverages, and processed foods; bans of extremely harmful food additives; limits on food ingredients linked to less serious but problematic health conditions; the establishment of higher standards for school lunches and other government assistance programs, including the elimination of the distribution of unhealthy foods through the Women, Infants and Children Nutrition Program (WIC); government-sponsored efforts to increase access to healthy food in all communities through financial support for grocery stores in underserved areas; minimum healthy food requirements for stores that are the sole purveyors of produce in food deserts; government funding for farmers markets, community supported agriculture programs, and urban agriculture; the building of playgrounds, recreation centers, and parks in depressed neighborhoods accompanied by efforts to keep these spaces safe for children and youth to play; and tangible support for traditional agriculture in Hawai'i and Puerto Rico.

Although altering many of the factors responsible for health disparities requires social movements and change at the highest level of politics, it is possible that greater awareness of the structural determinants of food choice would bring the United States closer to meaningful structural reform. Therefore, education through media and other forms of popular culture about these problems from a critical race and class perspective is important. Coalition building across social justice groups is also essential to the formation of a broader, critical food justice movement. to the extent that labeling can do some good, it should be clear and direct. Finally, where food consumers lack choice, the government's responsibility is not merely to provide information, but to implement change until that choice comes into being.

Notes

1 *See generally* Archon Fung et al., THE POLITICAL ECONOMY OF TRANSPARENCY: WHAT MAKES DISCLOSURE POLICIES EFFECTIVE? 16 (2004); Gerhard Schiefer & Jivka Deiters, TRANSPARENCY FOR SUSTAINABILITY IN THE FOOD CHAIN: CHALLENGES AND RESEARCH NEEDS (2013); Laura E. Derr, *When Food is Poison: The History, Consequences and Limitations of the Food Allergen Labeling and Consumer Protection Act of 2004*, 61 FOOD DRUG L.J. 65 (2006). Groups that advocate for transparency in the food system, with a recent emphasis on GMO labeling, include: Food Integrity Now, Just Label It, Food Democracy Now, Massachusetts Right to Know GMOs, Project Transparent Food, Center for Food Safety, Project on Government Oversight, Non GMO Project, Food Integrity Campaign, Right to Know GMO, and Food and Water Watch. *See, e.g.*, Lydia Zuraw, *Food Industry Association Plans to Make GRAS More Transparent*, FOOD SAFETY NEWS (Aug. 29, 2014), http://www.foodsafetynews.com/2014/08/gma-plans-to-make-gras-more-transparent/#.VFPpS8npdrV. Michelle Obama's " Let's Move" campaign also incorporates nutrition labeling. *See* A.J. Pearlman, *Helping Families Make Healthier Choices: FDA to Update Nutrition Facts Label*, LET'S MOVE BLOG (Feb. 27, 2014), http://www.letsmove.gov/blog/2014/02/27/helping-families-make-healthier-choices-fda-update-nutrition-facts-label.

2 *See e.g.*, Snejana Farberov, *Genesis of a National Plague: How Modern America's Obesity Epidemic Began in the 1950s and How Charting the Weight Loss Struggles of a 205lb Aspiring Nurse Helped Bring the Problem to the Forefront*, DAILY MAIL, July 19, 2013, *available at* http://www.dailymail.co.uk/

news/article-2371051/How-modern-Americas-obesity-epidemic-began-1950s.html; *An Epidemic of Obesity: U.S. Obesity Trends,* The Nutrition Source, Harvard School of Public Health, http://www.hsph.harvard.edu/nutritionsource/an-epidemic-of-obesity/ (last visited March 23, 2015); OBESITY (Gerald Litwack ed., Amsterdam: Elsevier Academic Press, 2013); OBESITY (Scott Barbour, ed., Farmington Hills, MI: Greenhaven Press, 2011); MABEL BLADES, OBESITY, Bradford Emerald Group Publishing (2005); ALEXANDRA A. BREWIS, OBESITY, Piscataway, N.J.: Rutgers University Press (2010); Adam Gilden Tsai and Thomas A. Wadden, *Obesity,* 159 ANNALS INTERNAL MED. ITC3-1-ITC3-15 (2013); David W. Haslam and W. Phillip T. James, *Obesity,* 366 LANCET 1197–1209 (2005); Susan Z. Yanovski and Zack A. Yanovski, *Obesity,* 346 NEW ENGLAND J. MED. 591–602 (2002); Richard Barnett, *Obesity,* 366 LANCET 984 (2005); David Arterburn, *Obesity,* 66 AM. FAM. PHYSICIAN 1279–80 (2002); Michael Rosenbaum, et al., 337 NEW ENGLAND J. MED 396–407 (1997); Per Björntorp, *Obesity,* 350 LANCET 423–26 (1997); F. SASSI, OBESITY AND THE ECONOMICS OF PREVENTION: FIT NOT FAT, Paris: Organisation for Economic Co-operation and Development (2010); A.H. BARNETT AND SUDHESH KUMAR, OBESITY AND DIABETES, Hoboken, N.J.: John Wiley & Sons (2004); JEFFERY KOPLAN, ET AL., PREVENTING CHILDHOOD OBESITY: HEALTH IN THE BALANCE, Washington, DC: National Academies Press (2005); EXPERT PANEL ON THE IDENTIFICATION, EVALUATION, AND TREATMENT OF OVERWEIGHT AND OBESITY IN ADULTS (U.S.), CLINICAL GUIDELINES ON THE IDENTIFICATION, EVALUATION, AND TREATMENT OF OVERWEIGHT AND OBESITY IN ADULTS: THE EVIDENCE REPORT, Bethesda, M.D.: National Institutes of Health, National Heart, Lung, and Blood Institute (1998); JEFFERY KOPLAN, PROGRESS IN PREVENTING CHILDHOOD OBESITY: HOW DO WE MEASURE UP?, Washington, D.C.: National Academies Press (2007).

3 *See* Takehiro Sugiyami & Martin F. Shapiro, *The Growing Socioeconomic Disparity in Dietary Quality: Mind the Gap,* 174 JAMA INTERNAL MED. 1595, 1595–96 (2014).

4 Kiyah Duffey et al., *Differential Associations of Fast Food and Restaurant Food Consumption With 3-y Change in Body Mass Index: The Coronary Artery Risk Development in Young Adults Study,* 85 AM. J. CLINICAL NUTRITION 201, 201 (2007).

5 *See generally* Shanthy A. Bowman & Bryan T. Vinyard, *Fast Food Consumption of U.S. Adults: Impact on Energy and Nutrient Intakes and Overweight Status,* 23 J. AM. C. NUTRITION 163 (2004); Duffey et al., *supra* note 4, at 201; S.A. French et al., *Fast Food Restaurant Use Among Women in the Pound of Prevention Study: Dietary, Behavioral and Demographic Correlates,* 24 INT'L J. OBESITY 1353 (2000); Megan A. McCrory et al., *Overeating in America: Association Between Restaurant Food Consumption and Body Fatness in Healthy Adult Men and Women Ages 19 to 80,* 7 OBESITY RES. 564 (1999); Mark A. Pereira et al., *Fast-Food Habits, Weight Gain, and Insulin Resistance (the CARDIA Study): 15-Year Prospective Analysis,* 365 LANCET 36 (2005); Jessie A. Satia et al., *Eating at Fast-Food Restaurants Is Associated with Dietary Intake: Demographic, Psychosocial and Behavioural Factors Among African Americans in North Carolina,* 7 PUB. HEALTH NUTRITION 1089 (2004); O. M. Thompson et al., *Food Purchased away from Home As a Predictor of Change in BMI Z-Score Among Girls,* 28 INT'L J. OBESITY 282 (2004).

6 *See Menu and Vending Machines Labeling Requirements,* FDA, http://www.fda.gov/Food/IngredientsPackagingLabeling/LabelingNutrition/ucm217762.htm (last updated Mar. 12, 2015). A

chain restaurant is one that has twenty or more locations. *See id.* The requirements also apply to vending machines operators with more than twenty machines and allows for restaurants or vendors with fewer than twenty locations to register for voluntary regulation. *See id.* Other nutrient information must be provided to consumers upon written request. In 2014, coverage expanded to movie theatres and grocery stores. *See* Food Labeling; Nutrition Labeling of Standard Menu Items in Restaurants and Similar Retail Food Establishments, 79 Fed. Reg. 71,156, 71,157 (Dec. 1, 2014) (to be codified at 21 C.F.R. pt. 11, 101).

7 *See* Food Labeling; Nutrition Labeling of Standard Menu Items in Restaurants and Similar Retail Food Establishments, 79 Fed. Reg. at 71,229.

8 FDA, NUTRITIONAL LABELING AND EDUCATION ACT (NLEA) REQUIREMENTS (8/94–2/95) 17 (1994), *available at* http://www.fda.gov/iceci/inspections/inspectionguides/ucm074948. htm; FDA, GUIDANCE FOR INDUSTRY: A FOOD LABELING GUIDE (7. NUTRITION LABELING; QUESTIONS G1 THROUGH P8) 2 (2013), *available at* http://www.fda.gov/Food/GuidanceRegulation/ GuidanceDocumentsRegulatoryInformation/LabelingNutritio n/ucm064894.htm.

9 FDA, GUIDANCE FOR INDUSTRY, *supra* note 8, at 2–3.

10 Sabrina Tavernise, *New F.D.A. Nutrition Labels Would Make 'Serving Sizes' Reflect Actual Servings*, N.Y. TIMES (Feb. 27, 2014), http://www.nytimes.com/2014/02/27/health/new-fda-nutrition-labels-would-make-serving-sizes-reflect-actual-servings.html.

11 *See id.*

12 *See, e.g.*, Bryan Bollinger et al., *Calorie Posting in Chain Restaurants* 2 (Nat'l Bureau of Econ. Research, Working Paper No. 15,648, 2010) (observing a 6% drop in calories per transaction at Starbucks locations that posted nutritional information, but suggesting this would only have a small impact on obesity, although it may encourage restaurants to offer more low calorie options or accustom consumes to calorie counting); LISA MANCINO & JEAN KINSEY, USDA, IS DIETARY KNOWLEDGE ENOUGH? HUNGER, STRESS, AND OTHER ROADBLOCKS TO HEALTHY EATING 2–4 (2008), *available at* http://www.ers.usda.gov/publications/err-economic-research-report/err62.aspx#.UyON3YXpdrU (finding that eating away from home and with long period between meals reduces the influence of cognitive dietary information). *See generally* Brian Elbel et al., *Calorie Labeling and Food Choices: A First Look at the Effects on Low-Income People in New York City*, 28 HEALTH AFF. W1110 (2009), *available at* http://www.ncbi.nlm.nih.gov/pubmed/19808705; Brian Elbel et al., *Child and Adolescent Fast-Food Choice and the Influence of Calorie Labeling: A Natural Experiment*, 35 INT'L J. OBESITY 493 (2011) [hereinafter *Child and Adolescent Fast-Food Choice*]; Rosanna Mentzer Morrison et al., USDA, *Will Calorie Labeling in Restaurants Make a Difference?*, USDA (Mar. 11, 2011), http://www.ers.usda. gov/amber-waves/2011-march/will-calorie-labeling.aspx#.UyN6d4XpdrW.

13 Elbel, *Child and Adolescent Fast-Food Choice, supra* note 12, at 496–97.

14 *See, e.g.*, Keith Wilcox et al., *Vicarious Goal Fulfillment: When the Mere Presence of a Healthy Option Leads To an Ironically Indulgent Decision*, 36 J. CONSUMER RES. 380, 381 (2009); Jessica Wisdom et al., *Promoting Healthy Choices: Information Versus Convenience*, 2 AM. ECON. J.: APPLIED ECON. 164, 165 (2010).

15 Wisdom, *supra* note 14, at 164.

16 *Id.* at 170.

17 Wilcox, *supra* note 14, at 382.

18 *Id.* at 381.

19 *See* Morrison, *supra* note 12; Jayachandran N. Variyam, *Do Nutrition Labels Improve Dietary Outcomes?*, 17 HEALTH ECON. 695, 701, 704 (2008).

20 *See* JAYACHANDRAN N. VARIYAM, NUTRITION LABELING IN THE FOOD-AWAY-FROM-HOME SECTOR: AN ECONOMIC ASSESSMENT, USDA, ERS (2005), *available at* http://webarchives.cdlib.org/sw1tx36512/http:/www.ers.usda.gov/Publications/ERR4; Wisdom, *supra* note 14, at 164.

21 *See* Judy A. Driskell et al., *Using Nutrition Labeling As a Potential Tool for Changing Eating Habits of University Dining Hall Patrons*, 108 J. AM. DIETETIC ASS'N 2071, 2072 (2008); Ranjita Misra, *Knowledge, Attitudes, and Label Use Among College Students*, 107 J. AM. DIETETIC ASS'N 2130, 2131 (2007).

22 *See* Jacqueline I. Aaron et al., *Paradoxical Effect of a Nutrition Labeling Scheme in a Student Cafeteria*, 15 NUTRITION RES. 1251, 1256 (1995); Martha T. Conklin et al., *College Students' Use of Point of Selection Nutrition Information*, 20 TOPICS CLINICAL NUTRITION 97, 98 (2005); Lisa J. Harnack et al., *Effects of Calorie Labeling and Value Size Pricing on Fast Food Meal Choices: Results from an Experimental Trial*, 5 INT'L J. BEHAV. NUTRITION & PHYSICAL ACTIVITY 1, 3 (2008).

23 Elise Golan et al., *Food Policy: Check the List of Ingredients*, USDA AMBER WAVES (June 2009), *available at* http://webarchives.cdlib.org/sw1tx36512/http:/www.ers.usda.gov/AmberWaves/June09/Features/FoodPolicy.htm.

24 *See* Lisa Mancino et al., *Getting Consumers to Eat More Whole-Grains: The Role of Policy, Information, and Food Manufacturers*, 33 FOOD POL'Y 489, 494 (2008).

25 *See* KEYSTONE CTR., THE KEYSTONE FORUM ON AWAY-FROM-HOME FOODS: OPPORTUNITIES FOR PREVENTING WEIGHT GAIN AND OBESITY 73 (2006), *available at* http://archive.oxha.org/knowledge/publications/us_keystone-center-obesity-forum_may-2006.pdf ("Between 1991 (before the implementation of the NLEA) and 1995 (after implementation), the number of available fat-modified cheese products tripled, and the market share for fat-modified cookies increased from zero percent of the market to 15%.").

26 *See* Sara N. Bleich et al., *Calorie Changes in Chain Restaurant Menu Items*, 48 AM. J. PREVENTIVE MED. 70, 73 (2015).

27 *See id.* at 75.

28 *See, e.g.*, Michael Pollan, *Omnivore's Solution*, Otis Lecture at Bates College (Oct. 27, 2008), *available at* http://www.bates.edu/food/foods-importance/omnivores-solution.

29 *See generally* NINA TEICHOLZ, THE BIG FAT SURPRISE: WHY BUTTER, MEAT AND CHEESE BELONG IN A HEALTHY DIET (2014).

30 *See Can Changes in Nutrition Labeling Help Consumers Make Better Food Choices?*, ELSEVIER (Jan. 23, 2013), http://www.elsevier.com/about/press-releases/research-and-journals/can-changes-in-nutrition-labeling-help-consumers-make-better-food-choices; Amy Lando & Serena Lo,

Single-Larger-Portion-Size and Dual-Column Nutrition Labeling May Help Consumers Make More Healthful Food Choices, 113 J. ACAD. NUTRITION & DIETETICS 241 (2013), *available at* http://www.sciencedirect.com.eres.library.manoa.hawaii.edu/science/article/pii/S2212267212018187; *Nutrition Facts Food Labels Are Too Confusing for Most People, FDA Researchers Say*, N.Y. DAILY NEWS (Jan. 24, 2013), http://www.nydailynews.com/life-style/health/food-labels-confuse-people-fda-study-article-1.1246816 (reporting on an FDA study recommending that labels state the nutritional content per package instead of per serving to reduce consumer confusion).

31 *See* Lando & Lo, *supra* note 30, at 244.

32 *See* David A. Kessler, *Toward More Comprehensive Food Labeling*, 371 NEW ENG. J. MED. 193, 194 (2014).

33 *See* Sara N. Bleich et al., *Reducing Sugar-Sweetened Beverage Consumption by Providing Caloric Information: How Black Adolescents Alter Their Purchases and Whether the Effects Persist*, 104 AM. J. PUB. HEALTH 2417, 2417 (2014).

34 *See* Sara N. Bleich et al., *Diet-Beverage Consumption and Caloric Intake Among US Adults, Overall and by Body Weight*, 104 AM. J. PUB. HEALTH, e72, e72 (2014); Sara N. Bleich et al., *supra* note 33, at 2417; *see also I Have To Walk How Many Miles to Burn Off This Soda?*, JOHNS HOPKINS BLOOMBERG SCH. PUB. HEALTH (Oct. 16, 2014), http://www.jhsph.edu/news/news-releases/2014/i-have%20to-walk-how-many-miles%20to-burn-off-this-soda.html. It is still problematic, however, that almost 90% of teenagers entering the store purchased an unhealthy sweetened beverage.

35 *See* Sue McGreevey, Mass. Gen. Hosp., *Enlightened Eating: Color-Coded Labels, Rearranged Items Encourage Healthy Choices in Study*, HARV. GAZETTE (Jan. 19, 2012), http://news.harvard.edu/gazette/story/2012/01/enlightened-eating.

36 *Id.*

37 *Id.*

38 *Id.*

39 *See, e.g.*, NICOLE LARSON & MARY STORY, ROBERT WOOD JOHNSON FOUND., MENU LABELING: DOES PROVIDING NUTRITION INFORMATION AT THE POINT OF PURCHASE AFFECT CONSUMER BEHAVIOR? 1, 3 (2009) ("Although consumers want nutrition information to be available, several other factors, aside from nutrition concerns, influence their menu selections. Most notably, food prices, taste and convenience are frequently reported as important influences on menu selections, and these factors are often at odds with healthful eating."); *see also* Melissa A. Z. Knoll, *The Role of Behavioral Economics and Behavioral Decision Making in Americans' Retirement Savings Decisions*, 70 SOC. SEC. BULL. 1, 2 (2010), *available at* http://www.ssa.gov/policy/docs/ssb/v70n4/v70n4p1.html (noting in the context of retirement savings that "[e]ven if decision makers had complete and accurate information … empirical findings suggest that they would still make suboptimal savings decisions as a result of issues related to the second category, heuristics and biases").

40 *See* DAVID R. JUST ET AL., USDA, COULD BEHAVIORAL ECONOMICS HELP IMPROVE DIET QUALITY FOR NUTRITION ASSISTANCE PARTICIPANTS? 14–15 (2007), *available at* http://www.ers.usda.gov/

publications/err-economic-research-report/err43.aspx#.UyNeyoXpdrV; Nanette Stroebele & John M. DeCastro, *Effect of Ambience on Food Intake and Food Choice*, 20 NUTRITION 821, 821 (2004).

41 Julie S. Downs et al., *Strategies for Promoting Healthier Food Choices*, 99 AM. ECON. REV.: PAPERS & PROCEEDINGS 159, 159 (2009), http://www-personal.umich.edu/~prestos/Downloads/DC/pdfs/Downs_Sept22_Downsetal2009.pdf.

42 *See* MICHAEL MOSS, SALT SUGAR FAT: HOW THE FOOD GIANTS HOOKED US xxv–xxvi (2013).

43 *See* Kelly Gurley Lambert et al., *Food-Related Stimuli Increase Desire to Eat in Hungry and Satiated Human Subjects*, 10 CURRENT PSYCHOL.: RES. & REVS. 297, 297–98 (1991), *available at* http://link.springer.com/article/10.1007%2FBF02686902#page-1.

44 *Id.*

45 *See generally* Cheryl L. Albright et al., *Restaurant Menu Labeling: Impact of Nutrition Information on Entree Sales and Patron Attitudes,* 17 HEALTH EDUC. Q. 157 (1990); Harnack et al., *supra* note 22, at 1 (finding that including calorie information and value size pricing did not significantly impact fast food meal choices); Jane Kolodinsky et al., *The Use of Nutritional Labels by College Students in a Food-Court Setting*, 57 J. AM. C. HEALTH 297 (2008) (finding that price, convenience, calories, fat, and nutrition labels play roles in food purchases); Amy M. Lando & Judith Labiner-Wolfe, *Helping Consumers Make More Healthful Food Choices: Consumer Views on Modifying Food Labels and Providing Point-of-Purchase Nutrition Information at Quick-Service Restaurants*, 39 J. NUTRITION EDUC. & BEHAV. 157 (2007) (finding that more studies are necessary to determine whether alternative presentations of nutrition information would be helpful); Maureen O'Dougherty et al., *Nutrition Labeling and Value Size Pricing at Fast-Food Restaurants: A Consumer Perspective*, 20 AM. J. HEALTH PROMOTION 247 (2006).

46 *See* Andrea Freeman, *Fast Food: Oppression Through Poor Nutrition*, 95 CALIF. L. REV. 2221, 2226 (2007) ("While the growth of fast food in poor urban neighborhoods has increased steadily, supermarkets stocking fresh, high-quality food have simultaneously relocated to the more spacious and affluent suburbs.").

47 *See* Sarah Treuhaft & Allison Karpyn, *The Grocery Gap: Who Has Access to Healthy Food and Why it Matters*, FOOD TRUST 8, http://thefoodtrust.org/uploads/media_items/grocerygap.original.pdf ("Residents in many urban areas (including Seattle, Central and South Los Angeles, and East Austin, Texas) have few transportation options to reach supermarkets. Inadequate transportation can be a major challenge for rural residents, given the long distances to stores."); *see also id.* at 21 ("Until more systemic solutions are instituted, transportation barriers to fresh food markets need to be removed. Community groups and planners should evaluate existing transportation routes and improve coordination of bus routes, bus stops, and schedules or add vanpools or shuttles to maximize transit access to grocery stores and farmers' markets.").

48 *See generally* BROOKINGS INST., THE PRICE IS WRONG: GETTING THE MARKET RIGHT FOR WORKING FAMILIES IN PHILADELPHIA 24 (2005) (explaining what causes higher grocery prices in Philadelphia); Erik Eckholm, *Study Documents 'Ghetto Tax' Being Paid by the Urban Poor*, N.Y. TIMES (July 19, 2006), http://www.nytimes.com/2006/07/19/us/19poor.html?_r=0 (discussing added costs that low income communities often pay for essential goods and services).

49 *See* Andrea Freeman, *Behavioral Economics and Food Policy: The Limits of Nudging, in* BEHAVIORAL ECONOMICS, LAW & HEALTH POLICY (forthcoming Fall 2016) (on file with author.) Ingredients banned in other countries but still legal and commonly used here include petroleum-based artificial dyes, olestra, brominated vegetable oil, potassium bromate, azodicarbonimide, butylated hydroxy-anisole (BHA) and butylated hydroxytoluene (BHT), synthetic growth hormones rBGH and rBST, and arsenic. Susanna Kim, *11 Food Ingredients Banned Outside the U.S. that We Eat*, ABC NEWS (June 26, 2013), http://abcnews.go.com/Lifestyle/Food/11-foods-banned-us/story?id=19457237#10.

50 *See* Freeman, *Fast Food: Oppression Through Poor Nutrition, supra* note 46, at 2225.

51 The USDA is responsible for both agricultural commodities and the federal nutrition programs, including school lunchrooms. *See* Andrea Freeman, *Farm Subsidies and Food Oppression*, 38 SEATTLE U. L. REV.__(forthcoming 2015); Juliana F.W. Cohen et al., *Impact of the New U.S. Department of Agriculture School Meal Standards on Food Selection, Consumption, and Waste*, 46 AM. J. PREVENTIVE MED. 388, 392 (2014).

52 *See* U.S. CENSUS BUREAU, LIVING IN NEAR POVERTY IN THE UNITED STATES: 1966–2012 (2014), *available at* https://www.census.gov/prod/2014pubs/p60-248.pdf; *How Many People Are Poor?*, UC DAVIS CTR. FOR POVERTY RES., http://poverty.ucdavis.edu/faq/how-many-people-are-poor (last visited May 14, 2015).

53 Andrea Freeman, *Transparency for Food Consumers & Food Oppression* 33, n. 90, *in* UCLA-Harvard Food Law and Policy Conference, Transparency in the Global Food System: What Information and to What Ends? (Oct. 24, 2014) (unpublished article), *available at* https://www.law.ucla.edu/~/media/Files/UCLA/Law/Pages/Publications/RES_PUB_Panel%203Oct2014.ash x [hereinafter *Transparency for Food Consumers & Food Oppression*] (internal citation omitted) ("While only 9.7% of whites lived below the poverty line in 2012, 27.2% of Blacks, 25.6% of Latinos, and 11.7% of Asian Americans did."); *id.* (internal citation omitted) ("In 2013, 26% of Black households and 24% of Latino house-holds had higher rates of food insecurity than the national average."). People who have ever received food stamps through the Supplemental Nutrition Assistance Program are 31% Black, 22% Latino, 18% other, and 15% white. *See id.* (citing Rich Morin, *The Politics and Demographics of Food Stamp Recipients*, PEW RES. CTR. (July 12, 2013), http://www.pewresearch.org/fact-tank/2013/07/12/the-politics-and-demographics-of-food-stamp-recipients). Additionally, "Black women and children make up 19.8% of WIC participants and only 12.6% of the population; Latinas represent 41.5% of WIC recipients but only 16.3% of the population." *Id.; see also* USDA, WIC PARTICIPANT AND PROGRAM CHARACTERISTICS 2012 FINAL REPORT 1, 27 (2013), *available at* http://www.fns.usda.gov/sites/default/files/WICPC2012.pdf [hereinafter WIC PARTICIPANT REPORT].

54 Freeman, *Transparency for Food Consumers & Food Oppression, supra* note 53, at 25; Andrea Freeman, *The Unbearable Whiteness of Milk: Food Oppression and the USDA*, U.C. IRVINE L. REV. 1251, 1253 (2013).

55 *See* Andrea Freeman, *"First Food" Justice: Racial Disparities in Infant Feeding As Food Oppression*, 83 FORDHAM L. REV. 3053, 3054 (2015).

56 *See* Chanjin Chung & Samuel L. Myers, Jr., *Do the Poor Pay More for Food? An Analysis of Grocery Store Availability and Food Price Disparities*, 33 J. CONSUMER AFF. 276, 276 (1999); Kimberlé Crenshaw,

Mapping the Margins: Intersectionality, Identity Politics, and Violence Against Women of Color, 43 STAN. L. REV. 1241, 1241 (1991); Freeman, *Fast Food*, *supra* note 46, at 2228; Angela Harris, *Race and Essentialism in Feminist Legal Theory*, 42 STAN. L. REV. 581, 581–616 (1990).

57 *See* Office of Disease Prevention & Health Promotion, *Disparities*, HEALTHYPEOPLE.GOV, http://www.healthypeople.gov/2020/about/foundation-health-measures/Disparities (last updated May 14, 2015).

58 Adam Benforado et al., *Broken Scales: Obesity and Justice in America*, 53 EMORY L.J. 1645, 1659 (2004).

59 *Id.* at 1658–68.

60 When grouping people by race in the context of health disparities, I do so with an awareness that these disparities arise from social factors, not to suggest that there is any biological basis for racial grouping. *See generally* DOROTHY ROBERTS, FATAL INVENTION: HOW SCIENCE, POLITICS, AND BIG BUSINESS RECREATE RACE IN THE TWENTY-FIRST CENTURY 64–66 (2011) (noting that among multiple genetic studies, "none support dividing the species into discrete, genetically determined racial categories"); Duana Fullwiley, *Race and Genetics: Attempts to Define the Relationship*, 2 BIOSOCIETIES 221, 224 (2007) (describing the "myriad problems" that arise when "racial generalizations" are drawn from genetic data); Ian F. Haney López, *The Social Construction of Race: Some Observations on Illusion, Fabrication, and Choice*, 29 HARV. C.R.-C.L. L. REV. 1, 13–14 (1994) (describing the history behind racialized groups); William M. Richman, *Genetic Residues of Ancient Migrations: An End to Biological Essentialism and the Reification of Race*, 68 U. PITT. L. REV. 387, 388 n.3 (2006) (explaining differences between racialized groups).

61 *See generally* AGENCY FOR HEALTHCARE RESEARCH & QUALITY, DISPARITIES IN HEALTH CARE QUALITY AMONG RACIAL AND ETHNIC MINORITY GROUPS: SELECTED FINDINGS FROM THE 2010 NATIONAL HEALTHCARE QUALITY AND DISPARITIES REPORTS 1 (2011), *available at* http://www.ahrq.gov/qual/nhqrdr10/nhqrdrminority10.htm (providing detailed statistics regarding racial groups and health status); *Race, Ethnicity, and the Health of Americans: ASA Series on How Race and Ethnicity Matter*, AM. SOCIOLOGICAL ASS'N (2005), *available at* http://www.asanet.org/images/research/docs/pdf/race_ethnicity_health.pdf (explaining how race plays a role in health status).

62 *See, e.g.*, *Adult Obesity Facts*, CDC, http://www.cdc.gov/obesity/data/adult.html (last updated Sept. 9, 2014).

63 *See, e.g.*, Alvaro Alonso et al., *Dairy Intake and Changes in Blood Pressure over 9 Years: The ARIC Study*, 63 EUR. J. CLINICAL NUTRITION 1272, 1274 (2009).

64 *See, e.g.*, Edward A. Chow et al., *The Disparate Impact of Diabetes on Racial/Ethnic Minority Populations*, 30 CLINICAL DIABETES 130, 130 (2012); Rafael Pérez-Escamilla & Predrag Putnik, *The Role of Acculturation in Nutrition, Lifestyle, and Incidence of Type 2 Diabetes Among Latinos*, 137 J. NUTRITION 860, 862 (2007).

65 *See, e.g.*, *Who Gets Angina?*, SPEAK FROM THE HEART, http://www.speakfromtheheart.com/who-gets-angina.aspx (last visited May 14, 2015).

66 Freeman, *Transparency for Food Consumers & Food Oppression*, *supra* note 53, at 24; *see, e.g.*, AM. CANCER SOC'Y, CANCER FACTS & FIGURES FOR AFRICAN AMERICANS 2011–2012 1, 16 (2011), *available*

http://www.cancer.org/acs/groups/content/@epidemiologysurveilance/documents/document/acspc-027765.pdf; *Cervical Cancer Rates by Race and Ethnicity*, CDC, http://www.cdc.gov/cancer/cervical/statistics/race.htm (last updated Aug. 27, 2014).

67 Freeman, *Transparency for Food Consumers & Food Oppression, supra* note 53, at 25; *see, e.g.*, LAURIE KAYE ABRAHAM, MAMA MIGHT BE BETTER OFF DEAD: THE FAILURE OF HEALTH CARE IN URBAN AMERICA 179–97 (1993); Robert D. Bullard et al., *Toxic Wastes and Race at Twenty: Why Race Still Matters After All of These Years*, 38 ENVTL. L. 371, 371 (2008); Michael D. Cabana & Glenn Flores, *The Role of Clinical Practice Guidelines in Enhancing Quality and Reducing Racial/Ethnic Disparities in Paediatrics*, 3 PAEDIATRIC RESPIRATORY REVS. 52, 52 (2002); Kevin Fiscella et al., *Inequality in Quality: Addressing Socioeconomic, Racial, and Ethnic Disparities in Health Care*, 283 JAMA 2579, 2579 (2000); Glenn Flores et al., *The Impact of Ethnicity, Family Income, and Parental Education on Children's Health and Use of Health Services*, 89 AM. J. PUB. HEALTH 1066, 1067 (1999); David M.K.I. Liu & Christian K. Alameda, *Social Determinants of Health for Native Hawaiian Children and Adolescents*, 70 HAW. MED. J. 11 Supp. 2 (Nov. 2011); Michael Massoglia, *Incarceration, Health, and Racial Disparities in Health*, 42 L. & SOC'Y REV. 275, 285 n.6 (2008); Barbara A. Noah, *Racial Disparities in the Delivery of Health Care*, 35 SAN DIEGO L. REV. 135, 138 (1998); Sidney D. Watson, *Race, Ethnicity and Hospital Care: The Need for Racial and Ethnic Data*, 30 J. HEALTH L. 125, 125 (1997); Michael Weitzman et al., *Black and White Middle Class Children Who Have Private Health Insurance in the United States*, 104 PEDIATRICS 151, 151 (1999); Mark B. Wenneker & Arnold M. Epstein, *Racial Inequalities in the Use of Procedures for Patients with Ischemic Heart Disease in Massachusetts*, 261 JAMA 253, 253 (1989); David R. Williams & Toni D. Rucker, *Understanding and Addressing Racial Disparities in Health Care*, 21 HEALTH CARE FINANCING REV. 75, 75 (2000).

68 *See* Ctr. for Responsive Politics, *Influence & Lobbying: Food & Beverage*, OPENSECRETS.ORG, http://www.opensecrets.org/industries/indus.php?ind=N01 (last visited May 14, 2015). In the 2008 campaign cycle, food and beverage companies donated over $16 million to political candidates. In 2013–14, the top campaign contributors in these industries were the National Restaurant Association, Coca-Cola, McDonald's, Darden Restaurants (including the Olive Garden), Pepsi, Bloomin' Brands (including Outback Steakhouse), CKE restaurants (including Carl's Jr. and Hardee's), Wendy's and the American Beverage Association. *See id.*

69 In 2014, the industry spent over $15.7 million on lobbying. The top lobbyists were Coca-Cola, Pepsi, the National Restaurant Association, McDonald's and Mars. *See id.*

70 *See generally* Ctr. for Responsive Politics, *Revolving Door*, OPENSECRETS.ORG, https://www.opensecrets.org/revolving/index.php (last visited May 14, 2015) (explaining how a revolving door forms and functions).

71 *See* MARION NESTLE, FOOD POLITICS: HOW THE FOOD INDUSTRY INFLUENCES NUTRITION AND HEALTH 48, 126 (2007).

72 *See* Mary Clare Jalonick, *Pizza Is a Vegetable? Congress Says Yes*, NBC NEWS (Nov. 15, 2011), http://www.nbcnews.com/id/45306416/ns/health-diet_and_nutrition/t/pizza-vegetable-congress-says-yes/#.VCn3AxbpdrU ("Food companies that produce frozen pizzas for schools, the salt industry and potato

growers requested the changes, and some conservatives in Congress say the federal government shouldn't bet telling children what to eat.").

73 *See* Freeman, *Farm Subsidies and Food Oppression*, *supra* note 51.

74 For example, on the island of Kaua'i in Hawai'i, the mayor vetoed a law regulating pesticide use after the city council passed the controversial bill by a vote of six to one, despite substantial lobbying efforts by the affected corporations, Syngenta Hawaii, DuPont Pioneer, Dow AgroSciences and BASF. *See* Natasha Lennard, *How the Monsanto Protection Act Snuck into Law*, SALON (Mar. 27, 2013, 4:44 PM), http://www.salon.com/2013/03/27/how_the_monsanto_protection_act_snuck_into_law. *See generally State & County QuickFacts: Kaua'i County, Hawai'i*, U.S. CENSUS BUREAU (Feb. 5, 2015), http://quickfacts.census.gov/qfd/states/15/15007.html. The Kaua'i ordinance also sought to protect its residents from potential health hazards from genetically modified (GM) crops. *See Kaua'i Mayor Vetoes Popular Ordinance Safeguarding Public from Pesticides*, EARTHJUSTICE.ORG (Oct. 31, 2013), http://earthjustice.org/news/press/2013/kaua-i-mayor-vetoes-popular-ordinance-safeguarding-public-from-pesticides. Large agricultural corporations have been very successful at blocking local and federal regulation of genetically modified organisms (GMOs). In March 2013, President Obama signed into law the Farmer Assurance Provision, also deemed the 'Monsanto Protection Act' as section 735 of H.R. 933, the Consolidated and Further Continuing Appropriations Act, 2013. *See* Consolidated and Further Continuing Appropriations Act, 2013, Pub. L. No. 113–6, § 735, 127 Stat. 198, 231–32 (2013). The provision allows major agricultural corporations to bypass standard regulatory requirements regarding new GM crops by instructing the Secretary of Agriculture to "immediately grant temporary permit(s) or temporary deregulation" upon a farmer, grower, farm operator or producer's request. *Id.* at 232. The provision eliminates judicial review, even upon a finding that a crop poses health harms. *See id.*

75 *See* William Saletan, *Don't Touch Anything But My Junk*, SLATE (Apr. 5, 2011), http://www.slate.com/articles/health_and_science/human_nature/2011/04/dont_touch_anything_but_my_junk.html; *Menu Labeling*, STATE OF OBESITY, http://stateofobesity.org/menu-labeling (last visited May 14, 2015).

76 *See* Tavernise, *supra* note 10 (stating that Kessler's changes have faced opposition, especially his push to place nutrition labels on the front of food items).

77 *See infra* pp. 14–15.

78 *See* JULIE GUTHMAN, WEIGHING IN: OBESITY, FOOD JUSTICE, AND THE LIMITS OF CAPITALISM 52–55 (2011).

79 *See generally* Benforado, *supra* note 58, at 1689–1742.

80 *See* Elizabeth Fee & Nancy Krieger, *Understanding AIDS: Historical Interpretations and the Limits of Biomedical Individualism*, 83 AM. J. PUB. HEALTH 1477, 1478–79 (1993).

81 See Alice Mah, *Lessons from Love Canal: Toxic Expertise and Environmental Justice*, RESILIENCE (Aug. 9, 2013), http://www.resilience.org/stories/2013-08-09/lessons-from-love-canal-toxic-expertise-and-environmental-justice; *Cancer Alley, Louisiana*, POLLUTION ISSUES, http://www.pollutionissues.com/Br-Co/Cancer-Alley-Louisiana.html (last visited May 14, 2015).

82 *See* Greenberg et al., *Portrayals of Overweight and Obese Individuals on Commercial Television*, 93 AM. J. PUB. HEALTH 1342, 1342 (2003); *see also* Gregory Fouts & Kimberley Burggraf, *Television Situation Comedies: Female Weight, Male Negative Comments, and Audience Reactions*, 42 SEX ROLES 925, 927 (2000); Susan Himes & J. Kevin Thompson, *Fat Stigmatization in Television Shows and Movies: A Content Analysis*, 15 OBESITY 712, 713 (2007).

83 *See e.g.*, Sonita Moss, The Big C's *Big Black Problem*, JEZEBEL (Jan. 17, 2012), http://jezebel.com/5876914/the-big-cs-big-black-problem; Tami Winfrey Harris, *When Will* Glee *Stop Ignoring Race?*, RACIALICIOUS (May 4, 2011), http://www.racialicious.com/2011/05/04/when-will-glee-stop-ignoring-race; *Sassy Black Woman*, TV TROPES, http://tvtropes.org/pmwiki/pmwiki.php/Main/SassyBlackWoman (last visited May 14, 2015).

84 *What's Happening!!*, IMDB, http://www.imdb.com/title/tt0074071 (last visited May 14, 2015) (starring Mabel King as "Mabel 'Mama' Thomas").

85 *Good Times*, IMDB, http://www.imdb.com/title/tt0070991/?ref_=fn_al_tt_1 (last visited May 14, 2015) (starring Esther Rolle as "Florida Evans").

86 *Gimme a Break!*, IMDB, http://www.imdb.com/title/tt0081869/?ref_=fn_al_tt_4 (last visited May 14, 2015) (starring Nell Carter as "Nellie Harper").

87 *How I Met Your Mother*, IMDB, http://www.imdb.com/title/tt0460649/?ref_=nm_flmg_act_6 (last visited May 14, 2015) (starring Sherri Shepherd as "Daphne").

88 *The Big C*, IMDB, http://www.imdb.com/title/tt1515193/?ref_=nv_sr_1 (last visited May 14, 2015) (starring Gabourey Sibide as "Andrea Jackson").

89 *Glee*, IMDB, http://www.imdb.com/title/tt1327801/?ref_=nv_sr_2 (last visited May 14, 2015) (starring Amber Riley as "Mercedes Jones").

90 *See Tongan American Aims to Eliminate Stereotypes, Promote Wellness Within Pacific Islander Community*, COMMUNITYHEALTHFORASIANAMERICANS (Jan. 7, 2011), http://www.chaaweb.org/news/20110165/tongan-american-aims-eliminate-stereotypes-promote-wellness-within-pacific-islander-co.

91 *Id.*

92 *Id.*

93 *See* Noa Emmett Aluli, *Prevalence of Obesity in a Native Hawaiian Population*, 53 AM. J. CLINICAL NUTRITION 1556S, 1559S (1991); Laurie D. McCubbin & Mapuana Antonio, *Discrimination and Obesity Among Native Hawaiians*, 71 HAW. J. MED. PUB. HEALTH 346, 346 (2012) (finding that discrimination is a risk factor for obesity in Native Hawaiians).

94 *See* ROBERT JI-SUN KU ET AL., EATING ASIAN AMERICA: A FOOD STUDIES READER 326 (2013) (stating that SPAM has particular importance due to its association with the American militarization of Hawaii); *see also* Noa Helela, *Ha*, GENIUS, http://genius.com/Noa-helela-ha-annotated (last visited May 14, 2015) ("We are boxed up/like a can of spam./Ingredients: ham, pork, precooked native people, separated chicken fat, suffocation, and sodium nitrate./Nutrition facts: happiness, air, self-respect 0 grams/bloody fists, alcohol, destruction,/It's over 9000!/Basically, nothing worth breathing./But I don't want to be an emergency food,/farm-raised in immersion schools/to preserve

the flavor of my native tongue,/and used in time of war,/so they can serve us up/in bite sized body bags.").

95 *See generally* ANGE-MARIE HANCOCK, THE POLITICS OF DISGUST: THE PUBLIC IDENTITY OF THE WELFARE QUEEN (2004); Rose Ernst, *Localizing the "Welfare Queen" Ten Years Later: Race, Gender, Place, and Welfare Rights*, 11 RACE, GENDER & CLASS 181 (2008); Carly Hayden Foster, *The Welfare Queen: Race, Gender, Class, and Public Opinion*, 15 RACE, GENDER & CLASS 162 (2008); Ange-Marie Hancock, *Contemporary Welfare Reform and the Public Identity of the "Welfare Queen,"* 10 RACE, GENDER & CLASS 31 (2003); Karen Johnson, *Myth of the Welfare Queen*, 25 ESSENCE 42 (1995); Premilla Nadasen, *From Widow to "Welfare Queen:" Welfare and the Politics of Race*, 1 BLACK WOMEN, GENDER & FAMILIES 52 (2007).

Chapter 8: **Discussion Questions**

1   What is the mutual aid approach to health care, and how does it differ from actuarial fairness?

   a.   How can public health law reduce health disparities?

2   Explain the relationship between socioeconomic status and life expectancy.

   a.   How do health disparities impact mental health?

3   Describe the impact of gender and socioeconomic status on dietary choices.

   a.   Do you think simplifying nutritional labels by requiring overall caloric content improve choices?

4   Describe the conflict between how consumers typically choose food (based on convenience, taste, and price), while nutrition labeling focuses on education and willpower.

   a.   What do you think is the most important change to food policy: increasing convenience and availability, improving the taste, or reducing the costs of healthy foods? Why?

5   List three factors that impact obesity other than personal dietary choices.

   a.   How can food policy reduce health disparities and improve American health outcomes?

BEHAVIORAL CHANGE
AND HEALTH POLICY

What Would Your Future Self Say? Using Motivational Interviewing to Affect Behaviour Change

Alison Firth

Based on a workshop delivered to RSPH members in February 2015 by Neal Gething, Registered Psychologist at Empowerment Training Consultancy, this article explores the technique of motivational interviewing and how it can be used to change behaviour.

> *We cannot change anything until we accept it.*
> *Condemnation does not liberate, it oppresses.*
> *—Carl Jung*

Before you start reading, think of a behaviour that you would like to change. If you can, write it down and describe it, so you can easily come back to it as you are reading through this article. An important part of motivational interviewing is to be able to first apply the technique to yourself: once you've found the trick to changing your own behaviours, you can then use this knowledge to help transform others.

Motivation, in simple terms, is the desire to change something. Motivational interviewing is a person-centred counselling approach that focuses on collaboratively eliciting, and subsequently strengthening, an individual's motivation to change. Rather than focusing on the negative battle, the technique encourages the individual to focus on what they are good at, who they are now—their needs, desires and goals—and the person they will turn into—their future self. Ultimately, motivational interviewing is about change, and the three principles that underlie all change: everything is a state of mind; state of mind is habit; and habits can change. We all learn things by habit, for example, how we sign our name and which arm our watch is on. Motivational interviewing focuses on finding these habits and discovering what it is that blocks you from getting up and doing what you know is right, that is, from changing your behaviour.

The Essence of Motivational Interviewing

Pause here and think about how compassionate you are towards yourself—what do you say to yourself when you think about the behaviour you are going to change? What motivates you?

'It's not your fault, but it is your problem.'

Change is the responsibility of the individual, and it is important to remember that you cannot force behaviour change in others: in order to change a behaviour, you need to own your own problem. The role of the motivational interviewer is to be a supportive companion who focuses on bringing the conversation back to change, and on listening to the person rather than the problem.

The first step is discovering who the client is (the present self) and facilitating them in looking at who they are when their problem owns them, beginning to engage the habit mind. The key here is developing a discrepancy with who/ where an individual is now compared to who/ where they want to be, which brings you to the second step—discovering who the client wants to be (desired future self). Here, it is important to focus on keeping statements positive: on 'be this' rather than 'don't be that'. This is an important stage in giving the mind the right information for change to happen and recognising the barriers that might get in the way of your future self:

The key here is developing a discrepancy with who/where an individual is now compared to who/where they want to be

'How dare you ask me to change, you don't know what I've been through.'

Spending time on feelings of ambivalence is necessary here as it is common for uncertainty to cause fluctuation through a range of emotions, including fear, anger, grief, guilt, shame and helplessness, leading to internal power struggles. Avoid letting this power become the focus of the discussion as it can cause individuals to fight back—this can lead to arguments, which should be avoided. It is important to remain focused on discovering and understanding the desired future self: through maximising the desire for change, the perceived ability to change and the actual ability to change will increase.

What Would Your Future Self Say?

Every time the problem is mentioned, ask the individual this question: establishing and focusing on the future self and driving towards it are the key to motivational interviewing. Collaborative and change-focused empathy is important here: displaying compassion and affirming an individual's struggle. Any behaviour that relates to the future self should be focused on and expanded: for example, if the future self is judging the current self, this needs to remain the focus until the relationship becomes a positive one:

'How do I accommodate the behaviour into my future self?'

The final step is goal setting: securing a commitment to change. Goal setting within motivational interviewing is slightly different—it is about cultivating change based on the values that have been drawn out from investigating your present self and your desired future self—rather than setting goals just to tick boxes. Goal setting to secure change includes the following: the changes I plan to make are, the reasons I want to make these changes are, future actions are, I will know I am changing when and I will know when I'm regressing when.

Conclusion

Motivational interviewing is a key behaviour change technique used by psychotherapists, occupational health doctors and general practitioners (GPs) in their day-to-day work with clients. As this article has explored, the technique makes use of short-term, solution-focused strategies to help individuals overcome behaviours and actions that may be impeding their health and wellbeing. This is achieved through the key principles: understanding what motivates you by focusing on the self and your values rather than on the problem, identifying the barriers to change and identifying how these barriers can be overcome by setting up a dialogue between the present self and the future self.

Thinking back to the behaviour that you identified at the start, what would your future self say?

Reference

Miller WR, Rollnick S. *Motivational Interviewing: Helping People Change*, 3rd edn. New York: The Guildford Press, 2012.

Beyond Genetic Determinism

David W. Chapman

Advances in genetic research have been hailed in many quarters as harbingers of a new Golden Age, an age in which cancer, congenital diseases, and the sometimes drastic treatments that accompanied them will be a dim memory of a brutal age—much the way we think of the practices of blistering and bloodletting in the eighteenth century. Indeed, we are already beginning to see the benefits of advances in genetics in the treatment of many diseases. Still, there are many who find genetic advances—from cloning to gene therapies—to be unsettling. And these questions are far from theoretical, as can be seen in Kevin Davies' description of genetic pre-selection in his book on *Cracking the Genome*:

> News that a woman with an early-onset hereditary form of Alzheimer's disease screened her embryos using in vitro fertilization to prevent her newborn child from inheriting the faulty genes sparked fears of the "slippery slope" to designer babies. Today, the technology is being used to screen non-fatal, adult-onset diseases such as cancer and Alzheimer's. Tomorrow, could it be used to screen personality, physique, or sexual orientation?[1]

As this incident reveals, genetic science is rapidly moving from the science fiction of Huxley's *Brave New World* to the reality of genetic selection and alteration.

Leaving aside the issue of genetic manipulation for the moment, how does our awareness of genetic information call into question the very notion of what it means to be human? Are we more than the sum of our genetic information? Humans have traditionally attempted to define themselves through their origins. The book of Genesis attempts to find a higher purpose in human life through its divine beginnings: "And the Lord God formed man of the dust of the ground, and breathed into his nostrils the breath of life; and man became a living soul."[2] Does the new "book of Genes" (our genetic code), eliminate the God-breathed "life" from our genetic dust and, thereby, lessen our basic human dignity? As Gordon Wenham writes in describing the significance of this passage:

> Man is more than a God-shaped piece of earth. He has within him the gift
> of life that was given by God himself. The biblical writer was not alone
> in rejecting a reductionist view of man which sees him as simply an in-
> teresting collection of chemicals and electrical impulses [or genetically
> determined tissues, we might add].[3]

To reject the notion of the divine value of human life is to remove the moral foundation for ethical behavior for many people. Furthermore, to understand our genetic makeup is no substitute for understanding what it means to be human. Those looking for some mark of distinction in our genetic structure are sure to be disappointed.

Indeed, one of the great surprises of the Human Genome Project was the simplicity of the decoded DNA. There are approximately 20,000 to 25,000 genes that carry all the information needed to convey every aspect of the human body's function and appearance.[4] Before the project was completed, scientists had expected to uncover at least 100,000 genes. It turns out that the humble field mouse, Robert Burns' "wee, sleekit, cow'rin, tim'rous beastie,"[5] had about the same number of genes as the poet himself.

In fact, the genome of a human is not much more complicated than that of a fruitfly (approximately 13,000 genes) or a roundworm (19,000 genes). And what of the plant world? We fall a bit behind the *Arabidopsis thaliana* (thale cress) with its 25,000 genes.[6] I'm not sure what to make of the fact that I may be less complicated genetically than the salad I eat.

So, what are we to conclude from the latest results of the genetic sweepstakes? We humans have typically taken our superiority over other species for granted. Our vast civilizations, gleaming cities, and towering monuments dominate the landscape. We have poetry, philosophy, art, and music. We are the creators of the I Ching and the Pieta, Machu Picchu and the Messiah. Like Shakespeare's Caesar, we "bestride the narrow world like a Colossus."[7] It has been hard on our collective ego to find ourselves in a dead heat with rodents on the gene count.

Even if we can live with the disappointing results of these genetic comparisons (it is now a well established fact that we share 96% of our genetic code with chimpanzees[8]), some of us may be slightly uncomfortable with the idea that a genetic blueprint is determining not only our physical traits, but the outcome of our lives. Popular psychology now tends to attribute every human decision to genetic destiny. If you are overweight, it may not be due to your eating habits, but to genetic predispositions toward obesity. If you struggle with anger management, you may well be genetically predisposed to violent outbursts. If you are unfaithful to your spouse, you are heeding the evolutionary call to increase your offspring.[9] To paraphrase the Bard, our destiny lies "not in our stars, but in our cells."

Let me hasten to add that serious scientists do not typically promote a worldview with a genetic escape clause from human responsibility. Biologists are in the business of describing the structure and function of living organisms; they are generally content to leave the "oughts" of human behavior to philosophers and priests. Still, the results of biological research often run headlong into the deepest moral and spiritual questions of the ages. The contest between "soul" and "appetite" described by Plato, or that of "spirit" and "flesh" bemoaned by St. Paul, are the classical manifestations of this problem.

In the *Phaedrus*, Plato famously uses the image of a chariot driver to describe the relationship between reason, appetite, and spirit:

> Let us ... compare the soul to a winged charioteer and his team acting together. ... The ruling power within us men drives a pair of horses... one of these is fine and good and of noble stock, and the other the opposite in every way. So in our case the task of the charioteer is necessarily a difficult and unpleasant business.[10]

Plato elaborates on these ideas in *The Republic*, where he notes that individuals prosper when the reasoning part (the charioteer in the analogy) holds reign over the spirited part (the good horse) and the appetite (the obstinate horse):

> It is proper for the reasoning part to rule, because it is wise and has to use forethought for the whole soul; and proper for the high-spirited part to be its ally and subject... These two, then, thus trained and educated, will truly learn their own business; then they will preside over the desiring part.[11]

In setting up this tug-of-war between the rational self and physical desire, Plato is only recognizing a common mental phenomenon—the internal conflict that humans inevitably experience when choosing between actions that may feel good, but which are harmful to themselves or others. We hear this same conflict echoed in Jesus' reprimand to his sleeping disciples that the "spirit is willing, but the flesh is weak."[12] Paul writes of his own internal conflict in his first letter to the Corinthians: "I do not understand my own actions. For I do not do what I want, but I do the very thing I hate."[13] And this is the same idea captured in the common plea for people to "listen to their better angels."

Although Plato understood the "desiring part" of man to encompass a variety of physical and psychological desires (particularly the ambition to rule over others in *The Republic*), we might well include genetic predispositions in that category today. Of course, many of the physical consequences of our DNA structure can't be controlled (although, as noted earlier, scientists are working toward genetic manipulation). In the meantime, we know that certain genetic abnormalities do increase the risk for cancer and other diseases. Angelina Jolie's highly publicized decision to have a double mastectomy when her BRCA1 gene put her at high risk for breast cancer certainly illustrates the new awareness of the connection between genetic information and health decisions.

It is important, however, to distinguish between the physical consequences of our genetic structures, whether we are considering our height, eye color, or the propensity for certain cancers, and the influence of our genetic predispositions on moral decision making. Plato's concept of the soul as the charioteer reminds us that we cannot simply point to our genetic predispositions as the reason for our actions. We have the ability as human beings to make rational and ethical choices that go against the "desiring part" of our natures. Aristotle takes the same line of reasoning in the *Nicomachean Ethics*, when he notes that a virtuous life is based on the conscious decision to choose the right course: "For we praise the rational principle of the continent man and of the incontinent, and the part of their soul that has such a principle, since it urges them aright and towards the best objects; but there is found in them also another natural element besides the rational principle, which fights against and resists that principle"[14]

Thus, Plato and Aristotle might recognize that some people are more inclined to drink to excess than others; and today we might suspect that there are certain genetic structures that may incline individuals towards alcoholism. However, the classical view holds that one should not simply submit to desire, but that one should "fight against and resist" that behavior. This is a principle widely recognized in law when we do not excuse illegal actions (driving under the influence, for instance) because of personal predispositions (genetic or otherwise). But perhaps new scientific developments may take some of the inevitability out of the genetic equation. It has been assumed until recently that most genetic information was "hardwired" into our nature over vast stretches of time. The actions of the individual (i.e., to subordinate natural desires to the rational principle) seemed to matter little to the genetic heritage that would be passed along to the next generation.

However, scientists have long been puzzled by the differences present in identical twins. Why would one twin suffer from a debilitating disease and the other be perfectly normal? If the genetic code is the same, what causes the differentiation? The answer apparently lies in the way the genetic code is expressed. It is possible, for instance, for a gene to be switched "on" in one twin and "off" in the other. The mechanism for this—the genetic software, if you will—comes through the epigenetic markers that surround the genome. Although not actually part of the DNA strand, epigenetics (literally, "on top of" the gene), not only account for differences in twins, but can also help explain the complexity of human characteristics despite the relatively small number of genes.

Scientists are only beginning to understand the nature of these epigenetic markers. They include methyl molecules that attach directly to the gene and histone proteins that condense chromosomes and prevent genes from being expressed.[15] Early studies have shown that there can be significant environmental factors in the development or loss of these epigenetic structures. Many scientists are beginning to acknowledge that the Human Genome Project—once thought to be the end-all and be-all of genetic discoveries—was only the tip of the genomic iceberg.

The implication for such studies in the health professions goes without saying. Laboratory studies are already providing evidence that these epigenetic markers can be manipulated with extraordinary outcomes, enabling rats with a propensity toward plus-sizes to produce offspring that are shopping in the petite boutiques. Understanding these epigenetic markers holds great promises for treating all kinds of diseases, from diabetes to cancer.

However, from a philosophical standpoint, epigenetics seems to reinforce the classical view that virtuous actions must be pursued over and against the desiring part of our natures. Unlike the genetic code, which is relatively stable and generally only changes over many generations, epigenetic markers can be influenced by the health of the parents. One study, for example, has shown that if your grandfather went hungry as a young man it might have a statistical correlation with your own life expectancy.[16] Such effects include not only unavoidable catastrophes (famines, epidemics), but also voluntary behaviors. For instance, a nurturing parent may actually strengthen the epigenetic well being of his or her children. Conversely, a biological parent with a history of smoking or drug abuse could pass along this damage to the next generation. As Marcus Pembrey from University College-London once remarked, "You live your life as a sort of guardian of your genome."[17]

The shift from the victim of genetic necessity to the guardian of our genome is not a trifling matter. It strengthens the importance of human choice; for our choices affect not only ourselves, but also generations to come. And while the maze of ethical questions created by genetic research—from cloning to genetic engineering—will not soon be resolved, the study of epigenetics provides evidence that genetic coding is not a one-way street. We are both influencing and being influenced by our genetic structures. For the humanist who feels a bit beleaguered by constant reference to evolutionary destinies and genetic determination—sometimes uttered with a dogmatism that would have put John Calvin to shame—the growing scientific evidence supporting the importance of epigenetic markers is like a fresh philosophical breeze. We may float on a tide of genetic predispositions, but we can still claim, "I am the master of my fate. I am the captain of my soul (and cell)."[18]

Notes

1 Kevin Davies, *Cracking the Code* (Simon and Schuster, 2001), xviii.

2 Genesis 2:7 (King James Version).

3 Gordon Wenham, Genesis 1–15. *Word Biblical Commentary*. Vol. I. (Word Incorporated, 1987), 60.

4 U.S. Department of Energy Genome Program. "How Many Genes Are in the Human Genome?" Accessed at http://www.ornl.gov/hgmis.

5 Robert Burns, "To a Mouse." Line 1.

6 U.S. Department of Energy Genome Program. "Functional and Comparative Genomics Fact Sheet." Accessed at http://www.ornl.gov/sci/techresources/Human_Genome/faq/compgen.shtml.

7 William Shakespeare, *Julius Caesar*. Act I, Scene II, Lines 135–36.

8 Stefan Lovgren, "Chimps, Humans 96 Percent the Same, Gene Study Finds" *National Geographic News*. August 31, 2005. Accessed at http://news.nationalgeographic.com/news/pf/87202973.html.

9 Many examples of genetic predispositions can be found in J. Craig Venter, *A Life Decoded* (Viking, 2007). For instance, severe depression is associated with a shortened form of the serotonin transfer gene, known as 5-HTTLPR (329) and the dopamine receptor 4 gene may have some influence on alcohol and drug addictions.

10 Walter Hamilton, trans., *Phaedrus* (New York: Penguin 1973), 50–51.

11 W.H.D. Rouse, trans., *The Republic*, Book IV. In *Great Dialogues of Plato* (New York: Mentor, 1984), 242.

12 Matthew 26:41 NRSV.

13 Romans 7:15 NRSV.

14 Richard McKeon, trans. *Nicomachean Ethics*. In *The Basic Works of Aristotle* (New York: Random House, 1941), 951.

15 Carl Zimmer, "The Rest of the Genome." *New York Times*. Nov. 11, 2008. Accessed at www. newyork-times.com.

16 "Ghost in Your Genes," NOVA. PBS. October 16, 2007.

17 Ibid.

18 William Ernest Henley. "Invictus." Accessed at http://www.poetryfoundation.org/poem/182194.

Chapter 9: **Discussion Questions**

1   List the three principles that underlie all change.

    a.   How does motivational interviewing seek to reduce ambivalence and increase desire for behavioral change?

2   How has motivational interviewing been used in health care?

    a.   Do you believe it is an effective tool? Explain.

3   How can motivational interviewing be used in public health efforts to reduce chronic conditions?

    a.   Decisional rulers can be used to ask patients, "On a scale of zero to ten, how likely are you to make a change?" Interviewers then focus on increasing change talk centering on why they didn't choose zero. How does this promote the principles of motivational interviewing?

4   Define genetic determinism.

    a.   What other factors besides genetics affect your health?

5   The field of epigenetics revealed that behavioral choices not only affect one's current health, but choices today can also affect the health of several future generations; should health policies focus on the health of current or future generations? Explain.

    a.   How has knowledge of genetics changed health care policy within your lifetime?

CHAPTER 10

ENVIRONMENTAL HEALTH POLICY

Integration of Social Determinants of Community Preparedness and Resiliency in 21st Century Emergency Management Planning

Paul A. Biedrzycki and Raisa Koltun

Introduction

The recent release by the Obama Administration of Presidential Policy Directive 8 (PPD 8), also referred to as the National Preparedness Directive, highlights a key imperative that speaks strongly and encourages the adoption and practice of a more comprehensive as well as community-oriented focus toward strengthening national emergency preparedness and resiliency.[1] Furthermore, the recent release of the *Whole Community Approach to Emergency Management: Principles, Themes, and Pathways for Action* by the Federal Emergency Management Agency (FEMA) underscores federal commitment in promoting the inclusion and engagement of diverse stakeholders in the overall community preparedness and planning process, recognizing the role of inherent and unique community-based social dynamics, networks, and informal leadership that can be leveraged to strengthen community resiliency.[2]

Both of these initiatives provide the opportunity and conceptual framework to establish a more community-focused approach to emergency management by willingly inviting to the table a wide array of key stakeholders, including citizens as legitimate and equitable partners and assets in the process. In essence, both PPD 8 and FEMA's whole of community philosophy represent an emerging trend and new modality for the emergency management discipline in incorporating socioeconomic conditions

Paul A. Biedrzycki and Raisa Koltun, "Integration of Social Determinants of Community Preparedness and Resiliency in 21st Century Emergency Management Planning," *Homeland Security Affairs*, vol. 8, no. 1, pp. 1-7. Copyright © 2012 by Naval Postgraduate School, Center for Homeland Defense and Security. Reprinted with permission. Provided by ProQuest LLC.

and more meaningful community participation at the planning and preparedness core. As such, it will also demand a fundamentally new emphasis on re-establishing or improving community relationships and most importantly, an authentic and genuine trust between government and citizenry.

This essay will outline this new modality in two interrelated parts—the concept of examining various social determinants of preparedness and community resiliency and the importance of fostering better community inclusion and trust. Three case studies are presented to exemplify the need for this shift in approach. The purpose of this essay is to advance these concepts and advocate inclusion into modern emergency management practice. This can only enhance preparation and nation-wide resiliency in the twenty-first century given the breadth and scope of natural and man-made threats to the country and global community as evident by recent historical events such as Hurricane Katrina, the British Petroleum Gulf Oil Spill, and the 2009 H1N1 Pandemic.

What are Social Determinants of Community Preparedness and Resiliency?

Social determinants of emergency preparedness and resiliency can best be thought of in the context of those dynamics or factors that influence the vulnerability of a community as it responds to and recovers from an emergency. Such factors are unique and vary greatly between communities but can be categorized into several domains. This variation in community social dynamics is not randomly distributed and is largely due to inequities in the ownership and distribution of resources, wealth, and opportunity. These in and of themselves can account for many disparities in outcomes between communities that are often seen and indeed magnified in the aftermath of a catastrophic event such as Hurricane Katrina in 2005.

Identifying social determinants of emergency preparedness and resiliency then can be viewed as a function of the socio-economics of a community (e.g., mean income, percent savings, education levels, unemployment rates); environmental infrastructure (e.g., housing availability, crime rates, suboptimal geographic locations); and other intangible but nevertheless important community attributes (e.g., degree of social cohesion, predominance of family/neighborhood structure, and level of community engagement). Communities with high levels of poverty become the most vulnerable to the impact of disasters in terms of lacking adequate preparedness and being at highest risk for adverse consequences. This is primarily due to government and related system failures in addressing appropriate and timely response and recovery necessary to seed and foster a culture of resiliency within this population.

Currently, underlying social and economic considerations relevant and unique to a given community are generally not fully integrated within traditional emergency management planning activities or approaches. Consideration of such data such as unemployment rates, high school graduation rates, social capital, and crime statistics do not readily find their way into discussions involving the emergency management paradigm of preparedness, mitigation, response, and recovery. Indeed, emergency planning is often conducted as "one size fits all" and only very recently—in the aftermath of Katrina—has attention been cast on the functional and cultural dimensions of communities. Even then, the discourse has been limited to issues of mobility or achieving basic cultural competency around ethnic group communication and outreach. Much of this approach may be enabled and driven by resource availability; however, it is our contention that a deeper understanding of the above social determinants is lacking in emergency management training, discipline, practice, and strategies.

Instead, we suggest that communities need to be thought of as unique organisms representing a network replete with informal leadership, communication conduits, and a sense of identity and purpose that is dynamic, constantly evolving, and based on economic, social and political shifts in its sands. As such, disparities in income, health, and education along with varying levels of social cohesion and civic engagement are part of a landscape that both shapes and anticipates human behaviors including those around emergency preparedness and level of resiliency toward catastrophic events. The silo of emergency management as a government-centric and uni-dimensional planning model that currently meets the needs of only a subset of the population is no longer viable nor is it appropriate to meet the needs of twenty-first century disaster preparedness around diverse threats. Neither is it a prescription for successful achievement of community resiliency as called for in PPD 8 or as a fundamental outcome of the "whole of community" tenet being promoted by FEMA as the lead federal disaster preparedness agency.

The "Whole of Community" and Importance of Inclusion and Trust

Understanding the underlying social determinants of a particular community is paramount to the successful engagement of its members and subsequent shared ownership and participation in a range of issues from public works to public health. However, engagement and inclusion of community is often reduced to simple invitations to participate in pro forma processes already developed by government entities and typically directed through reactionary administrative policy. Emergency management agencies at federal, state, and local levels are therefore expected, as a matter of good practice, to engage the community in ways that are not only ineffective but lack formal evaluation mechanisms to gauge success. These agencies, faced with the unenviable task of planning for the unexpected and low probability event, seldom generate sufficient community interest and momentum to create realistic plans. The outcome of such endeavors is plans that do not reflect community input in a way that maximizes citizenry buy-in or clarifies roles and responsibilities. Engaging the "whole of community" in a comprehensive, genuine, and authentic way, while complex, can pay dividends in achieving community resiliency. Furthermore, it is only through meaningful inclusion of the broader community and development of mutual trust that an accurate understanding and integration of underlying social determinants can occur.

Engaging the community entails more than an invitation to the discussion. Inclusion must acknowledge and emphasize community knowledge and other assets, as well as enact a truly collaborative process between all stakeholders. This requires early and sincere outreach, reflective listening, demonstrating patience in relationship-building, acknowledging deficits, practicing transparency in process, sharing the true rationale behind policy, and equitable evaluation of progress toward mutually agreeable goals.

Government emergency management agencies must learn to let go of the need to control and micromanage community preparedness activities and instead find ways to incentivize citizen participation to ensure a creative flow of ideas during problem solving as well as enable community ownership of solutions. Too often government entities, albeit well intentioned, are subconsciously prescriptive in approach and mentality in what is a supposedly objective assessment and analysis of perceived gaps in preparedness planning or capabilities. This can become obvious to key members of a community and quickly derail trust and create suspicion in terms of underlying motives. Collaboration with the community should entail government at the periphery and not the center and must include the ebb and flow of input in a timely and constructive manner so that trust, attentiveness to mutually agreed upon outcomes and a win-win environment is created and maintained.

Adopting the above attitude and approach toward improved community inclusion by government emergency management agencies will not only result in enhanced trust, but also a better calibrated response to catastrophic events through better anticipation of community needs as well as availability and deployment of community assets when needed. An added benefit is the impact on resiliency and the ability of the community as a whole to mitigate the consequences of such events through more strategic coordination and collaboration across the whole of community sectors, disciplines and citizenry.

Why it is Essential to Consider Social Determinants of Community Preparedness and Resiliency

Three examples of historically important events of national scope and prominence can serve to highlight the advantages of considering community social determinants and inclusion in the planning phase of emergency preparedness. In each instance, a failure to adequately consider this level of community dynamic and effects on the long-term impact of the disaster resulted in a less than optimal response that included significant adverse health, economic, and social consequences and failure to build or strengthen community resiliency.

Example No. 1: Hurricane Katrina

Considered by many to be one of the greatest failures of post 9/11 national preparedness efforts (especially in the context of being an "anticipated emergency event"), the 2005 landfall of Hurricane Katrina continues to plague New Orleans and the surrounding region not only with remnants of physical impact but by citizen emotional scarring. Revisiting the Katrina experience by the media, academics, first responders, and the general public has done little to dispel distrust and cynicism regarding the real or perceived pitfalls in local, state, and federal government emergency planning and response. In particular, stories of "individuals left behind," "neighborhoods ignored," and "populations excluded," suggest a planning and response model out of touch with community rhythm and cadence at a very fundamental level. In addition to the expected political finger pointing across both sides of the partisan aisle in an effort to diffuse blame, emergency management preparedness planning post-Katrina has not been sufficiently recalibrated to meaningfully include and accommodate special populations, meet community functional needs, and improve cultural attenuation to foster a level of self-sufficiency and resiliency.

New Orleans even before Katrina was a poverty-stricken city, plagued by social factors that put certain neighborhoods at much higher risk than others for hurricane damage. Residents from higher poverty neighborhoods were less likely to rapidly or easily evacuate prior to the hurricane coming ashore.[3] Although the media placed blame on these communities through the lens of a lack of individual responsibility, in reality, deficits in planning necessary infrastructure and resources to evacuate resulted in the most severe damage to these communities. This was most evident in news reports that depicted deteriorating medical surge and support as well as concerns regarding public safety during and after evacuation was declared by government authorities.

In essence, Hurricane Katrina uncovered many stark social ills that have existed for decades in New Orleans but became both acutely evident and exacerbated as the emergency unfolded. However, meaningful and authentic engagement of the community and advanced consideration and integration of various social determinants could have resulted in a very different historical account of the event. It is our belief that taking time for emergency managers to fully understand these social factors will make all the difference in the success of future local preparedness activities and recognized improvements in community trust and resiliency.

Example No. 2: British Petroleum Deepwater Horizon Disaster

The British Petroleum (BP) Deepwater Horizon oil rig disaster in 2010 had immediate implications for the surrounding environment including deposition of millions of gallons of crude oil on the shorelines and beaches of several states stretching from Louisiana to Florida. While media and first responder attention appropriately focused on control of the spill at the rig and related underwater infrastructure, longer-term response efforts quickly shifted to mitigating ecosystem impact and residual environmental contamination. However, issues have since emerged farther inland and among shoreline resident populations that speak loudly to the unanticipated social and economic disruption that is an equally important repercussion of the spill. These types and categories of impacts are seldom considered upfront in the typical emergency planning model or mindset. The response is often calibrated to the more immediate, easily understandable and tangible consequences of a disaster.

Indeed, offshore disasters such as the BP oil rig explosion in the Gulf can have significant and devastating effects far onshore. An article in the *New England Journal of Medicine* highlighting long-term health effects of the spill points toward a number of social phenomenon that are directly attributable to the incident months later.[4] These demonstrable psychosocial issues relate to chronic unemployment by individuals involved in the once robust Gulf fishing industry. Persons caught in a prolonged economic downturn in this regional economic mainstay have reported stress related gastrointestinal illness, unexplained back and leg pain, and difficulty sleeping. The fact that many of these workers quit high school and have few specific skills outside of the fishing industry should not be ignored. A better understanding of economic impact of such events must include consideration of workforce demographics and alternative employment placement programs to ease such transitions.

Equally significant were the authors' findings regarding an increase in community domestic violence cases and reports. While not suggesting that the number of abusers had actually increased, the hypothesis that extended unemployment placed abusers in the home environment was theorized. The question remains as to how we can better predict, plan, and prepare for such consequences within communities that are directly involved or peripheral to these types of disasters or emergency events. Achieving community resiliency as part of a national preparedness objective has a clear nexus with social determinants such as high school graduation and unemployment rates along with public health and safety trends.

Example No. 3: 2009 H1N1 Pandemic

The H1N1 pandemic in 2009 offers a number of insights into the importance of considering upstream social determinants and community dynamics in emergency preparedness planning and resiliency. The spread of novel disease within a population is of particular concern to public health officials who are immediately faced with characterizing the magnitude of disease spread, severity of illness, and efficacy of available medical countermeasures as well as non-pharmaceutical interventions such as social distancing and isolation and quarantine.

As school closure became the social distancing measure most readily implemented by local public health agencies early in the first phase of the pandemic, it became equally clear that the public were less eager to embrace such a maneuver due to the economic consequence that appeared to outweigh risk of infection from a flu strain that appeared not much different from seasonal epidemics. Loss of income, inability to place displaced children in alternative congregated childcare settings, and consideration of breakfast and lunch needs for many low-income public students quickly raised issues by parents and policymakers alike as to whether such social distancing measures were warranted. In Milwaukee, Wisconsin, public health officials ordered closure of twenty-one public and private schools within two weeks prior to rescinding the directive and abandoning the policy based on political and community economic considerations. This represented a light bulb moment for public health emergency planners and others who were married to standard pandemic plans that were not calibrated against severity of illness and unequivocally endorsed such measures for protection and preservation of the public's health.

In addition, it became apparent in Wisconsin and by the State Division of Public Health during the second wave of the pandemic that a disproportionate number of hospitalizations due to influenza complications were occurring among minority populations as compared to non-Hispanic white cohorts.[5] In the City of Milwaukee, this disparity in hospitalizations was seven times higher in African-American populations. A number of factors were hypothesized as contributing to this phenomenon including: higher prevalence of chronic disease in minority populations contributing to severity of influenza complications; access to and availability of early healthcare intervention in the community; continued reflection of low influenza vaccination rates within some minority populations; and inadequate educational outreach and awareness building in terms achieving cultural competency in message content, format, and method of delivery.

A closer examination of social influences within populations, especially around economic status and healthcare behavior, may have provided valuable insight on more measured and targeted interventions and prevention strategies. However, it is often easier and more convenient for government agencies to develop strategies that are uniformly standardized across a large geographic region to maximize deployment and allocation of resources with little effort or thought to critically evaluate outcomes at the individual community level during the response.

Conclusion: Redefining "The Way Forward"

These three examples offer several lessons on the need to identify and consider integration of social determinants within future emergency preparedness efforts in order to improve response and achieve community resiliency. First, many ill-effects of disasters can be linked to inadequate planning—specifically in regards to incorporating existing economic, social, and health impacts that define a community's daily reality into the preparedness equation. Second, through the use of proper community inclusion and trust building throughout every facet of the emergency planning model (preparedness, mitigation, response, and recovery), many post-emergency consequences could be better predicted and responded to in a manner that strengthens community self-sufficiency and encourages resiliency. Translating both of these important components into modern emergency management practice will achieve a robust and successful model of national preparedness and resiliency—the ultimate goal of PPD8 and philosophical tenet of the FEMA "Whole of Community" strategic approach.

There are certainly examples in other disaster response analyses where emergency management agencies have successfully engaged community organizations in the planning process. Often these included community health promoters, community activists, organizers, and others who have built community trust, are trained to understand community dynamics, and are best situated to implement an effective response through their already established social networks. Further research and evaluation is needed to demonstrate the effectiveness and outcomes of these partnerships, as well as best practices for implementation.

Unique communities require unique solutions to what can be complex planning models forwarded by emergency management agencies. Therefore, a less prescriptive approach by government agencies and more guiding and consulting roles need to be adopted to integrate creative solutions and problem solving by the community. This will strengthen trust between the community and government agencies as well as attract atypical stakeholders to the discussion forum. Sustaining this level of constructive dialogue becomes paramount and stimulates further evolution of discussion including a more diverse array of effective solutions around planning, response, and recovery.

It is incumbent upon emergency management and homeland security professionals to not only incentivize and improve active involvement of nontraditional stakeholders in the planning process but to also consider and incorporate social determinants as previously suggested. Federal workgroups assigned the task of creating and leveraging "Whole of Community" must reflect the diversity of communities in such forums and pursue outcomes based on creating an environment of empathy and trust. This requires authenticity in leadership by federal authorities as well as state and local emergency management agencies to partner with communities to discern relevant social determinants that are the key to moving forward in successful emergency preparedness and community resiliency in the twenty-first century.

Notes

1 Barack Obama, *Presidential Policy Directive/PPD-8: National Preparedness*. (Washington, DC: US Department of Homeland Security, March 30, 2011), http://www.dhs.gov/xabout/laws/gc_1215444247124.shtm.

2 Federal Emergency Management Agency (FEMA) *A Whole Community Approach to Emergency Management: Principles, Themes, and Pathways for Action* (Washington, DC: FEMA, December 2011), http://www.fema.gov/about/wholecommunity.shtm.

3 Richard M. Zoraster, "Vulnerable Populations: Hurricane Katrina as a Case Study," Prehospital Disaster Medicine 25, no. 1 (2010): 74–78.

4 Bernard D. Goldstein, Howard J. Osofsky, and Maureen Y. Lichtveld, "Current Concepts: The Gulf Oil Spill," *New England Journal of Medicine* 364, no. 14 (April 2011): 1334–1348.

5 A.S. Chitnis, S.A. Truelove, J.K. Druckenmiller, R.T. Heffernan, and J.P. Davis, "Epidemiologic and Clinical Features Among Patients Hospitalized in Wisconsin with 2009 H1N1 Influenza A Virus Infections, April to August 2009," Wisconsin Medical Journal 109, no. 4 (August 2010): 201–208.

Ecological Public Health and Climate Change Policy

George P. Morris

Abstract

The fact that health and disease are products of a complex interaction of factors has long been recognized in public health circles. More recently, the term 'ecological public health' has been used to characterize an era underpinned by the paradigm that, when it comes to health and well-being, 'everything matters'. The challenge for policy makers is one of navigating this complexity to deliver better health and greater equality in health. Recent work in Scotland has been concerned to develop a strategic approach to environment and health. This seeks to embrace complexity within that agenda and recognize a more subtle relationship between health and place but remain practical and relevant to a more traditional hazard-focused environmental health approach. The Good Places, Better Health initiative is underpinned by a new problem-framing approach using a conceptual model developed for that purpose. This requires consideration of a wider social, behavioural etc, context. The approach is also used to configure the core systems of the strategy which gather relevant intelligence, subject it to a process of evaluation and direct its outputs to a broad policy constituency extending beyond health and environment. This paper highlights that an approach, conceived and developed to deliver better health and greater equality in health through action on physical environment, also speaks to a wider public health agenda. Specifically it offers a way to help bridge a gap between paradigm and policy in public health. The author considers that with development, a systems-based approach with close attention to problem-framing/situational modelling may prove useful in orchestrating what is a necessarily complex policy response to mitigate and adapt to climate change.

Keywords ecological; public health; climate; systems

Introduction

It is difficult now to imagine a time when public health professionals did not define health in an inclusive way or speak of the interaction of many influences in its creation and destruction. This broader view of health and its determinants (and arguably, the first steps towards a modern ecological perspective) began with the work of Lalonde[1] in the 1970s whose aspiration was to identify upstream approaches to stem healthcare costs in Canada. In repetition, analysis and refinement, the causal complexity implicit in the ecological perspective has become a cliché of discourse in public health and is acknowledged throughout the contemporary literature.[2,3,4] While politicians and the media may be drawn towards more individualistic and proximal explanations and responses, the public health constituency converges around a conviction that aspects of our social and physical environment, our behaviour and that of others, interact continuously with genetic factors throughout life to determine morbidity and longevity. This perspective pervades teaching and training in public health and the structures through which it seeks to deliver. The 21st century has been termed an 'era of ecological public health'[4,5,6] and is underpinned by the paradigm that, when it comes to health and well-being 'everything matters'.[7] Individual and population health may have always been the product of interaction between many factors, but few would deny that cultural change, globalization and a sea change in the area of communications have each greatly added to causal complexity in public health. The most compelling reason of all for acclaiming a new public health era may simply be to create the sense of urgency necessary to generate new ways of responding to the contemporary public health challenge—to make explicit that with so much still to be done, 'more of the same' cannot deliver progress on the scale and with the speed required.

The defining complexity of the ecological public health era, or more accurately, the rather ineffective policy response to it, is nowhere better illustrated than in the stubborn inequalities in health that exist between different socio-economic groups across the world,[8] within countries and even within our UK towns and cities.[9,10,11] Stark differences in health and well-being are not simply a question of 'money in the bank' but neither can they be satisfactorily explained by individual, social or other variables operating through relationships of simple 'cause and effect' to damage health and well-being. A key message of the ecological era is that health and health inequality are never solely about behaviour, place or social context, offering a clue as to why targeted policies so often fail to deliver anticipated outcomes.

The task of developing an appropriate public health policy approach is daunting. If 'everything matters', then, by extension, many constituencies must be engaged to deliver the desired outcomes. Success demands much more than acceptance of a complex reality and pleas for interdisciplinary working. An unprecedented gap is now apparent between paradigm and policy, and bridging it is likely to require a fundamental rethink of how things are done. Part of the answer must lie in organization—in adopting more strategic approaches that use co-ordinated systems and structures to capture evidence, to evaluate it and direct the messages that emerge to appropriate policy constituencies.[12] However, at a more fundamental level there is a need to frame public health problems to truly reflect the ecological perspective, while remaining pragmatic and policy-focused. The approach to problem framing must capture interconnectivity across the public health agenda and between public health and the many other complex policy agendas. So many intractable contemporary policy challenges are intractable precisely because they are products of this complex interplay of social, economic, physical and behavioural factors applying at both individual and societal level. It may be convenient and indeed logical to label, for example, health inequality or the obesity epidemic as 'public health' problems as long as we recognize an infinitely wider policy context when framing the problems and seeking solutions. Although it is too soon to judge its utility for policy, the Foresight work—*Tackling Obesity: Future Choice*[13]—reflects this approach in its use of modelling and in its application of systems thinking. In a similar vein, it may be convenient, and again logical, to label environmental justice, sustainability or the challenges of preserving and enhancing the natural and built environments as 'environmental' problems, provided that the interconnectivity with a much wider policy context, including public health, is made explicit. In this way the necessary cross-cutting policy response is more likely to be developed.

For all the above reasons, ecological perspectives on policy are indicated, but for many people the greatest imperative for seeking new approaches to policy is climate change.

Initially characterized as an environment/energy issue, climate change and the response to it will impact on almost every aspect of life and almost every sphere of public policy. The interconnections with public health and public health policy are widely discussed.[14,15] Direct health effects from increasing temperatures and extreme weather events are confidently predicted, as are indirect health effects on health in one country from climate change in another. Health effects, many of which may be positive—sometimes termed 'co-benefits'—are also likely to flow from adaptation but particularly from national policies to mitigate global climate change. The challenge of climate change is the challenge of complexity writ large and the policy response must be sophisticated and carefully orchestrated.

By any interpretation, the concept of ecological public health introduced above ought to embrace biological complexity, the ecological complexity of society and the interconnections between the two. Arguably, the boundaries of ecological public health could be set still wider to include the subjective world of individual human beings (where matters such as ethics, norms, aspirations and values apply) and also the inter-subjective world of culture. Forging the correct policy approach for the ecological public health era is the defining task of the discipline today and shares many intellectual and practical challenges with the task of creating a sophisticated policy response to climate change with which it is intertwined. By extension, approaches and tools that make us more effective in developing policy in ecological public health must offer pointers to better orchestrate the potentially even more complex policy response to climate change.

The idea that problem framing using conceptual models may be used to address complex policy challenges is not new. There are various examples from the field of public health. Precedent can be found in the observations of Evans and Stoddart.[2] With their 'socio-ecological model of health', developed in the early 1990s, they sought to provide a tool to allow the many factors that have a bearing on health and well-being to be illustrated schematically. They proposed a model to map the complexity of health and its determinants and to assemble the requisite evidence to inform policy and action.

From Paradigms to Policies in An Ecological Era—A Case Study From Scotland

When seeking a 'smarter', more strategic approach to environmental health in Scotland, Morris *et al*[12] were drawn to the earlier insights of Evans and Stoddart and specifically the implicit policy relevance of their approach to problem framing using a conceptual model. Evans and Stoddart had made the capacity of their model, the Socio-Ecological Model of Health, to present evidence in a way that would make its implications more apparent; a test of its usefulness.[2] Morris *et al* had a similar aspiration but enjoyed the luxury of a rather narrower focus. They were less concerned to model an entire system but rather to present a generic approach to answering policy-relevant questions in physical environment and human health. The purity of any model was seen as secondary to its utility in underpinning policy and its delivery. They argued that the right model should support, and to a degree configure, the component systems and structures they considered would be necessary to give effect to a strategic approach to environment and health. These, they considered to relate to intelligence, its evaluation and the operation of the 'levers of change'. To achieve this, and for individuals and organizations to understand their role and exert influence (which seemed central to delivering policies in complex situations), it was argued that a model must represent not only causation but also interventions in the form of policies and actions. To exclude the input of policy from the representation of causal processes, would be to disregard an important factor with the potential to bear upon the outcome. To do so would undermine the analytical capacity of a model and significantly diminish its capacity to support strategy. However, a model must represent the key variables and the interaction between them without becoming burdened by complexity. It ought to be a practical tool, characterized by simplicity but, when applied to a particular issue, its outputs must be in a form amenable to being taken up by the policy constituency.[12]

The model that emerged was a modified version of one first developed to configure an environmental health information system for a World Health Organization (WHO) European

Region initiative on environment and human health.[16] The WHO model—DPSEEA (an abbreviation of the different elements within the model)—provides a simple structure to consider the ways in which aspects of the environment impact on health; the ways in which these environments are created; and actions that are or might be taken at different points on a chain or network of causation to ameliorate outcome. A simple adaptation of the model produced Modified DPSEEA, which additionally requires consideration of the issues that influence whether individuals are exposed to particular environmental factors and whether these exposures subsequently lead to health effects. These so-called 'contextual factors' can also be targets for policies and actions to deliver a better health outcome.[12] The Modified DPSEEA model (Figure 10.2.1) can be used to elucidate the determinants of both positive and negative health effects.

To populate Modified DPSEEA for a particular issue, it is possible to enter the model at any point. For example, one could start with an environmental 'state' or a health 'effect'. The latter requires immediate consideration of the environmental 'exposures' that may influence the effect and the 'contexts' that determine exposure and the risk of an observable health effect. It is necessary to consider the environmental states that lead to exposures; the man-made 'pressures' (or modifiers) that result in these states; and the social, political, economic, commercial and other anthropogenic 'drivers' that create these pressures. It is also necessary when populating the model for a specific issue to include actions, usually policies, and their points of impact, either on the chain of causation or on context.[12]

Populating the model to represent the environmental contributions to a particular health effect often highlights that more than one environmental factor is involved. This will generate multiple chains. In a similar vein, a particular environmental state can be created by more than one pressure, thus introducing the possibility of branching chains. Additional health effects may also be identified leading from different parts of the populated model as it develops. Thus, the Modified DPSEEA model, when applied to a particular issue often comprises multiple chains

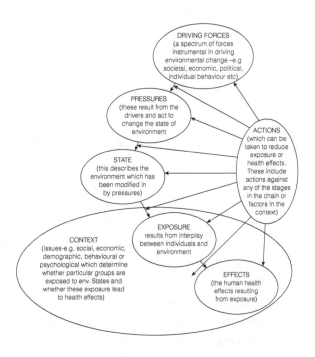

Figure 10.2.1 Modified DPSEEA

Source: Morris et al[12]

which may be branched. Figure 10.2.2 shows an example of multiple chains in a specimen model populated using the example of scald injuries.

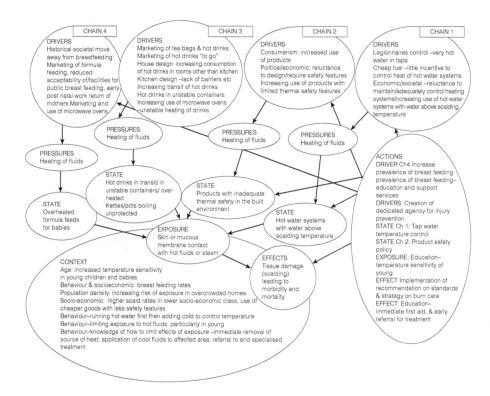

Figure 10.2.2   Modified DPSEEA applied to scalds (specimen only)

Applying the Approach in Practice

In publishing ideas for a strategic approach to environment and health centring on close attention problem framing, and delivered through carefully developed systems, Morris *et al* were working to support an earlier statement of intent by the Scottish Government to create a 'strategic framework for environment and health'. The ideas for a new approach in this field had been generated during extensive dialogue within government and beyond, which highlighted a desire to move beyond the prevailing rather narrow, compartmentalized and hazard-focused environmental health ethos to one that recognized a wider potential for environmental change in promoting positive health and well-being. Linked to this was a wish to reflect not only the more complex reality but a greater subtlety in the relationship between environment and health wherein, among other things, greater account was taken of a psychosocial dimension. This latter issue was considered to have particular relevance to the health inequalities agenda.[12]

Morris *et al* had observed that the process of applying the Modified DPSEEA model to an issue could produce a 'helicopter view' illustrating more comprehensively the situation within which policies on environment and health must be developed and implemented. Indeed, another term for the approach might be 'situational modelling' and a key benefit demonstrated through extensive piloting of the approach was a capacity to engage a wide stakeholder constituency.

December 2008 saw the launch in Scotland of a major strategic policy initiative, Good Places, Better Health.[17] The policy is being rolled out through a process that begins with problem framing using the Modified DPSEEA model in workshops with relevant stakeholders. The decision to launch the policy followed consultation among stakeholders and successful piloting of the Modified DPSEEA approach for a range of environment and human health issues in various settings across the UK.

A three-year prototype phase focusing on a limited number of priorities is now under way.[17] It applies the analytical techniques and develops the structures in relation to four health outcomes (asthma; unintentional injury; obesity; mental health and well-being) in children of eight years and under, and a parallel priority relating to sustainable homes and their immediate environs. The experience of populating Modified DPSEEA in stakeholder workshops prior to and since the launch of Good Places, Better Health affirms the utility of the analytical approach. Some learning points are emerging, which are now refining the process. Among these is the necessity to engage a wide spectrum of relevant stakeholders in workshops; the benefits of validating and refining the populated Modified DPSEEA 'maps' in 'secondary' workshops and by reference to a wider literature. To this end, the prototype phase of Good Places, Better Health is supported by a major research project funded by the Scottish government and involving a consortium of key academic interests. The Environmental Determinants of Public Health in Scotland (EDPHiS) project,[18] in addition to validating and refining the populated models produced in stakeholder workshops, applies the insights of, and extrapolates from, a wider literature to a Scottish context and as far as possible attempts to quantify the impacts of existing and promising policy interventions.

An interesting development relates to how the outputs from problem-framing workshops are held. It has been found convenient to enter the tabular information that lies behind the situational models a relational database. This confers obvious benefit in terms of access but critically the database can be interrogated to reveal, for example, policies and actions that have the potential to impact on different policy areas.

Informing Policy

The problem framing conducted in stakeholder workshops; the research element provided through EDPHiS; the work to bring forward information in the form of data about the environment, health and other factors; and a further work package providing insights into good and promising practice at local level, together constitute the intelligence stream. Those responsible

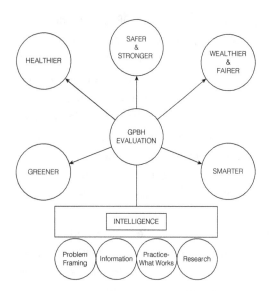

Figure 10.2.3 Intelligence to policy and the cross-cutting dividend

for each component of the intelligence stream make up the Good Places, Better Health Intelligence Partnership. Intelligence is regarded as the first core system of the initiative and part of a conduit flowing from intelligence to policy.[17] Figure 10.2.3 illustrates this progression by showing the individual components of the intelligence system and how these are directed through expert evaluation (the second core system of Good Places, Better Health) to inform policy areas within government. The specific policy areas are represented under broad headings that reflect the National Objectives of the Scottish Government (Figure 10.2.4). However, the intention is clear. In keeping with the cross-cutting aspirations of Good Places, Better Health, messages from evaluation are directed not solely to health or environmental policy interests, but to the policy constituencies most appropriate to operate the levers of change. These might relate to transport, planning, communities, environmental protection, health improvement, building standards, social policy, justice etc. Unsurprisingly perhaps, the need to secure the optimal functioning of the 'levers of change' is the function of the third core system of Good Places, Better Health.

Intelligence to Policy and the Cross-Cutting Dividend

The messages from evaluation for potential action across the policy constituency might concern the following:

- Lack of data about a key variable
- Insufficient core knowledge (indicating a need for epidemiological or biomedical research or for evaluation)
- A discernable policy void
- Efficacy of existing policy
- A promising policy option (with potential for significant or crosscutting impact)
- The need for wider dissemination of identified good and promising practice

However, a very important overarching message for those who create policy, and indeed for those who deliver it, will be about the interconnectivity of agendas and how this can be exploited.

The necessary 'reach' to impact at policy level is being facilitated by a carefully conceived governance structure, but also through other recent developments in the Scottish Government, including the development of the Government's five strategic objectives (Box 10.2.1).

Box 10.2.1

Among the first actions of the incoming administration on taking office in May 2007 was to align the Scottish government around five strategic objectives. The aspiration was for a Scotland that is:

- Wealthier and fairer
- Smarter
- Healthier
- Safer and stronger
- Greener

These national objectives are being pursued through a smaller ministerial team matched to a simpler structure of directorates within the Scottish government. Each directorate carries responsibility for delivery of each of the five national objectives and the overarching National Purpose of Sustainable Economic Growth. It is considered that the corporate responsibility to deliver on each of the national objectives can only help to create an appetite for the messages emerging from the evaluation processes within the Good Places, Better Health initiative.

Lessons Learned and Wider Implications

This paper offers an account from conception to inception of a policy initiative relating to environment and human health in Scotland (population approximately 5 million). At the time of writing, the Good Places, Better Health initiative has been in place in prototype form for only a short time and, while a commitment to project evaluation exists, this is understandably some way off. By any interpretation it is inappropriate to draw firm conclusions, still less any that can be generalized. However, against the background of urgency occasioned by climate change, some tentative observations on the process and based on experience to date are perhaps admissible.

The public health challenge is presented above as one of embracing and navigating complexity. The contemporary 'environment and health challenge' is a scarcely less complex subset of it. In reality, public health cannot effectively respond to either without adopting a more ecological approach. Each must bridge the gap between a paradigm that says 'everything matters' and the sophisticated cross-cutting policy response which that implies.

Throughout the analysis, discussion and stakeholder consultation leading to the launch of Good Places, Better Health, certain criteria have emerged that appear synonymous with success in delivering the right approach on policy. The modern, strategic approach must speak to a wider ecological public health agenda—i.e. it must:

- Match policy much more closely to the paradigm 'everything matters'
- Reflect a much more subtle and complex relationship between places and human health and well-being than is captured by the current emphasis on infections, allergens and physical hazards acting through simple relationships of cause and effect
- Identify the synergies and antagonisms in policies and actions addressing a number of the key contemporary agendas of government
- Align *short-* and *long*-term goals
- Explicitly link *local* action to *national* and *global* outcomes

These criteria are the ideological touchstones for the Good Places, Better Health initiative and success in fulfilling them may in the long term be the true measure of success for the work. They demonstrably resonate with the generic aspirations of ecological public health and may well be among the more important characteristics of a coherent, well-orchestrated policy response to climate change.

The Scottish approach has extolled the virtues of problem framing with reference to all the factors that have a bearing upon the issue as a means to navigate complexity (including existing policies and actions) when framing any issue. Only then, it is argued, can the approach achieve full analytical potential and support the vital bridge to a wide policy constituency and to the other complex cross-cutting agendas of government. This thinking has informed the development of Modified DPSEEA as a problem-framing tool.

It seems particularly relevant that framing environmental health problems with reference to the axis of place and health is proving useful not only in linking to a wider public health agenda but also other complex challenges of government. Perhaps this is so because many of these have at their core the axis of people and place. This is certainly true of climate change.

At the heart of Good Places, Better Health lie three core systems. How these are configured and the governance arrangements that oversee and coordinate them are central to the operation of policy. Together they provide the conduit through which to assemble the wider public/

environmental health intelligence and direct it, through expert evaluation, to deliver pragmatic and policy-relevant messages to the policy constituencies. In short, the systems and the governance structures are just as important in bridging the gap between paradigm and policy as a more ecological and enlightened approach to problem framing.

In conclusion, even on the limited evidence available thus far from implementation of Good Places, Better Health, the new approach offers a promising way to navigate complexity to produce better environmental health and, we would submit, better public health policy. It is attuned to the Era of Ecological Public Health, but if an appropriate conceptual model can be developed, a similar approach can surely facilitate the orchestration of a more coherent approach to climate change policy.

Acknowledgements

The author acknowledges the continuing work and helpful comments from the Good Places, Better Health team (past and present) within Scottish Government. Particular thanks are also due to Dr Sheila Beck of NHS Health Scotland and Professor Phil Hanlon, University of Glasgow for their commitment to this theme of work and helpful comments on the manuscript.

References

1 Lalonde M. A New perspective on the Health of Canadians. Ministry of Supply and Services, Government of Canada, Ottawa 1974. Available at: www.hc-sc.gc.ca/hcs-sss/com/fed/lalonde-eng.php (accessed 19 October 2009)

2 Evans R, Stoddart G. Producing health, consuming healthcare. In: Evans R, Barer M, Marmor I, editors. Why are Some People Healthy and Others Not? (pp 27–64). New York: Aldine De Gruyter, 1994

3 Reniscow K. Embracing chaos and complexity: A quantum change for public health. *American Journal of Public Health* 2008; 98: 1382–1389

4 Lang T, Raynor G. Overcoming policy cacophony on obesity: An ecological public health framework for policymakers. *Obesity Reviews* 2007; 8 (Suppl 1) 165–181

5 McLaren L, Hawe P. Ecological perspectives in health research. *Journal of Epidemiology and Community Health* 2005; 59: 6–14

6 Arya N, Howard J, Isaacs S, McAllister ML, Murphy S, Rapport D, Waltner-Toews D. Time for an ecosystem approach to public health? Lessons from two infectious disease outbreaks in Canada. *Global Public Health* 2009; 1: 31–49

7 Whyte B. Views of Health in Glasgow (DVD). Glasgow: Centre for Population Health, 2009

8   Commission on the Social Determinants of Health. Closing the Gap in a Generation: Health Equity through Action on the Social Determinants of Health. Final Report of the Commission on Social Determinants of Health. Geneva: World Health Organization, 2008. Available at: www.who.int/social_determinants/thecommission/finalreport/en (accessed 19 October 2009)

9   Walsh D, Taulbut M, Hanlon P. The aftershock of Deindustrialization—Trends in Mortality in Scotland and Other Parts of Post-Industrial Europe. *European Journal of Public Health* doi:10.1093/eurpub/ckp063

10   Hanlon P, Walsh D, Whyte B. Let Glasgow Flourish. Glasgow: Centre for Population Health, 2006

11   Scottish Government. Equally Well: Report of the Ministerial Task Force on Health Inequalities. Edinburgh: Scottish Government 2008. Available at: www.scotland.gov.uk/Resource/Doc/229649/0062206.pdf (accessed 19 October 2009)

12   Morris GP, Beck SA, Hanlon P, Robertson R. Getting strategic about environment and health. *Public Heath* 2006; 120: 889–907

13   Department of Health. Foresight—Tackling Obesities—Future Choices. London: Department of Health, 2007. Available at: www.dh.gov.uk/en/Publichealth/Healthimprovement/Obesity/DH_079713 (accessed19October 2009)

14   Department of Health. Expert Group on Climate Change and Health in the UK. Health Effects of Climate Change. London: Department of Health, 2008

15   Griffith J, Stewart L. Sustaining a Healthy Future: Taking Action on Climate Change. London: Faculty of Public Health, 2008

16   World Health Organization. Environmental Health Indicators for Europe: A Pilot Indicator-Based Report. Copenhagen: World Health Organization, 2004. Available at: www.euro.who.int/document/eehc/ebakdoc04.pdf (accessed 19 October 2009)

17   Scottish Government. Good Places Better Health: A New Approach to Environment and Health in Scotland—Implementation Plan. Edinburgh: Scottish Government, 2008. Available at: www.scotland.gov.uk/Resource/Doc/254447/0075343.pdf (accessed 19 October 2009)

18   Environmental Determinants of Public Health in Scotland. Available at: www.edphis.org (accessed 19 October 2009)

Chapter 10: **Discussion Questions**

1   List two indicators of environmental infrastructure within a community.

   a.   List two indicators of socioeconomic status within a community.

2   How did the social determinants of community preparedness affect population health after the British Petroleum Deep Water Horizon disaster?

   a.   Give an example of a negative health care outcome after the disaster and a health policy change that could stave it off if (when) another disaster occurs in the future.

3   Compare the after effects of Hurricane Katrina and the H1N1 disaster.

   a.   How were the communities similar and different?

4   List three determinants of health in addition to hereditary disease.

   a.   What does the World Health Organization's acronym DPSEEA stand for?

5   Describe the driving forces, pressures, states, exposure, effects, and actions related to developing a local health policy aimed at an important goal, such as reducing pediatric deaths due to consumption of e-cigarette fluid.

   a.   Explain further by drawing your own DPSEEA model.

CHAPTER 11

PATIENT SAFETY
AND HEALTH POLICY

Ethics

A Foundation for Quality

William A. Nelson

A *strong ethical framework helps determine organizational success.*
A question rarely, if ever, raised in executive ethics training is, "Is ethics important for healthcare organizations?" The participants' presence suggests an interest in and commitment to the importance of ethics.

But while no executive would ever indicate that ethical values are unimportant, do executives regularly acknowledge, demonstrate and ensure ethical values are the foundation and framework for today's healthcare organizations? If staff were surveyed, would they report that ethical values serve as the organization's foundation and framework?

Ethical Values as the Organization's Foundation

Basic ethics principles that make up our common morality, including respect for patients, acting in patients' best interest, avoiding bringing harm to patients and treating patients in a fair and equitable manner, serve as the foundation for healthcare values. These values are generally captured in the organization's mission and values statements.

In thinking about the importance of values as the organization's foundation, consider the construction of a home. After the building site is cleared and the concrete forms have been placed, the cement is poured, creating the concrete foundation. The foundation becomes the base that will support the load of the structure; its contents and all that occurs within it will rest on that foundation. Similarly, achieving a healthcare organization's purpose depends on having a strong foundation. But rather than a concrete foundation, the hospital or health system's foundation is its ethics.

Ethical Values as the Organization's Framework

Ethical values also serve as the organization's framework. In a building, the framework gives shape to the various activities and functions within the structure. Analogously, ethical values frame the guidelines for the organization's operations. They guide staff in how to "live out" that foundation in its overall culture and administrative and clinical practices, which ultimately affects patient encounters.

Do executives regularly acknowledge, demonstrate and ensure ethical values are the foundation and framework for today's healthcare organizations?

The culture should reflect organizational values in the behaviors of all individual staff members and in organizationwide actions. For example, clinical practices should consistently reflect organizational values such as promoting patient self-determination in end-of-life decision making. Management decisions should be based on and reflect the organization's values as well, such as in crafting physician compensation guidelines in a manner that avoids conflicts of interest.

Applying ethical values as the foundation and framework for today's healthcare organizations can be particularly challenging because of economic tensions so common in the delivery of care. For example, do you purchase a new CT scanner because it will generate a larger revenue stream or because evidence supports the belief that the scanner will improve patient care? Which is the real, underlying rationale for the potential purchase? Does it correlate with the organization's values? Professor Kurt Darr, in *Ethics in Health Services Management* (Health Professions Press, 2004), reminds executives that when considering such a purchase, "Health service organizations are social enterprises with an economic dimension rather than an economic enterprise with a social dimension."

When ethics challenges arise in either the clinical or administrative setting, ethical reasoning can serve as a useful tool in addressing the conflict, highlighting a second role of ethical values in the organizations framework. Regarding the example of resource allocation noted earlier, healthcare executives need to recognize that such decisions raise ethical questions and must be considered within the context of the organization's values.

Ethics resources, such as an ethics committee member or a healthcare ethicist who can effectively facilitate ethics reflection, need to be available and should have a seat at the table when such decisions are being made. The process can decrease the presence of an organization's values-practice gap and ensure organizational values serve as the foundation and framework—not just words on some document.

The Ethics, Quality and Value Linkage

Recognizing ethical values as the foundation and framework for healthcare organizations is direcdy tied to the quest for quality and value in the delivery of care. The pursuit of quality and value is based on the application of ethics principles and values, including autonomy, beneficence, nonmaleficence, and social and distributive justice. These basic ethics principles are the foundation for the Institute of Medicine's (IOM) six aims for improving healthcare, as proposed in its landmark report *Crossing the Quality Chasm* (National Academies Press, 2001): patient-centered, effective, safe, efficient, timely and equitable.

Ethics values provide the underlying reasons that quality aims and economic value are essential for healthcare organizations. The same ethics values that serve as the foundation and framework for healthcare serve as the basis of quality goals. When facilities seek to fulfill the IOM's six quality aims, they are also seeking to provide ethics-grounded healthcare. The chart below (adapted from "Preventing Ethics Conflicts and Improving Healthcare Quality," Nelson and colleagues, *Quality and Safety in Health Care,* 2010) highlights the linkage between ethical values, quality and economic value.

Ethics Principles	Applications of Ethics Values to Quality Care	IOM's Quality Aims
Autonomy	Support, facilitate and respect patient self-determination; promote the consistent application of a shared decision-making process	Patient-centered
Beneficence	Ensure beneficial patient healthcare is uniformly implemented; make certain the patient's best interest is paramount	Effective, safe, timely, patient-centered
Nonmaleficence	Avoid and protect the patient from actions that cause harm	Safe, effective, patient-centered
Social and distributive justice	Provide fair allocation of resources to support the patient's best interest, impartial distribution of the benefits and burdens related to delivery of healthcare, and equitable access to healthcare services	Equitable, efficient, patient-centered

The connection between quality and ethics becomes apparent when ethics conflicts occur or quality issues arise. When organizational quality is compromised, ethics norms or standards of practice are frequently violated or eroded. For example, when healthcare professionals provide nonbeneficial or futile care, they erode the organization's quality aims of providing only effective, patient-centered care, which correspond to the ethical norms of providing only beneficial patient care and avoiding actions that can cause harm. Additionally, in such situations, physician decisions can waste organization or third-party economic resources because the margin of benefit per unit of expenditure lacks value.

Similarly, when ethics issues occur, quality aims and care can be compromised. For example, when healthcare professionals willfully ignore patient decisions or do not provide full, open and truthful information regarding an invasive procedure to a terminally ill patient, or when they fail to disclose an adverse event, the quality standard of patient-centered care is not met, nor is the ethical standard of respecting self-determination. In these examples you can see that synergy between ethics, quality and value reinforces the need for executives to recognize the importance of ethical values to healthcare organizations.

Characteristics of Organizations With an Ethics-Grounded Foundation and Framework

Several general characteristics in healthcare organizations reflect the recognition of ethical values serving as the organization's foundation and framework.

Ethical leadership—The organization's leadership acknowledges and consistently demonstrates the importance of ethics in his or her decisions and actions. Leadership expects that managers and supervisors serve as ethics role models to the staff they are directing. Leaders support and use ethics resources and mechanisms.

Integrated mission and ethical values—The mission and ethical values are clearly understood by all staff and serve as the driver for the organization's actions.

Ethics culture and practice—The organizational values are recognized and integrated into the daily actions and behavior of all staff The values provide identity to the staff and the organization and are consistently embodied in all clinical and administrative practices.

Effective ethics programs linked with the quality program—The organization has an effective ethics program that is comprehensive, staff and leadership supported and respected, and that addresses administrative and clinical ethics issues in a system-oriented, reactive and proactive manner. Rather than operating in a silo, the program is linked to quality improvement, patient safety and compliance to ultimately foster and ensure quality patient care. Healthcare leaders need to be serious about the importance of ethics to their organizations—it is not just window dressing. Ensuring that your organization has an ethics-grounded foundation and framework can be a primary factor in determining whether your organization successfully provides value and quality of care to the community it serves.

Interview with Lucian Leape, MD, HFACHE, Adjunct Professor of Health Policy, Department of Health Policy and Management, Harvard School of Public Health

Kyle L. Grazier

Before joining the faculty at Harvard School of Public Health in 1988, Lucian Leape, MD, HFACHE, was professor of surgery and chief of pediatric surgery at Tufts University School of Medicine and the New England Medical Center. Dr. Leape is internationally recognized as a leader in the patient safety movement, starting with the 1994 publication of his seminal article, "Error in Medicine," in *JAMA*. He has published more than 130 papers on the topics of care quality and patient safety.

An outspoken advocate of making patient safety a national priority and the nonpunitive systems approach to preventing medical errors, Dr. Leape has testified many times before the U.S. Congress and has served on various public and private boards and committees. He was one of the founders of the National Patient Safety Foundation, the Massachusetts Coalition for the Prevention of Medical Error, and the Harvard Kennedy School Executive Session on Medical Error. In addition, he was a member of the Institute of Medicine's Committee on Quality of Health Care in America, which produced the influential reports *To Err Is Human* and *Crossing the Quality Chasm*.

He is the recipient of multiple honors, including the Alfred I. duPont Award for Excellence in Children's Health Care from the Nemours organization, the John M. Eisenberg Patient Safety and Quality Award from the Joint Commission and the National Quality Forum, the Distinguished Service Award from the American Pediatric Surgical Association, the Avedis Donabedian Healthcare Quality Award from the American Public Health Association, an Investigator Award in Health Policy Research from the Robert Wood Johnson Foundation, and an honorary fellowship in the Royal

College of Physicians and Surgeons of Canada. In addition, he has been honored with leadership awards from the American Society of Health-Systems Pharmacists, the American Pharmacists Association, and the Institute for Safe Medication Practices. In 2006, *Modem Healthcare* named him one of the 30 people who have had the most impact on healthcare in the past 30 years. In 2007, the National Patient Safety Foundation established the Lucian Leape Institute to advance strategic thinking in patient safety.

Dr. Leape is a graduate of Cornell University and Harvard Medical School. He trained in surgery at Massachusetts General Hospital and in pediatric surgery at Boston Children's Hospital.

Dr. Crazier: *What motivated you to leave 20 years of clinical practice as a pediatric surgeon for a career that is focused exclusively on health policy?*

Dr. Leape: There is no simple answer. I was getting more and more frustrated and fed up about the way healthcare was being run. It became time to quit complaining, roll up my sleeves, and do something. Taking care of patients, particularly performing surgery, was very satisfying. I was able to cure people one by one, and each person was very grateful for that. But I could spend my whole life practicing medicine and only make an impact on a few thousand people. With health policy, on the other hand, I can help millions of people by motivating positive changes to the healthcare system.

Dr. Grazier: *In 1994, JAMA published your paper entitled "Error in Medicine." In 2008, that paper continues to influence policymaking. How do you explain this impact?*

Dr. Leape: A lot of factors are at play. Part of it is that I wrote about the right thing at the right time. Many people outside of healthcare don't understand that doctors and nurses really don't like to hurt people. They take their jobs seriously, and they have high personal and professional standards. When things go wrong, they take the errors personally and suffer terrible feelings of shame and guilt. The message that it isn't all their fault resonated with a lot of people.

The other part is that we established the fact that medical injuries can be reduced by changing systems. We learned concepts from human factors engineering, sociology, and psychology that were applicable to healthcare. Once we proved that those concepts could work, people became enthusiastic. Clinicians were unhappy with the status quo and the accidental harm they were causing. They welcomed the opportunity to try something different.

Dr. Grazier: *There has been significant progress toward reducing medical errors in a relatively short time.*

Dr. Leape: True, but what we hear most commonly is, "Why are we not moving faster?" Of course, that is a good question. In 1999, the IOM [Institute of Medicine] issued a report, *To Err Is Human,* that called for a national effort to reduce serious injury by 50 percent in five years. That was eight years ago, and we haven't seen a massive national initiative, not at the federal level.

What has developed, however, is a grassroots effort—an almost entirely voluntary movement started by a lot of people wanting to do a lot of good things.

Dr. Grazier: *Do you foresee a national effort?*

Dr. Leape: I do. The pressure at the federal level continues to mount, as it becomes even more apparent that a regulatory body has to be involved to set national standards and to ensure that best-practice methods are disseminated. Once we know what to do to keep people safe and to provide high-quality care, there is no moral justification for not ensuring that every caregiver follows those same proven methods.

Certainly, a lack of resources and leadership plagues efforts at the national level. It is pretty disgraceful that Britain, Denmark, and smaller countries are investing so much more into patient safety initiatives than we are in the United States. What has been most disappointing to those of us involved in this issue is that we haven't really convinced the vast majority of hospital and health system CEOs [chief executive officers] to make safety the first priority in their organizations. Part of the reason for this is that the American healthcare system puts so much emphasis on the business of medicine. As a consequence, the primary focus is the fiscal stability of the organization, and success is measured by the robust bottom line and market share. Safety always loses out in that equation. Whether the industry is aviation, nuclear power, or healthcare, the same principle applies: If the first objective is production, then safety is always second.

Since the IOM report was published—when the IOM said we ought to redesign healthcare to fix the problem—a lot of specific, tested, and validated safe practices have emerged that every hospital ought to implement. For example, the Institute for Healthcare Improvement initiated the 100,000 Lives Campaign that urged hospitals to implement six safe practices. Similarly, the National Quality Forum developed a list of 30 practices aimed at reducing errors. Therefore, healthcare organizations can no longer say that they don't know what to do, because we obviously have figured out what to do. Many organizations also say they can't afford to put these practices into operation, which isn't so. The main reason for these excuses is that the American healthcare system has not made safety its number one priority.

Dr. Grazier: *Isn't there a clear economic benefit for providing safe care?*

Dr. Leape: Evidence in favor of following safe practices has been emerging. The economic benefits are very impressive. For example, preventing a central-line bloodstream infection translates to a saving of somewhere between $15,000 and $40,000 per patient. With that amount, a healthcare organization can pay for an awful lot of safe care. From a marketing standpoint, it is certainly advantageous to publicize that your hospital is a safe hospital. Aside from these financial benefits, providing safe care is simply the right thing to do.

Dr. Grazier: *What other incentives are available to promote safety as a priority?*

Dr. Leape: Linking compensation to outcomes has gained a lot of interest. Many organizations are in the midst of experimenting with pay for performance. Specifically, Medicare has announced recently that it will no longer pay for outcomes on certain kinds of serious preventable events. The next frontier for this could be the limitation on more common preventable events. Other payers will participate in this trend, and the list of limitations will expand.

As an extension to pay for performance, we could see payers withholding payment when patients develop hospital-acquired infections. That amounts to a lot of withheld money because such infections are prevalent, and that will get the organizations' attention and motivate them to move in the right direction. Dozens of hospitals have succeeded in totally eliminating central-line infections and ventilator-associated pneumonia, and incidents of surgical-site infections have greatly decreased as well. Therefore, it is obvious that these infections can be prevented, and it makes sense for payers not to recompense for preventable practices that hurt people.

Dr. Grazier: *What do you prescribe for a healthier healthcare system in the future?*

Dr. Leape: The future of patient safety and healthcare quality improvement is tightly linked to the overall decisions we make now. The United States is spending twice as much on healthcare as the average European country. But we are getting poorer results and leaving 47 million people without a way to pay for basic care.

Healthcare is steadily climbing to the top of the domestic agenda for financial reasons. Solving these cost problems, however, requires quantum changes. These changes relate to improving the quality of care and maximizing patient safety. One fundamental step we can take is to quit paying for individual services and specific procedures or tests. Comprehensive, coordinated, integrated, continuous care is a better alternative, because it puts the emphasis on teamwork and multidisciplinary work. Another step that may be advantageous is to evaluate the way we finance healthcare. Orthopedic surgeons make, on average, $450,000 a year, while many primary care doctors earn $120,000 annually. That disparity in income certainly sends a loud, clear message: We put more emphasis on services than on care. Until we realize this connection, we cannot realize big improvements.

Dr. Grazier: *Do you think this shift in emphasis will require a single-payer scheme?*

Dr. Leape: That would be the easiest, most efficient, and cheapest way to go, but this system is possible through commercial insurance companies, as long as standard rules are established and followed. Basic rules may include paying physician groups, not individual physicians; prohibiting cancellation of insurance; and not basing the premiums on experience rating. Such a system will require heavy regulation, and this is perhaps why nobody wants to recommend it.

Dr. Grazier: *What lessons can healthcare executives and managers learn from your patient safety work?*

Dr. Leape: There are several lessons. First, human errors are secondary to the primary failures in the system. All errors are the result of system breakdowns; therefore, the system has to be redesigned. Enough evidence supports this fact, but it remains difficult for people to believe it, thinking that the person is the one who made the horrible mistake. Changing systems is difficult because it requires changing embedded human mind-set and behavior. Managers must really understand this driving force behind patient safety.

Second, everyone in the organization has to be held accountable. This is a lesson from high-reliability organizations and industries, such as aviation, nuclear power, chemical manufacturing, and businesses that have intrinsically hazardous processes. The idea here is that individuals have to follow the rules and to take personal responsibility so that they are not just implementing safe practices, they are also spotting hazards and preventing them. Accountability is absolutely crucial to a culture of safety.

There is a misconception about what a nonpunitive environment entails. In a nonpunitive environment, people are not punished if they make an error as a result of a lack of resources or circumstances beyond their control. If people caused an error because of misconduct—such as deliberately breaking a rule for personal gain, intentionally not following protocols, or purposely trying to hurt somebody—they should be punished. That kind of behavior cannot be tolerated. We need to separate these two human causes of harm. Occurrence of an error in itself is not bad because it allows for an opportunity to understand what is wrong with the system.

Third, change happens at the bottom, but it starts at the top. The leader must articulate the vision, stimulate other people to carry it out, provide necessary resources, and set an example. Over and over again, we have observed process and quality improvement efforts implemented but ultimately fail because the CEO did not lend support to the initiatives. A subset of leadership support is physician participation. In healthcare, not much can get done without physicians, and any patient safety effort is not possible without their involvement. Most physicians are independent contractors, not employees, so they can take the position of not following or adopting a system that they don't agree with. We must end the current scheme of physicians as independent contractors. They must be part of the healthcare team and, as such, will have to lead and be involved.

Finally, the key success factors in a safety effort are teamwork and respect, two basic ideas that are too often lacking in medicine. People have to be trained to work in teams and to respect others on the team.

Dr. Grazier: *What role should patients play?*

Dr. Leape: Patients have to be much more a part of the action now than ever before. First, we need to get used to the idea that they have the right to know everything about their condition.

Hospital policy should require transparency and honesty, as doctors, hospitals, and health systems have no right to keep secrets from patients. When errors occur, the caregivers and the organization have to share the information with, apologize to, and compensate the patient. These are some of the things we recommend to CEOs and other leaders. Some leaders are making great strides toward this end, and some others have had major success. In some hospitals, patients are involved in all planning activities. They serve on committees, review boards, and other groups. Patients bring a voice that is otherwise missing in healthcare, and, of course, this perspective is probably the most important of all.

The Path to Continuously Learning Health Care

Robert Saunders and Mark D. Smith

The United States has a timely opportunity—and pressing need—to build a smart health care system that provides best care at lower cost. Here's how.

Health care in the United States has experienced an explosion in biomedical knowledge, dramatic innovations in therapies and surgical procedures, and expanded capacity to manage conditions that previously were debilitating or fatal— and ever more exciting clinical capabilities are on the horizon. Yet, paradoxically, health care is falling short on basic dimensions of quality, outcomes, cost, and equity. Actions that could improve the health care system's performance—developing knowledge, organizing and translating new information into medical evidence, applying the new evidence to patient care—are marred by significant shortcomings and inefficiencies that result in missed opportunities, waste, and harm to patients.

The human and economic impacts are great. An estimated 75,000 deaths could have been averted in 2005 alone if every state had delivered care on par with the best performing state. Current waste—an estimated $750 billion in unnecessary health spending in 2009—diverts valuable and limited resources from productive use.

It is important to note that individual physicians, nurses, technicians, pharmacists, and others involved in patient care work diligently to provide high-quality, compassionate care to their patients. The problem is not that they are not working hard enough. Rather, it is that the health care system does not adequately support them in their work. The system lags in adjusting to new discoveries, disseminating data in real

Robert Saunders and Mark D. Smith, "The Path to Continuously Learning Health Care," *Issues in Science and Technology*, vol. 29, no. 3, pp. 27-36. Copyright © 2013 by Issues in Science and Technology. Reprinted with permission. Provided by ProQuest LLC. All rights reserved.

time, organizing and coordinating the enormous volume of research and recommendations, and providing incentives for choosing the smartest route to health, not just the newest, shiniest—and often most expensive—tool. These broader issues prevent clinicians from providing the best care to their patients and limit their ability to continuously learn and improve.

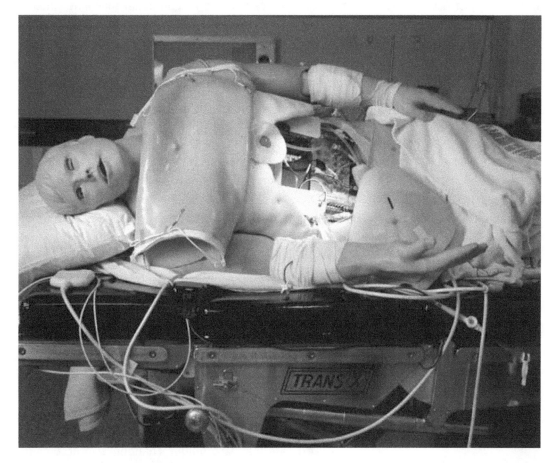

JUSTINE COOPER, *Charles*, C-Print, 30 × 40 inches, 2007.

Justine Cooper

Australian-born and New York-based photographer Justine Cooper's *Terminal* series features large format photographs depicting medical robots and manikins. These sophisticated manikins, typically connected to computers, simulate living situations from crisis to childbirth. At once alien and familiar, they represent the feats of modern medical technology. Far from the public dissections of the 17th century, these private theaters play out imagined traumas for the benefit of doctors and surgeons honing their skills. In this landscape, the body of the patient is supplanted by creations that are neither virtual, nor real. At a time when medical intervention can be de-humanizing, when technology is criticized for removing us from reality, these images create a perverse inversion. Cooper found that the personnel charged with the care of the manikins had humanized these objects into subjects by naming them, dressing them in holiday attire and constructing a narrative through their care. These million-dollar manikins embody memories of daily life, offering up their injuries and procedures as rather austere visual diaries in the era of Second Life and the blogosphere. The *Terminal series*, dating from 2008, marks the beginning of Cooper's exploration of medical robots and manikins. Her *Living In Sim* series, created the following year, presents the real and imaginary lives of manikins via blog, video soap opera, installation, and photographs.

Cooper's artwork investigates the intersections between culture, science, and medicine. She moves between many forms of media including animation, video, installation, and photography, as well as medical imaging technologies such as MRI, DNA sequencing, ultrasound, and scanning electron microscopy. Her work has been internationally recognized and exhibited in more than sixty shows and screenings, including the New Museum of Contemporary Art, New York; the NTT InterCommunication Center, Tokyo; the Singapore Museum of Art; the Netherlands Institute for Media Art; the George Pompidou Centre, Paris; Kwang Ju Biennale, Korea, and the International Center of Photography, New York. Cooper's artwork is held in public and private collections including the Metropolitan Museum of Art, the Powerhouse Museum (Sydney), the Queensland Art Gallery, and the Australian Center for the Moving Image.

The shortcomings are especially apparent when considering how other industries routinely operate compared with many aspects of health care. Builders rely on blueprints to coordinate the work of carpenters, electricians, and plumbers. Banks offer customers financial records that are updated in real time. Automobile manufacturers produce thousands of vehicles that are standardized at their core, while tailored at the margins. Although health care may face unique challenges in accommodating many competing priorities and human factors, the health care system could learn from these other industries how to better meet specific needs, expand choices, and shave costs.

The bottom line is that the nation, and its citizens, would be better served by a more nimble health care system that is consistently reliable and that constantly, systematically, and seamlessly improves. In short, the nation needs health care that learns by avoiding past mistakes and adopting new-found successes.

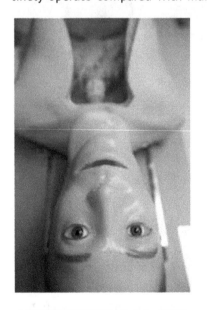

JUSTINE COOPER, *Ready,* 2009.

A Vision—And a Pathway

The Institute of Medicine has provided a roadmap for reaching this goal. It is detailed in *Best Care at Lower Cost: The Path to Continuously Learning Health Care in America*, a report released in September 2012. The good news is that opportunities for improving health care exist that were not available just a decade ago. Vast computational power is increasingly affordable and widely available, and connectivity allows information to be accessed in real time virtually anywhere by professionals and patients, permitting unprecedented diffusion of information cheaply, quickly, and on demand. Human and organizational capabilities offer expanded ways to improve the reliability and efficiency of health care. And health care organizations and providers increasingly recognize that effective care must be delivered by collaborative teams of clinicians, each member playing a vital role.

Yet simply acknowledging such opportunities does not necessarily result in putting them to good use. Indeed, building a learning health care system within current clinical environments requires overcoming substantial challenges. Clinicians routinely report moderate or high levels of stress, feel there is not enough time to meet their patients' needs, and find their work environments chaotic. They struggle to deliver care while confronting inefficient workflows, administrative burdens, and uncoordinated systems, preventing them from focusing on additional tasks and initiatives, even those that have important goals for improving care.

Given such real-world impediments, crafting and implementing initiatives that focus merely on incremental improvements and add to a clinician's daily workload are unlikely to succeed in fundamentally improving health care. Significant change can occur only if the environment, context, and systems in which health care professionals practice are reconfigured to support learning and improvement.

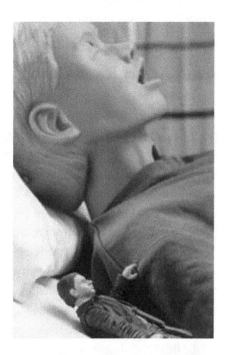

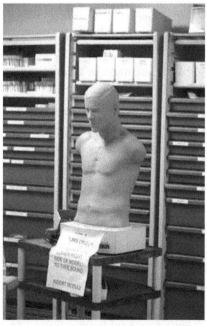

JUSTINE COOPER, *Action Figures* **(top), and** *Turn On Box* **(below), 2009.**

Realizing these objectives will require efforts in four main areas: generating and using real-time knowledge to improve outcomes; engaging patients, families, and communities; achieving high-value care; and creating a new culture of care.

Advancing Real-Time Knowledge

Although unprecedented levels of information are available, clinicians and patients often lack practical access to guidance that is relevant, timely, and useful for the circumstances at hand. For example, of the clinical guidelines for the nine most common chronic conditions, fewer than half address the issues of patients who experience two or more of the conditions at the same time, even though 75 million patients fit this category. Bridging gaps in how knowledge is gathered and used will require applying computing capabilities and analytic approaches to develop real-time insights from routine patient care and then using new technological tools to disseminate the emerging knowledge.

One key step will be to strengthen the digital infrastructure of the health care system to better capture data on clinical care and patient outcomes, on the care delivery process, and on the costs of care. Data should be digitally collected, compiled, and protected as reliable and accessible resources for managing care, assessing results, improving processes, strengthening public health, and generating new knowledge.

Large quantities of clinical data are now generated every day in the regular process of care, but most of the information remains locked inside paper records that are difficult to access, transfer, and query. Digital systems have the potential to turn each of those bothersome traits on its head. Care must be taken, however, to integrate the new electronic methods seamlessly into providers' daily workflow so as not to disrupt the clinical routine.

To complement the development of better digital systems, efforts are needed to promote expanded access to data and expanded data sharing. The idea is that the capacity for learning experiences increases exponentially when a system can draw knowledge from multiple sources. In one promising example, called distributed data networks, each participating organization stores its information locally, often in a common format. When a researcher seeks to answer a specific research question, all of the organizations in the network execute identical computer programs that analyze the data, create a summary from each site, and share those summaries with the entire network. In other efforts to expand data collection and access, insurance companies and other payer groups, health care delivery organizations, and companies that make medical products should be encouraged to contribute data to ongoing and new research efforts. And patients can play an important role by fully participating in self-reporting systems designed to gather data on patient outcomes, and by using new communication tools, such as personal portals, to better manage and record their own care.

Beyond technical matters, various legal and regulatory restrictions can be barriers to re-al-time learning and improvement. The privacy and security rules under the Health Insurance Portability and Accountability Act (HIPAA) pose particular challenges. In several surveys, re-searchers have reported that the rules increase the time and cost of research, impede collabo-ration among researchers, and make it difficult to recruit volunteers for studies. Protecting patient privacy is, of course, the basic starting point. But the current rules, with their inconsistent interpretation, offer a relatively limited security advantage to patients while impeding health research and the improvement of care. HHS is cur-rently reviewing HIPAA rules, along with the policies of various institutional review boards that oversee research at many lo-cations, with respect to actual or perceived regulatory impediments to the use of clinical data.

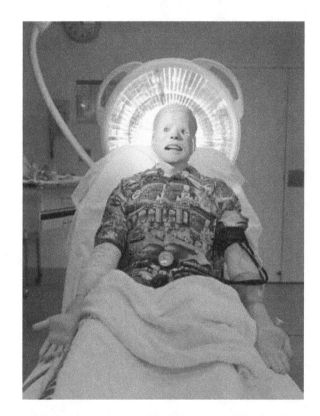

As more and better data become avail-able, the obvious job will be to identify and adopt improved approaches for de-livering accurate information to clinicians and patients in a timely manner. This will require making decision support tools and knowledge management systems routine features of health care delivery. Accelerating their use requires developing tools that deliver reliable, current clinical knowledge, in a clear and understandable format, to providers at the point of care, in addition to incentives that encourage the use of these tools. This also requires a shift in health professional education to teach skills for engaging in lifelong learning on how best to deliver safe care in an interdis-ciplinary environment. Furthermore, there are still multiple poorly understood barri-ers to dissemination and use of scientific evidence at the point of care. Addressing

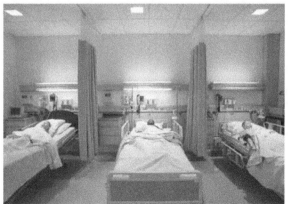

JUSTINE COOPER, *Peter* (top), C-Print, 30 × 40 inches, 2007, and *The Ward* (below), 2009.

these barriers will require additional research and the development of practical tools that can improve the usefulness and accessibility of such data for clinicians and patients.

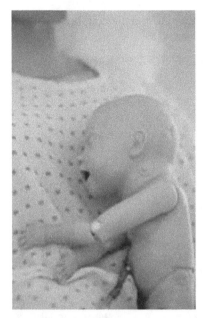

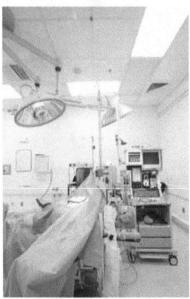

JUSTINE COOPER, *Bonding* (top), C-print, 20 × 30 inches, 2009, and *Eyes Wide Shut* (bottom), 2009.

Empowering Patients

An effective, efficient, and continuously learning system requires patients who are actively engaged in their own care. Clinicians supply information and advice based on their scientific expertise in treatment and their best assessment of potential outcomes, while patients, their families, and other caregivers bring personal knowledge on the suitability—or lack thereof—of different treatments for the patient's circumstances and preferences. Both perspectives are needed to select the right care. Of course, providing what has come to be called "patient-centered" care does not mean that providers simply agree to every patient request. Rather, it entails meaningful awareness, discussion, and engagement among patient, family, and the care team on the evidence, risks and benefits, options, and decisions in play.

The structure, incentives, and culture of the current health care system, however, are poorly aligned to engage patients and respond to their needs—and patients are often insufficiently involved in their care decisions. Even when encouraged to play a role in decisions about their care, they often lack understandable, reliable information—from evidence on the efficacy and risks of different treatment options to information on the quality of different health care providers and organizations—that is customized to their needs, preferences, and health goals.

Patient-centered care takes on increasing importance in light of research that links such care to better health outcomes, lower costs, and customers—the patients themselves—who are happier with their experience, among other benefits. With these rewards in mind, health care providers and organizations will need to draw on a full toolkit of actions.

Providers should begin by placing a higher premium on involving patients in their own health care to the extent that patients choose, encouraging them and their families to be active participants. From this base, clinicians should employ high-quality, reliable tools and skills that are customized to a patient's situation to aid in shared decision making. New technologies offer opportunities for clinicians to engage patients by meeting them where they are, rather than in traditional clinical settings. Further efforts may include providing new online sources of information and assisting patients in managing their own health—options that highlight the need for health professionals to assume new roles in partnering with patients.

Several actions can increase patient centeredness more broadly. First, there is a need for new tools that can assist individuals in managing their health and health care. Furthermore, public and private payers can promote and measure patient-centered care through payment models, contracting policies, and public reporting programs. There are also gaps in our ability to measure patient-centered care, which will require the development of a reliable set of measures of patient-centeredness for consistent use across the health care system. These measures can be used both to incentivize patient centered care and to assist organizations as they measure their improvement.

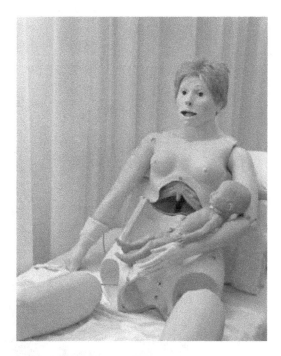

JUSTINE COOPER, *Mandy*, C-Print, 30 × 40 inches, 2007

Fostering High-Value Care

Health care payment policies strongly influence how care is delivered, whether new scientific knowledge and insights about best care are diffused broadly, and whether improvement initiatives succeed. The prevailing approach to paying for health care, based predominantly on paying set fees for individual services and products, encourages wasteful and ineffective care. New models of paying for care and organizing care delivery are emerging to improve quality and value. Although evidence is conflicting on which models work best and under what circumstances, it is clear that a learning health care system would incorporate incentives aligned to encourage continuous improvement, identify and reduce waste, and reward high-value care.

Health care delivery organizations and clinicians should fully and effectively employ digital systems that capture patient care experiences reliably and consistently.

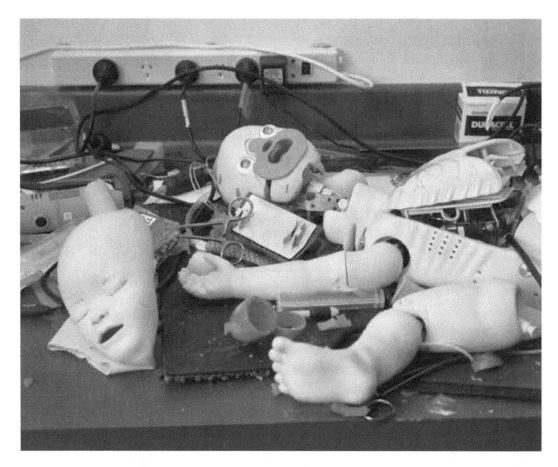

JUSTINE COOPER, *Sally*, C-Print, 30 × 40 inches, 2007.

The system would also be transparent. It would systematically monitor the safety, quality, processes, costs, and outcomes of care and make the information available for clinicians, patients, and families to use in making informed choices. This type of information on health care options, quality, price, and outcomes can then spur conversations among individuals and health care providers to promote informed decision making.

Multiple strategies exist for increasing the value of health care. Health care delivery organizations can use systems engineering tools and process improvement methods to eliminate inefficiencies, remove unnecessary burdens on clinicians and staff, enhance patient experience, and improve patient health outcomes. Furthermore, these organizations can reward continuous learning and improvement through internal practice incentives. For their part, public and private payers can adopt outcome- and value-oriented payment models and contracting policies that would support high-quality, team-based care focused on the needs and goals of patients and families. With an eye toward ongoing improvement, payment models, contracting policies, and benefit designs need to continuously refined to better reward high-value care that improves health outcomes.

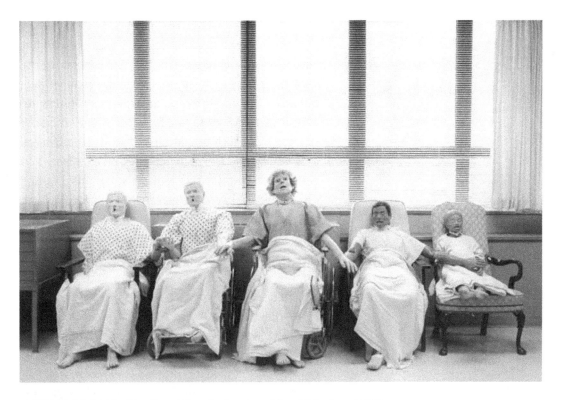

JUSTINE COOPER, *The Royal Family,* C-print, 26 × 40 inches, 2009.

Creating a New Culture

Although each step along the path to a learning health care system is important, none by itself is sufficient. Rather, the host of needed changes must be interwoven to achieve a common goal: health care organizations that are devoted at their very core to optimizing care delivery practices, continually improving the value achieved by care and streamlining processes to provide the best patient health outcomes. Reaching this point will require broad participation by patients, families, clinicians, care leaders, and those who support their work. Health care delivery organizations, however, will play an especially important role. Because of their size and care capacities, they can set an example for improvement across the health care system by using new practice methods, setting standards, and sharing resources and information with smaller facilities and individual care providers.

Although details may vary among organizations, some key concepts will remain constant. A learning health care organization harnesses its internal wisdom—staff expertise, patient feedback, financial data, and other knowledge—to improve its operation. It also engages continuous feedback loops monitoring internal practices, assessing what can be improved, testing and adjusting it response to data, and implementing its findings across the organization.

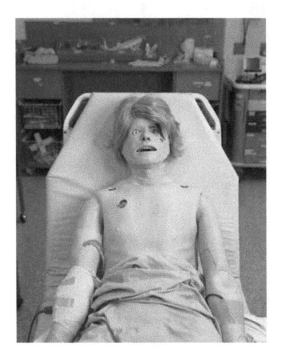

JUSTINE COOPER, *Wilbur*, C-Print, 30 × 40 inches, 2007.

Simply put, an organization that promotes continuous learning and improvement is one that makes the right thing easy to do. Its environment simplifies procedures and work-flows so that providers can operate at peak performance to care for patients, and embraces support tools, such as checklists, that make providers' jobs easier. This not only improves care delivery and patient outcomes; it also reduces stress on front-line care providers, improves job satisfaction, and prevents staff burnout.

Many organizations still struggle to implement such transformational system changes. They face both external obstacles, such as financial incentives that emphasize quantity of service over quality, and internal challenges to achieving constant improvement. To evolve successfully, health care organizations must develop a culture that supports improvement efforts, by adopting systematic problem-solving techniques, building operational models that encourage and reward sustained quality, and becoming transparent on costs and outcomes.

Leadership will be vital, as an organization's leadership and governance set the tone for the entire system. The visibility of leaders at the highest level makes them uniquely positioned to define the organization's quality goals, communicate these goals and gain acceptance from the staff, and make learning a priority. Leaders also have the ability to align activities to ensure that staff members have the necessary resources, time, and energy to accomplish the organization's goals. By defining and visibly emphasizing a vision that rewards continuous learning and improvement, leadership encourages an organization's disparate elements to work together toward a common end.

To complement leadership at the top, a continuously learning organization also requires leadership on the part of the managers and front-line workers who translate an expressed vision into practice. Middle managers play a crucial role in on-the-ground, day-to-day management of the units that, collectively, make up an organization. Unit leaders therefore must often challenge the prevailing mental models—deep-seated assumptions and ways of thinking about problems—and refocus attention on the barriers to learning and improvement. To this end, middle managers must be able to set priorities for improvement efforts, establish and implement continuous learning cycles, and foster a culture of respect among staff that empowers them to undertake continuous learning and improve patient care.

To promote continuous learning, health care organizations also need to adopt dedicated learning processes—mechanisms that help in constantly capturing knowledge and using the lessons to implement improvements. Achieving this type of systems-based problem solving requires an organizational culture that incentivizes experimentation among staff. While success is the goal, the system should recognize failure as key to the learning process and not penalize employees if their experiments are unsuccessful. Systems that continuously learn also need to be adept at transferring the knowledge they gain throughout the organization. Although each of these factors is important, it is the organization's operational model—the way it aligns goals, resources, and incentives—that makes learning actionable. In this way, an organization's operating model can promote continuous learning, help control variability and waste that do not con tribute to quality care, and recoup savings to invest in improving care processes and patient health, and make improvement sustainable.

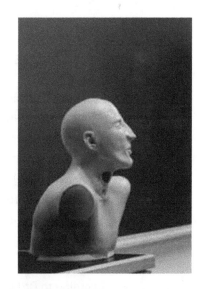

JUSTINE COOPER, *Smiling Man*, C-Print, 20 × 30 inches, 2009.

Pioneering health care organizations that successfully become continuously learning operations—fully or even partially—should also take the lead in diffusing the lessons learned more broadly. In this way, they not only can stand as beacons of opportunity, but also can provide the type of granular, hard-won information that can encourage and speed similar transformations across the entire health care system.

The entrenched challenges of the U.S. health care system demand a transformed approach. Left unchanged, health care will continue to underperform; cause unnecessary harm to patients; and strain national, state, community, and family budgets. The actions required to reverse current trends will be notable, substantial, sometime disruptive—and absolutely necessary.

The challenges are clear. But the imperatives are also clear, the changes are possible, and there are at least signs of success. Moving ahead, following the path to a continuously learning health care system, offers the prospect for best care at lower cost for individuals and society.

Chapter 11: **Discussion Questions**

1   What conflicts do health care organizations face when working to build ethics into the foundation of their organization?

   a. How do short-term and long-term finances play affect building an ethical foundation?

2   Explain how the Institute of Medicine's (IOM) quality aims [SEPTEE] relate to different ethical principles?

   a. What benefits and conflicts can occur when patients exercise their autonomy?

3   Describe incentives to improve patient safety.

   a. According to Dr. Lucian Leape, who should be held liable when errors occur? Why?

4   How can medical error be reduced by changing health policy in health care systems?

   a. What was the goal of the book *To Err Is Human*?

5   What does the path to continuously learning health care in America look like?

   a. What challenges do organizations face in adopting this path?

CHAPTER 12

HEALTH POLICY LEADERSHIP

Importance of Leaders with the Right Leadership Styles

Sattar Bawany

Introduction

> *"Research has found six distinct leadership styles, each springing from different components of emotional intelligence. The styles, taken individually, appear to have a direct and unique impact on the working atmosphere of a company, division, or team, and in turn, on its financial performance."*
>
> **—Daniel Goleman**
> **(Leadership That Gets Results, Harvard Business Review, March 2000)**

In essence, the heart of the leadership challenge that confronts today's leaders is learning how to lead in today's VUCA (volatile, uncertain, complex and ambiguous) business environment, allied with the needs to deal with scale and new organisational forms that often break with the traditional organisational models and structures within which many have learned their 'leadership trade'. So the basic assumption that past experience is the key for future leadership success is more open to scrutiny than ever.

At Centre for Executive Education (CEE) we believe that leadership is all about the ability to have impact and influence on your followers using the right leadership styles so as to engage them towards *achieving your organizational results* through both Ontological Humility and Servant Leadership approaches blended with elements of social intelligence competencies and socialised power.

Selecting the Right Leader for your Organization

Leaders come in a variety of colours, style and fashions. Picking the one you need when you need her is critical

You are the CEO of your organization and must select a new business leader. To succeed, all you have to do is figure out what makes a good leader, a debate that has been ongoing for centuries. You prefer not to wait centuries to make this decision. You have six reasonable candidates, and your organization needs leadership now.

You learn that there is a new study (Goleman, 2000) that may help, in two ways. First, it shows how leadership affects profitability. The equation goes like this: leadership directly affects the organization's climate. The quality of the climate accounts for about one third of profitability. Thus, the decision you make about the new leader has the potential to have a huge impact on your bottom line.

Climate is not an amorphous, feel-good word. It is used with precision as a comprehensive term to describe six important elements among workers:

- How flexible employees are in solving problems;
- The sense of responsibility employees feel to the organization;
- The kinds of standards employees have;
- The effectiveness of rewards the organization uses;
- The clarity workers have about the organization's mission and values;
- How committed employees feel to the common objectives.

Second, the study accesses how each of six leadership styles affects climate. As good luck sometimes has it, each of the leadership styles fits with one of your candidates.

The Coercive Leader: This person riles by fear. "My way or the highway." The leader takes charge and invites no contrary opinions. This style has the most detrimental impact on climate in this study.

The correlation between coercive leadership and climate is minus, .26, i.e., as coercion increases, quality of climate declines. But don't rule out your coercive candidate. This is the leadership style of choice when a company is in crisis. If your organization is in serious trouble, you may want to hire this person. Remember, though, that once the crisis resolves, coercive can create its own crisis unless your leader can shift to another style.

The Authoritative Leader: This leader has a powerful ability to articulate a mission and win people to it with enthusiasm. He makes a clear path for followers, cutting away confusion that exists in most organizations. Followers do not work at cross purposes because a commitment to a common vision is created. This leadership style has plus, .54 correlation with climate, the biggest correlation of any leadership style. As authoritative behaviours increase, so does the equality of the climate. This style will be particularly effective if your organization needs a new vision. Before making a final determination, however, look at the other styles, their impact, and when they work best.

The Affiliation Leader: This leader is a master at establishing positive relationships. Because the followers really like their leader, they are loyal, share information, and have high trust, all of which helps climate. The affiliative leader gives frequent positive feedback, helping to keep everyone on course. The correlation of this leadership style with climate is plus, .46. Consider your affiliative candidate if your organization primarily needs team harmony, improved morale, or if previous events created an atmosphere of mistrust. The downside of this style is that poor performance of followers is sometimes tolerated out of loyalty.

The Democratic Leader: This leader focuses on decision making by winning consensus. With consensus comes intense commitment to goals, strategies and tactics. Trust is a major feature of this leadership style as well. The correlation with climate is a healthy plus, .43. It works particularly well when the leader is genuinely not sure what to do and has talented employees who can and will make excellent input. In accessing your democratic candidate, consider the talent level of direct reports. If they have had time to grow into their jobs and work well as a team, the democratic candidate might be a good choice. Drawbacks of this style include that it works poorly during crisis that need rapid action.

The Pacesetter: This leader sets high performance standards for everyone, including himself. He walks the talk. This sounds admirable and has been widely believed to be effective. The data, however, indicate otherwise, with a minus, .25 correlation with climate. Why?

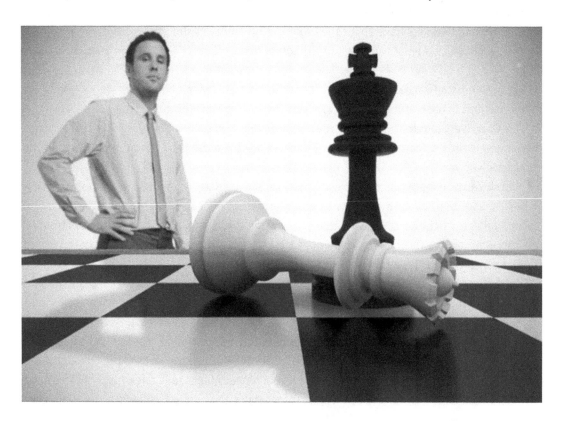

Pacesetters tend to have trouble trusting their followers. Their self-esteem rest on being smarter, faster and more thorough than everyone else. They unintentionally undermine the efforts and morale of those around them. Before dismissing your pacesetter candidate, however, look at the followers. If they are already highly motivated with strong technical skills, a pacesetter can be effective because their styles and competence already fit with the pacesetter's expectations.

The Coach: This leader develops people. He is able to recognize talent and how best to develop it. He offers developmental plans, including challenging assignments that push people to cultivate new skills. The leader can see the future and bring out the best in followers. This style has a plus, .42 correlation with climate. It works best when followers are receptive to personal growth. If your organization is characterized by individuals who are waiting for retirement, don't hire the coach candidate. If your employees are excited about learning, give the coach a good look. If you hire this candidate, recognize that coaching is time consuming, meaning that this leader will devote less time to other activities.

Conclusion

In making your decision, consider the fit between leadership style and the characteristics of your organization. Even more important, remember that things change. Take one more look at your six candidates. Look for flexibility. The very best leaders are those who have learned how to shift from one leadership style to another as circumstances demand. If one of your candidates shows evidence of being able to move smoothly among several of these six styles, that may tip the balance.

Since leaders lead people, the style with which you do it is important. It must truly represent you, fit with the situation, the results you wish to achieve and the people you hope will follow your lead. In truth, having a particular style is not as essential to being a leader as having a vision of what could exist, being committed to the vision, bringing great energy to realising that vision and having people to support you towards achieving the organizational results.

Radically Redesigning Patient Safety

Lea E. Radick

In 2004, Virginia Mason Medical Center, a 336-bed health system in Seattle, was approximately three years into deploying its production system when one of its patients, Mary McClinton, died from a preventable medical error.

The new production system—based on the Lean production process—was intended to identify and eliminate waste, improve quality and safety, and control cost. McClinton's death inspired VMMC to make safety its single organizational goal for the next three years, according to Gary S. Kaplan, MD, chairman and CEO of VMMC and an ACHE Member.

In 2002, the health system implemented a patient-safety alert system. The system also is based on Lean—or the Toyota Production System—in that all 6,000 VMMC employees are considered safety inspectors and are expected to signal an alert any time they see or hear something that causes a safety concern. Filing an alert notifies a patient safety specialist and a senior executive responsible for the process or area. In addition, the alert initiates an investigation with a goal of fixing the problem as quickly as possible.

"Protecting the safety of our patients was a singular focus for us, and I think the result has been a culture that now prioritizes safety above all else," Kaplan says.

The health system's production and patient safety alert systems represent just two ways VMMC has increased its focus on patient safety during the past decade. In addition to its efforts to standardize its processes, VMMC also has endeavored to ensure there is executive-level accountability for the safety of the health system's patients.

VMMC is one of several hospitals and health systems that have hardwired safety and high reliability into their organizations. These systems' efforts to improve patient safety, such as VMMC's standardization of its processes, mirror the Institute for Healthcare Improvement's 10 new rules for radical redesign in healthcare.

Rules for Radical Redesign in Healthcare

IHI's Leadership Alliance—a group of approximately 40 healthcare organizations committed to achieving the IHI's Triple Aim—developed the rules to address current challenges facing the healthcare field.

IHI—an independent, nonprofit organization based in Cambridge, Mass.—also developed the Triple Aim, which sets forth a framework for optimizing health system performance by simultaneously pursuing improvements in the patient experience, population health and healthcare costs.

IHI's rules for radical redesign are intended to apply to every dimension of quality, including patient safety, explained Derek M. Feeley, IHI's new president and CEO as of January of 2016.

"Our theory is that these radical redesign principles can be applied to any dimension of the Triple Aim," says Feeley, an ACHE Member.

Some hospitals and health systems, such as VMMC, intentionally employ the radical redesign concepts. "Every one of these radical redesign principles is alive and in operation here at Virginia Mason," says Kaplan, who serves as chairman of IHI's board of directors.

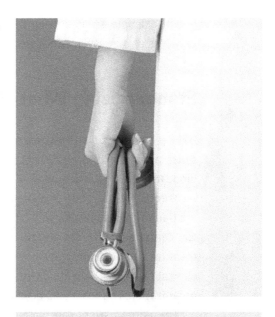

"I believe strongly that there's no more important work for us to do than to keep our patients safe."

—Gary S. Kaplan, MD
Virginia Mason Medical Center"

Other organizations, such as the University of Tennessee (Knoxville) Medical Center, a 581-bed, nonprofit academic medical center that has tried to standardize what makes sense to improve patient safety, have not directly invested in any of IHI's collaboratives—yearlong programs designed for organizations committed to achieving sustainable change within a specific topic area—to redesign healthcare.

However, "Everything that we did is parallel and consistent with the processes that they have advocated with the redesign," says Inga Himelright, senior vice president and chief quality officer for UTMC.

Both Feeley and his predecessor, Maureen A. Bisognano, HFACHE, who served as IHI's president and CEO until her retirement at the end of 2015, have identified several radical redesign rules that particularly apply to patient safety efforts.

For example, standardizing what makes sense and customizing to the individual "are at the very core of the way in which we think about how to make care safer," Feeley says.

Standardizing What Makes Sense

UTMC embarked on an initiative to improve both quality and safety by standardizing what makes sense after realizing in 2007 that it had the second- highest rate of central-line associated bloodstream infections among Tennessee hospitals, according to Joe Landsman, CEO, UTMC.

Through the creation of patient-care pathways—evidence-based, best practice standards that are tied to specific workflows—UTMC sought to reduce unwarranted clinical variation. The medical center began to develop the pathways in 2012 under the guidance of an interdisciplinary team for agreed-upon procedures. The team established guiding principles for the creation of clinical pathways, beginning with those focused on reducing the incidence of CLABSI within the organization. The team also developed processes for compliance management.

The initial patient-care pathway measures proved so successful that, by the end of 2014, the medical center was managing 68 percent of admitted patients through clinical pathways, according to Landsman.

Since the implementation of the pathways, UTMC has reduced its CLABSI numbers by 98.6 percent, from 72 incidences in 2008 to one in 2014. UTMC also has experienced a drop in its catheter-associated urinary tract infections, with reductions in acute care CAUTIs of 68 percent from 2011 to 2014, and a 75 percent reduction in critical care CAUTIs during the same period. Furthermore, use of the pathways has led to a significant reduction in the occurrence of surgical site infection rates in colon procedures, coronary artery bypass grafts, hysterectomies and C-sections.

"Our thinking is, if we're reducing complications, we should be reducing mortality," Landsman explains.

Bellin Health System in Green Bay, Wis.—an integrated healthcare delivery system composed of Bellin Hospital, an acute care, 167-bed multispecialty facility, and various other service centers—also has tried to standardize its processes in several ways, including through the implementation of an electronic event reporting system and video surveillance with video monitor technicians.

Bellin Health added video surveillance in 2010 to better monitor patients at high risk for falls. One of the contributing factors for patient falls and fall-related injuries is inadequate supervision and low staffing levels. Further, the use of bed and chair alarms is not effective with fast-moving patients, and the use of patient sitters is costly.

Bellin Health saved $448,000 in patient sitter costs in the first nine months after it implemented video surveillance, and the organization has logged more than 1,000 days since the last avoidable patient fall that resulted in an injury.

The electronic event reporting system resulted in a 50 percent increase in event reporting by staff within four months after its implementation, leading to improved analysis of events, enhanced identification of common themes and more focused improvement work.

10 Rules for Radical Redesign in Healthcare

Change the balance of power. Coproduce health and well-being in partnership with patients, families and communities.

Standardize what makes sense. Standardize what is possible to reduce unnecessary variation and increase the time available for individualized care.

Customize to the individual. Contextualize care to an individual's needs, values and preferences, guided by an understanding of what matters to the person in addition to asking, "What's the matter?"

Promote well-being. Focus on outcomes that matter the most to people, appreciating their happiness and well-being may not require healthcare.

Create joy in work. Cultivate and mobilize the pride and joy of the healthcare workforce.

Make it easy. Continually reduce waste and all non-value-added requirements and activities for patients, families and clinicians.

Move knowledge, not people. Exploit all helpful capacities of modern digital care and continually substitute better alternatives for visits and institutional stays. Meet people where they are — literally.

Collaborate and cooperate. Recognize the healthcare system is embedded in a network that extends beyond traditional walls. Eliminate siloes and tear down self-protective institutional or professional boundaries that impede flow and responsiveness.

Assume abundance. Use all the assets that can help optimize the social, economic and physical environment, especially those patients, families and communities bring.

Return the money. Use the money from healthcare savings for other public and private purposes.

Source: Institute for Healthcare Improvement.

University of Tennessee Medical Center Central-Line Associated Bloodstream Infection Events by Year

Priorities based on strategic initiatives and nationally recognized measures have produced advanced results for CLABSIs, with a reduction rate of 98.6 percent from 2008–2014.

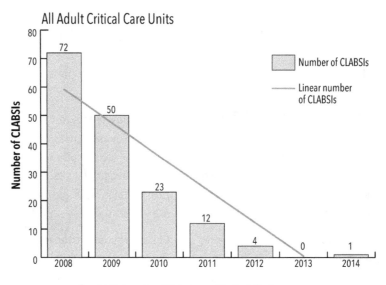

Source: University of Tennessee Medical Center.

Mercy Health, a vertically integrated health system based in Chesterfield, Mo., that cares for 1.2 million patients annually, has implemented a variety of patient-safety initiatives during the last decade to improve its culture of safety. These include developing an event-reporting system, adopting strategies and policies to improve professional behavior and establishing a systemwide adverse event management policy, among other measures.

> "Our theory is that these radical redesign principles can be applied to any dimension of the Triple Aim.
>
> —Derek M. Feeley
> Institute for Healthcare Improvement

Similar to Bellin Health, Mercy Health uses telesitters, which have the ability to monitor multiple patients who are at high risk of falling. Other methods to reduce falls include improvements in bedside rounding, expanded use of gait belts and the use of a fall-assessment tool embedded in Mercy Health's EHR. These efforts have reduced the organization's rate of falls with injury by nearly half between 2008 and 2015.

Furthermore, since launching a systematic approach to reducing mortality in its hospital settings in 2008, Mercy's mortality rates have declined from 1.75 percent in 2007 to 1.35 percent in 2015.

Customize to the Individual

Another radical redesign principle that is particularly applicable to improving patient safety is customizing care to the individual, according to Feeley.

"Reduce unnecessary variation, but at the same time understand what matters to the patient and customize the care to their requirements," Feeley says.

For example, hospitals in Singapore categorize patients by their medical and social complexity. When a patient's level of complexity in either of these areas increases, the hospital will assign a specific navigator or caregiver to that patient to help him or her navigate complex care situations, Bisognano explains. "In Singapore, there is a rule that states that the more complex the patient's illness, the fewer providers the patient will have to interact with," she says. "That's because it becomes unsafe when a patient is trying to navigate through five or six or 10 different providers to manage multiple prescriptions and coordinate their lives around orders from different specialists."

Change the Balance of Power

Changing the balance of power is about ensuring the patient's voice can be heard. To adhere to this rule, one must coproduce health and well-being in partnership with patients, families and communities.

VMMC emphasizes listening to patients through its family- activated safety alert team, which encourages patients and their family members to reach out to VMMC staff members whenever a concern arises. Staff members respond to such concerns 24 hours a day, seven days a week. The health system also engages with patients through rapid process improvement workshops, in which people who work on a particular process or are familiar with a certain problem focus on that issue and develop an improvement plan. VMMC employees participate in these continuous improvement events alongside selected patients and their families.

> "You can't overstate the fact that having everybody in the room is the magic here.
>
> —Jano Janoyan, DO
> University of Tennessee Medical Center"

Bellin Health adheres to the radical redesign concept of changing the balance of power by striving to maintain responsibility for safety among all staff involved in offering a service rather than putting this responsibility solely on the physician, according to health system president/CEO George F. Kerwin, FACHE.

For example, "There's a great deal of respect about what the surgeon does, and in an operating room, the surgeon's skill is still critical, no question about it," Kerwin says. "But there are other issues in an operating room that may require the surgical procedure to be coproduced by the surgeon, circulating staff, radiation technicians, anesthesiologists, the housekeeping team, the patient and the patient's family, who need to know how to care for that patient once the patient is discharged."

Creating Joy in Work

As healthcare organizations strive to improve the quality of care they provide and the safety of their patients, it is important that providers pay attention to their own well-being, too.

"I'm a big believer that you can't give what you don't have, and our patients need empathy and caring when they're undergoing acute problems," says Maureen A. Bisognano, HFACHE, former Institute for Healthcare Improvement president and CEO.

In *Managing Stress and Preventing Burnout in the Healthcare Workplace*, author Jonathan R.B. Halbesleben writes, "One of the more consistent findings in the literature is that stress, especially when it reaches the point of burnout, has a negative impact on job performance."

The notion of creating joy in work—one of the IHI's 10 rules for radical redesign in healthcare, which is defined as cultivating and mobilizing the pride and joy of the healthcare workforce—also has implications for patient safety, quality of care and the patient experience. This is an area that will require attention going forward, according to IHI president/CEO Derek M. Feeley.

"We hear a lot about clinical teams feeling [depressed] or under significant stress. If we can learn from some of the efforts of others to create a joyful workforce, that's going to pay a patient-safety dividend," says Feeley, also an ACHE Member.

Halbesleben defines stress as "a state of being that results from our evaluation of a specific situation. It is our response when we face a demand at work but do not feel we have sufficient resources to meet the demand." Burnout is defined as "an extreme response to work stress that occurs when we continually face stressors with which we are unable to fully cope."

Stress and burnout can have negative consequences for the individual and the organization for which he or she works. Individual consequences can include decreased performance, potentially problematic (and even dangerous) adjustments to work process, high turnover and poor health. On an organizational level, stress and burnout also can translate to higher turnover and increased healthcare costs.

Stress and burnout also can impact patients. "Stress among your employees significantly affects the quality of care they provide to their patients," writes Halbesleben. "It leads to medical errors, near misses (most of which are not reported) and lower patient satisfaction."

Healthcare leaders can help individual employees deal with their stress by enrolling them in time-management programs or providing them with additional vacation time when needed. Halbesleben also suggests incorporating action research, a style of research that can result in a customizable framework for addressing stress in healthcare facilities.

Leadership Principles

Although all of the aforementioned rules for radical redesign have played significant roles in hospital and health system efforts to improve patient safety, healthcare leaders agree it is particularly important to have leadership principles in place that support an environment of enhanced patient safety in hospitals and health systems. Closing the gap between "the front office and the frontline" is one such principle, according to Bisognano.

"When you're sitting in an executive suite, it's so easy to make decisions when you're looking at data alone or you're looking at an outlier case, without a clear understanding of the profound or complicating effects of what's happening on the frontlines," she says. To close the gap between perception and understanding, Bisognano encourages healthcare leaders to make the rounds and interview physicians, nurses and patients, talking with them about barriers to safety in the organization.

Another important leadership tool needed to create an environment of enhanced patient safety is interviewing a patient about his or her entire care journey, rather than simply asking how the patient is doing on a particular day.

When teaching leadership in health systems, Bisognano often begins by interviewing a patient at the front of the room. "I don't know who these patients are, but I can tell you that without exception, when I sit and interview a patient about his or her journey, it opens up the eyes of the leaders to things they never saw," she says.

Feeley also said leaders should have an authentic presence at the point of care so they can see "every care interaction and every measurement and result as an opportunity to learn."

Mercy Health is not only committed to improving patient safety, but also to educating its leaders. Each CEO of the health system's hospitals goes through a day and a half of training on the importance of patient safety and their role in patient safety, according to president/CEO Michael D. Connelly, FACHE.

When there is a significant safety event, team members at Mercy Health thoroughly review it. "If there is an outcome that needs to be communicated to the family, we want the CEO or a senior leader in the organization directly involved," Connelly explains. "We found that having the CEOs and significant leaders involved and actually communicating with families helps them [to be] more focused on the importance of patient safety."

Another leadership principle Mercy Health employs is to "examine every bad outcome and then look for process improvements," Connelly says.

After VMMC reemphasized its efforts to improve patient safety following the 2004 death of McClinton, all of its staff, including the health system's leaders and physicians, have had mistake-proofing training.

> *"We found that having the CEOs and significant leaders involved and actually communicating with families helps them [to be] more focused on the importance of patient safety.*
>
> *—Michael D. Connelly, FACHE Mercy Health"*

"This work is all of our work," Kaplan says of the importance of VMMC's senior executives undergoing safety training.

Furthermore, Kaplan says transparency and recognition also are important leadership principles. "We recognize and celebrate staff who speak up and report safety concerns," Kaplan says, adding VMMC gives out a monthly "Good Catch" award.

Accountability also is critical, Kaplan adds, noting VMMC holds its senior leaders accountable for safety events, too.

It is important staff members feel empowered and supported to raise concerns about patient safety, says Kerwin of Bellin Health. Also critical: celebrating successes and improvements in patient safety, clearly defining safe care as an operating principle within an organization's mission statement, defining safety and measuring it regularly.

Tackling Interdisciplinary Challenges

Healthcare leaders of various hospitals and health systems also cite the importance of an interdisciplinary approach to developing sustainable patient-safety initiatives. VMMC's rapid process improvement workshops, for example, bring together cross-functional teams that include professionals from numerous disciplines.

"You can't overstate the fact that having everybody in the room is the magic here," says Jano Janoyan, DO, medical director of UTMC and an ACHE Member. "It's about breaking down silos and saying, 'How do we work together across the continuum of care to make things better for the patient?'"

To work across disciplines in improving safety, team members must remain focused on defining causes of patient harm rather than pointing fingers. "What we've found is that team members from various disciplines want to get to the root of the problem; they aren't interested in beating each other up," Kerwin says.

"The opportunities for us to learn from each other are huge," Feeley says. "I think that's what leaders need to do if they're going to overcome these challenges: work on them together."

The Role of Senior Leaders in Radically Improving Safety

Ultimately, to drive sustainable improvements in patient safety, senior leaders must take ownership of the organization's safety agenda. They also must be effective at building the organizational will for change.

"More and more, there is a need for healthcare's senior leaders to reinforce a culture of safety in their organizations—to think about the values, attitudes and patterns of behavior that are going to drive safety and to create an environment that promotes high reliability and respect for one another," Bisognano says.

Senior leaders must embrace the work that goes into building a culture of safety for such a culture to be sustainable, Kaplan says. "This is our work. This is not work that we would delegate to others," he says. "We need to be visibly leading this work across our organizations so that we as senior leaders are setting the agenda and we can set the culture by our behaviors.

"I believe strongly that there's no more important work for us to do than to keep our patients safe."

Ethical Leadership in Uncertain Times

John M. Buell

When Ethical Leadership Is Put to the Test

Ethical erosion, according to Gilbert, is characterized by a series of small, sometimes unnoticed acts that erode ethical behavior, with each act providing a foundation for a more erosive act. Taken together, such acts can lead to significant and even disastrous consequences for both the organization and individuals.

"Ethical erosion is a slow, almost unnoticeable diminishment of values," Gilbert says. "When you let little wrongs continue, this makes it easier to slowly slide into committing wrongs of a larger scale."

Gilbert pointed to consumer health company Johnson & Johnson and the ways in which the company both lived up to its intentions and failed to during two crises 25 years apart.

Robert Wood Johnson II, who formerly served as president of Johnson & Johnson from 1932–1963, crafted the company's credo in 1943, just before Johnson & Johnson became a publicly traded company. The organization thought so highly of its credo that it engraved the credo onto a large piece of limestone that sits in the lobby at its headquarters in New Brunswick, NJ. The beginning of the credo states, "We believe our first responsibility is to the doctors, nurses and patients, to mothers and fathers and all others who use our products and services. In meeting their needs, everything we do must be of high quality."

Johnson & Johnson's credo was put to the test in 1982 during what became known as the Chicago Tylenol murders, in which seven people died after taking cyanide-laced Tylenol. Within 24 hours, the manufacturer pulled the product off every shelf in the country. "It was a no-brainer," Gilbert says. "They didn't wait. [Johnson & Johnson's] action came about because of their credo." It was learned that bottles on the store shelves had been tampered with.

In 2008, however, the manufacturer was faced again with another crisis—but this time, the company was slow to react to consumer complaints. Fortunately, no consumers suffered serious health problems. As a result of this incident and others, Johnson & Johnson's reputation suffered.

> *"Our promise is to our patients. The one thing we can do when it comes to ethics is make a commitment to patients that we will keep them at the center of what we do."*
>
> *—Darlene M. Stromstad, FACHE, Waterbury Hospital*

"It was a lesson for any organization proud of its values: Without vigilance, there is an ever-present risk of waiving them," Gilbert says.

So how can organizations make sure they are doing the right thing every day in these uncertain times? For Darlene M. Stromstad, FACHE, president and CEO of Waterbury (Conn.) Hospital, it's about never forgetting the organization's purpose.

"Our promise is to our patients," says Stromstad, who participated on an ethics panel during the program. "The one ethical thing we must do is to make a commitment to our patients that we will keep them at the center of everything we do."

Adds Joseph N. Mott, FACHE, vice president, health-care transformation, Intermountain Healthcare, Salt Lake City, who also participated on the panel: "Healthcare transformation is an ethical journey for Intermountain, and we believe that there is ample evidence pointing to overtreatment. Instances of over-treatment are not, generally, overt, but they do occur nonetheless. And knowing that overtreatment exists, we have a duty to search it out and redesign our processes to minimize it."

Gilbert advises organizations to harness the ethical wisdom they have by taking steps to ensure the organization maintains an ethical culture. *Ethical wisdom* is defined as the individual and collective knowledge, experience and good sense to make sound ethical decisions and judgments everywhere, every day.

For example, Barbara S. Ohm, FACHE, administrator, The Orthopedic Specialty Hospital, Intermountain Healthcare, Murray, Utah, says hospital and health system leaders should have practices in place that make it easy for staff to do the right thing.

"Not all [staff] will have the highest stages of ethical wisdom, but the ones who do should be encouraged to help develop the mission, vision and values of the organization," says Ohm, who also participated in the panel discussion.

The wisdom to do the right thing could come from anyone at any level of the organization, Gilbert says. That's why maintaining an ethical culture is an organization-wide effort.

The Fund for Innovation in Healthcare Leadership

The program "Ethical Leadership in Uncertain Times" was funded in part by the Fund for Innovation in Healthcare Leadership, a philanthropic initiative of the Foundation of the American College of Healthcare Executives. "The Journey to Value-Based Care for Population Health: Sharing, Scaling and Replicating to Accelerate Results," an article on the first of two Fund programs held in 2014, appeared in the January/February 2015 issue of *Healthcare Executive*.

The Fund was established in 2006 to bring innovation to the forefront of healthcare leadership by developing and enhancing its focus on future healthcare leaders, ethics and innovations in healthcare management. In its commitment to developing future leaders, the Fund also has provided scholarships for the Foundation of ACHE's Senior Executive and Executive Programs.

Since the Fund's inception, more than 2,100 generous donors have made contributions totaling more than $3.1 million. This support has enabled the Fund to strengthen the field of healthcare leadership by providing educational opportunities on important trends and issues.

For more information on the Fund, including ways to contribute, please visit **ache.org/Innovation** or contact Timothy R. Tlusty, vice president, Development, ACHE, at (312) 424–9305 or ttlusty@ache.org.

A Framework for An Ethical Culture

During his presentation, Gilbert shared five disciplines that can guide the development of an ethical culture in healthcare organizations.

Mindfulness. This can be described as simply being aware that something unethical might be going on or that a decision might be off. Mindfulness is the private voice of ethical wisdom. It is also "a time for reflection; to take a step back," Gilbert says.

Voice. This step entails bringing mindfulness into the public conversation and sharing ethical wisdom with colleagues and leaders. "What is the voice of the company?" Gilbert says. "Do people speak up when they see or hear a potentially unethical situation? Do they have an opportunity

"What is the voice of the company? Do people speak up when they see or hear a potentially unethical situation? Do they have an opportunity to speak up? Voice is important."

—*Jack A. Gilbert,*
EdD, FACHE,
Arizona State University

to speak up? Voice is important." When employees and leaders do not share ethical wisdom, an organization is at risk of repeating its mistakes.

Respect. This is a basic building block of an ethical culture. "We cannot move forward together unless we are willing to listen to each other," Gilbert says.

Tenacity. This is a central element in doing the right thing and sustaining an ethical focus. Tenacity is about a shared commitment to seeing difficult conversations through to their resolution, Gilbert says, recognizing that a perfect solution is not always attainable.

Legacy. Leaders that are mindful of their organization's values and legacy create a positive legacy for those who will follow. "Are we doing what we do just for today or for the future as well?" Gilbert says.

4 Disciplines of Ethical Leadership

Just as there are disciplines that foster an ethical culture, there also are disciplines that foster ethical leadership. Such disciplines are interconnected with the five disciplines of an ethical culture and set the tone for this culture.

Noble purpose. This is the calling of the healthcare organization as expressed in its vision, mission and values and by those who work for the organization, starting with its leaders. "This discipline is important because the business of the business of healthcare is caring," Gilbert says.

Ceaseless ambition. This is what transforms an organization's noble purpose into committed, bold goals and action. Ceaseless ambition is critical to preventing ethical erosion and to leveraging ethical wisdom. "Think of the 100,000 Lives Campaign, which later became the 5 Million Lives Campaign. With this initiative, the Institute for Healthcare Improvement set the bar high to create a challenge for change," Gilbert says.

Candor. Share the good, the bad and the ugly in a spirit of acknowledgment and engagement for the future.

Passion. A passion for healthcare's calling to care, combined with rational arguments regarding the need for ethical behavior drives change in healthcare organizations. "Passion reflects a true commitment to care, which can fade if it is not cultivated," Gilbert says.

Preventing ethical erosion and leveraging ethical wisdom within healthcare organizations are never-ending quests for healthcare leaders and staff—but they are endeavors that patients and their families depend upon.

Editor's note: For information on ACHE's many ethics resources, including the Code of Ethics and ACHE's Ethics Toolkit, visit **ache.org** and, under About ACHE, click on ACHE's Commitment to Ethics.

Chapter 12: **Discussion Questions**

1   What leadership style do you most identify with personally? Explain.

   a.   Give an example of a leader who exemplifies your selected style and include a quote by that leader to support your selection.

2   How can you discover which type of leader is best for your organization?

   a.   How does health care leadership differ from other industries?

3   Within the ten rules for the radical redesign of health care to improve patient safety, which three do you think are the most important and why?

4   Describe the importance of leadership in patient safety initiatives.

   a.   What leadership quality do you think is most important to achieve and maintain sustainable quality care? Why?

5   What is ethical erosion, and how can we avoid it?

   a.   How does the framework for an ethical culture differ from the disciplines for ethical leadership?